FROM DEMONS AND EVIL SPIRITS

TO CANCER GENES:

The Development of Concepts

Concerning the Causes of

Cancer and Carcinogenesis

Patrick J. Fitzgerald, M.D.

Production Editor: Dian Thomas
Production Assistant: Andrew Male
Copyeditor: Audrey Kahn
Graphics Editor: Ken Stringfellow

(Cover "Demon" figure courtesy of the British Museum.)

2000
Published by the American Registry of Pathology
Armed Forces Institute of Pathology
Washington, D.C. 20306-6000
ISBN 1-881041-71-9

From out of olde feldes, as men seyth,
Cometh al the newe corn, from yer to yere,
And out of olde bokes, in good feyth,
Cometh al this newe science that men lere.

Chaucer, Parliament of Foules

To: Helena
"Grandpie" Roche
Kathleen
Nancy
Geneva
Mary and Ernie
Mary Griggs Burke
Richard J. Mackool, M.D.

ACKNOWLEDGMENTS

In this study I became indebted to many persons and institutions, all of whom, unfortunately, cannot be named. For knowledge about human cancer I am obligated principally to the staff of Memorial Hospital, New York City, particularly to Dr. Fred W. Stewart and Dr. Frank W. Foote, former chairmen of the Department of Pathology. The latter dispensed their accumulated experience and wisdom about the pathology of cancer with patience and personal friendship; the years with them were unique, invaluable, and treasurable.

Dr. C.P. Rhoads, the first Director of Sloan-Kettering Institute, an inspiring leader and benefactor to so many young physicians and scientists, gave me my first opportunity to become involved in research. Others to whom I am indebted for their hospitality, scientific approach, and friendship are the late Professor Torbjörn Caspersson of the Karolinska Institutet, Stockholm, Sweden, and the late Professor Pierre Desnuelle of l'Université de Provence at Marseille. Most of all, I am indebted to Dr. Margery Ord and Dr. Lloyd Stocken of Oxford University.

Dr. H. Clarke Anderson, chairman of the Department of Pathology and Oncology, School of Medicine, the University of Kansas Medical Center, gave wholehearted encouragement and support to me while I was a member of the department. Dr. Robert Hudson, former chairman of the Department of the History of Medicine at the University of Kansas Medical Center graciously made available to me the facilities of the department and the library at the Kansas Medical Center.

Dr. John T. Ellis, late chairman of the Department of Pathology, Cornell University Medical College, enthusiastically supported the project from its inception and made available many facilities of the department, including photography, as well as other personal considerations. Dr. Daniel Knowles, the present chairman, has kindly continued support of the project.

I have been most fortunate to have as consultants Dr. Margery Ord and Dr. Lloyd Stocken of the Department of Biochemistry, Oxford University, personal friends and tutors for decades, including an exciting year with them at Oxford. Their constant gentle prodding over many years has been the spur which resulted in the completion of this book. Dr. Peter Nowell, Department of Pathology, University of Pennsylvania Medical School, has generously given much needed advice in the field of genetics and its relation to cancer. Dr. George Klein kindly gave advice on immunology and forwarded his chapter on the multistep development of tumors prior to its publication in Advances In Cancer Research.

An obvious debt is acknowledged to the medical historians, such as Fielding H. Garrison, Arturo Castiglioni, Henry E. Sigerist, Max Neuburger, and Charles Singer; the surgeon-historians Owen Wangensteen and Cushman Haagenson; and the medical scholars Saul Jarcho and Roy Porter, who furnished background settings. Esmond Long's *History of Pathology* was a necessary primer. Other stimulating writings of medical history were Dr. Guido Majno's *The Healing Hand,* and Dr. Leland Rather's *The Genesis Of Cancer. A Study In The History Of Ideas.* Rather's erudite exposition of the contributions of the German medical scientists of the 19th century and earlier studies on carcinogenesis are obligatory milestones for one interested in the history of ideas concerning the etiology of cancer. Recent remarkable advances in the cancer field suggested to me that such studies should be updated.

All oncologists owe a deep debt to the late Dr. Michael Shimkin of the National Institutes of Health, Bethesda, MD, for his devotion to the history of oncology, particularly for his graphic portrayal of many contributors to the cancer field as published in Cancer Research and in his book *Contrary to Nature* (Cancer Research, 1986;46:cover). The editors of Cancer Research, particularly Dr.

Sidney Weinhouse (Cancer Research, 1999;59:cover), continued this interest in cancer researchers and institutions. The translation of the first volume of Dr. Jacob Wolff's exhaustive studies of early cancer research was a gold mine of information.

Most of the library work has been conducted in the Samuel J. Wood Library, Cornell University Medical College. Dr. Robert M. Braude, Librarian, and his staff have given generous aid to the project for many years. The Interlibrary Loan Division, under Mr. Steven Bright and his staff, did yeoman work in obtaining books, journals, microfilms, and reprints. Ms. Anny Khoubesserian took charge of the arduous task of supervising the checking of references and other library services; their accuracy is the result of her faithful perseverance and experience in locating hard-to-find foreign references; and Ms. Helen-Ann Browne was of considerable help with her computer searches for information concerning many recent subjects pertinent to the study. The Medical Arts and Photography Division of Cornell University College of Medicine ably supplied photography. Dr. Doria Columbo kindly translated an article in Italian by Durante. Dr. Eric Myerhoff, former Director of the Library at Cornell, was very helpful in the early years of this study.

Mrs. Dorothy Marcinek played a vital role in deciphering my handwriting, correcting grammatical errors, checking the spelling and use of medical terms, and keeping a sharp eye out for inconsistencies and other mistakes. She was deeply interested in the project and maintained her enthusiasm for it even after moving to an adjacent state. She was a most important cog in the necessary logistics involved in book-making and, in addition, kept her sense of humor and was the spark that kept the process moving forward over a period of years.

Part of this study was written while on fellowships at St. Catherine's College, Oxford University; I am deeply grateful to the College for granting me a Fellowship (1968) and an Allen Christensen Visiting Fellowship (1990). I am also indebted to the Commonwealth Fund, New York City, and to the State University of New York for support during a year's sabbatical leave (1968) at the Department of Biochemistry, Oxford University.

I am greatly indebted to Dr. Donald West King, Executive Director, American Registry of Pathology, who has been enthusiastically interested in the project for some years and has accepted the responsibility of publishing it. The editorial staff, Ms. Dian Thomas, Mr. Andrew Male, and Ms. Audrey Kahn, have capably and graciously guided the book through the process of publication. I am indebted to the American Registry of Pathology, the Universities Associated for Research and Education in Pathology, and the Armed Forces Institute of Pathology for their support of the publication of this study.

INTRODUCTION

What I hope to do in this book is to outline, historically, the development of concepts concerning the process of carcinogenesis, including the agents believed to have caused cancer in the past. Prominent ideas about the subject held by physicians, biologists, scientists, or other individuals are discussed. The countless victims of cancer, as well as their friends and observers, probably held opinions about what instigated this affliction and how it progressed to death. Superstition, demonology, old wives' tales, speculations, religions, fear, folklore, hypotheses, theories, doctrines, and dogmas have all played a part in this conceptual history.

Only a few remarks about the incidence, diagnosis, treatment, or prevention of cancer are made here, and these are provided only to give the background necessary for an exploration of the thoughts expressed about the possible agents involved.

It might be thought that the story of cancer represents a depressing saga in that a satisfactory complete explanation of the disease has not been forthcoming. Yet in the past centuries there has been a slow, unfortunately depressingly slow, increase in our knowledge about the disease and what agents may cause it. In the latter half of the 20th century, particularly in the last few decades, astounding progress has taken place in elucidating the disease process. Cancer, a mystery for centuries, is now discussed in biochemical, biophysical, and genetic terms, and it is now possible to piece together a rational general picture of the cancer process.

The magnitude of the task of providing an acceptable survey of the many fields of cancer research is great when one considers the specialties of science and medicine now involved in it. Medical clinicians, biochemists, molecular biologists, geneticists, immunologists, radiobiologists, pathologists, epidemiologists, and many other specialty experts have played a role in recent cancer research. To simplify and make understandable the complex studies from those various fields, I have divided the text into four parts. The historical approach in parts I and II illustrates the limited knowledge of cancer that evolved from ancient times to a renaissance at the end of the 19th century. Part III concerns cancer research in the 20th century. So many contributors were involved in this that in order to keep a balanced perspective, each of the major specialties is considered individually, e.g., advances in biochemical carcinogenesis are discussed separately from those in viral or radiation carcinogenesis. Because of the rapid developments after World War II in molecular biology, cellular biology, microbial genetics, virology, and genetics, a summary of the most important developments in these fields, germane to cancer, is presented in part IV as a background for an appreciation of the present view of how normal cells are transformed into cancer cells.

Important individuals have been selected to represent prominent milestones in the development of cancer concepts. Regretfully, the important contributions of too many others in the intervals between these markers remain unmentioned.

It may appear that there has been a direct line of logical, step-by-step, steady progress in cancer research. However, advances more often have involved false starts, blind alleys, the revision or dropping of concepts after years of effort, or long periods of negative, frustrating experiments for investigators. Luck has played a part in some scientific advances. Investigators have had their hypotheses ignored for decades before they were finally proven correct. The human mind would prefer to review a logical steady progression of events, but the backward line-of-sight survey of the reviewer is not the route usually followed by human progress in medical and, probably, in all sciences.

It is obvious that no single author could master all the disciplines involved in cancer research, but, with the recent appearance of excellent books, reviews, and seminars on the history of many of the specialties, there is available today a plethora of authoritative information about this subject. I have borrowed heavily from such sources and have also imposed unduly upon friends and other scientists for advice regarding those areas in which they excel. This assistance, plus involvement in teaching, diagnosis, and research in the cancer field for over four decades, has been the background from which this study has emerged. The final text is mine, as is the responsibility for it.

I hope that I have presented a fair, representative, objective survey of the history of the most important ideas and concepts concerning the cause(s) of cancer and the development of the process of carcinogenesis.

The dénouement of the riddle of cancer appears to be at hand. It is a fascinating story.

Permission to use copyrighted illustrations has been granted by:

Academic Press:
Adv Can Res 1988;40:25–70. For figure 13-9 and table 13-1.
Chromosome Identification: Technique and Application in Biology and Medicine. Proceedings of the 23rd Nobel Symposium, Stockholm, Sweden, 1973. For figure 19-11.

American Association for Cancer Research:
Cancer Research 1990;50:2. For figures 20-4 and 20-5.
Cancer Research 1989;49:1620. For figure 21-3.

American Association for the Advancement of Science:
Science 1996;274:1652–1659. For figure 18-8.
Science 1996;274:948–953. For figure 21-7.
Science 1976;194:23–28. For figure 19-8.

Bantam Doubleday Dell:
Oedipus and Akhnaton, 1960. For figure 2-7.

British Museum of Art:
For figure 2-3.

Charles C. Thomas:
De Abditis Nonnullis ac Mirandis Morborum et Sanationum Causis, 1954. For figure 4-4.
W.C. Roentgen, 2nd ed., 1958. For figure 14-1.

Excerpta Medica:
J Am Coll Surg 1999;188:74–79. For figure 21-8.

Harvard University Press:
Medieval and Early Modern Science, Vol. 1, 1963. For figure 5-5.

The Indian Museum:
For figure 2-9.

John Wiley and Sons:
Am J Phys Anthropol 1923;6:218–329. For figure 2-13.
Cancer 1966;19:607–10. For figure 2-14.
Genes, 3rd ed., 1987. For figure 19-5.
Cancer Cytogenetics, 1987. For figure 19-10.
Principles of Genetics, 8th ed., 1991. For figure 21-1.

Jones & Bartlett:
Oncogenes, 1990. For figures 20-1 through 20-3, 20-7, 20-9, 20-10, 21-5 and 21-6.

Karger:
Paracelsus: an Introduction to Philosophical Medicine in the Era of the Renaissance, 1982. For figures 5-1 and 5-2.

Kegan Paul International:
Egyptian Mummies, 1991. For figure 2-6.

Lippincott Williams & Wilkins:
    CA Cancer J Clin 1977;27:172–81. For figure 12-1.
    Radiobiology for the Radiologist, 3rd ed., 1988. For figure 14-7.
    Virology, 2nd ed., 1988. For figure 15-1.
    Principles of Medical Genetics, 1990. For figure 18-19.
    The Origin of Malignant Tumors, 1929. For figure 19-7.
    Principles and Practices of Oncology, 1985. For figure 19-13.

Macmillan:
    The Cell in Development and Inheritance, 1896. For figure 18-14.

Massachusetts Institute of Technology Press:
    A Century of DNA: A History of the Discovery of the Structure and Function of the Genetic
        Substance, 1977. For figures 18-3 and 18-11.

Massachusetts Medical Society:
    N Engl J Med 1994;331:39–41. For figure 18-16.
    N Engl J Med 1993;329:1318–1327. For table 21-1.
    N Engl J Med 1994;331:931–933. For figure 19-14.
    N Engl J Med 1995;333:306–306. For figure 20-8.

McGraw-Hill:
    The Basic Science of Oncology, 2nd ed., 1992. For figures 13-5, 14-4, 14-5, and 14-6.

Mosby:
    Soft Tissue Tumors, 1983. For figure 10-14.
    Medical Radiobiology, 2nd ed., 1989. For figures 14-8, 14-10, and table 18-1.

The Nelson-Atkins Museum of Art
    For figures 2-8, 2-10, and 2-12.

The Nobel Foundation:
    Science 1975;189:347–58. For figure 18-13.

Oxford University Press:
    Early English Magic and Medicine, 1919–20. For figure 4-1.
    John Baptista van Helmont, 1982. For figure 6-1.
    Otto Warburg: Cell Physiologist Biochemist and Eccentric, 1981. For figure 13-6.
    A Short History of Scientific Ideas to 1900. For figure 19-1.

Parthenon Press:
    The Theory and Practice of Oncology, 1990. For figure 15-7.

Pergamon Press:
    Microscope. The Evolution of the Microscope, 1967. For figure 10-4.
    Oncogenic Viruses, 1983. For figures 13-4, 15-4, 15-6, and 15-9.

Scientific American Books:
    Molecular Cell Biology, 1986. For figures 18-6, 18-7, 18-18, and 19-12.

Scientific American Library:
   Viruses, 1992. For figures 15-2, 15-5, and 15-8.

Slatkine:
   Anatomies de Mondino dei Luzzi et de Guido de Vigevano, 1316, 1977. For figure 5-6.

Springer-Verlag:
   An Introduction to the Concept of Cancer Genes, 1988. For tables 15-1 and 15-2.
   Human Chromosomes: Structure, Behavior, Effects, 1993. For figures 19-3 and 20-6.

University of California Press:
   Andreas Vesalius of Brussels, 1514–1564, 1964. For figures 5-3, 5-4, and 5-7.

W.H. Freeman:
   Readings from American Scientific Magazine, 1991. For figures 16-1 through 16-5.

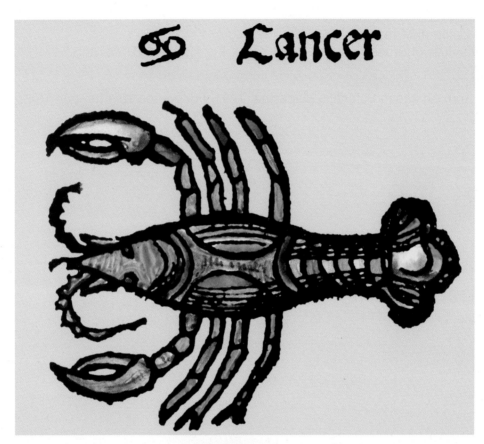

FRONTISPIECE

Sigil (a graphic symbol representing planets, signs of the zodiac, and other astrologic factors) of Cancer in the Astrorum Scientia of Leopold of Austria, 1489 edition. The crayfish was used as an astrologic symbol for Cancer prior to the 17th century; later the crab became the symbol. The figures that appear to be a horizontal 6 and 9 were also used as a symbol for Cancer. Their derivation is uncertain. (Fig. 76 from Goodman F. Zodiac Signs. London: Brian Trodd Pub. House, 1990:68.)

CONTENTS

❊ ❊ ❊

PART I
THE "LUMP" AND "ULCER" PERIOD
(PREHISTORIC TIMES TO AD 1800)

1
CANCER

In most of the industrialized countries of the world today, cancer is recognized as a common disease, particularly of the elderly, although infants and children are afflicted, but much less frequently. The extent of the disease is illustrated by its yearly toll of over 500,000 deaths in the United States. An accurate worldwide number of deaths caused by cancer is not known but it must be many millions per year.

Cancer has been recognized as a disease entity for centuries. Slowly, with time, more and more agents have been incriminated with or suggested to be involved in the cancerous process. Probably the most striking example, a relatively recent one, has been cigarette smoking and lung cancer. Even with this association the mechanism of action, how the carcinogen acts, is not known. The actual process that takes place in persons whose normal cells have become cancerous is still a mystery.

Since World War II great advances have been made in the diagnosis, description, and treatment of many cancers, with newer techniques in pathology, surgery, radiation therapy, and chemotherapy. There have been spectacular empirical results in the chemical treatment of some cancers such as leukemia, testicular tumors, and bone sarcomas; moderate advances in the treatment of other cases; and not much change with cancers of the lung, stomach, ovary, brain, and some other organs. With greater knowledge of the fundamental nature of cancer, it is likely that therapy will become more effective.

In regard to understanding the cancer process, there has been a relatively slow addition of significant information until recently. The advances in the basic sciences of biochemistry, virology, molecular biology, and genetics since World War II have led to revolutionary changes in concepts regarding the nature of cancer and its progression. But the long trail of the evolution of concepts of carcinogenesis still represents an unanswered challenge that has baffled mankind for centuries. A final explanation in modern scientific terms may be at hand.

THE GREEKS HAD A WORD FOR IT—"KARKINOS"

Credit for naming cancer has been accorded to a Greek physician, Hippocrates, who lived about 2,500 years ago. He introduced the word "karkinos" to describe a tumor of the breast in women which eventually caused the death of the patient. Karkinos, the Greek word for crab, was used because the appearance of advanced cancer of the human female breast was fancifully likened to that of a crab. The dilated blue veins adjacent to the cancer were thought to resemble the claws of the crab and the cancer itself was likened to the body of the animal. Other explanations for the use of the term were that the cancer's growth into the underlying tissue resembled a crab in its tenacious, unrelenting grip on the breast, or that cancer tissue was hard and resembled the shell of a crab (5,6). The name was also used for some ulcers of the skin that didn't heal and tumors of other organs. Later, the Latin word for crab, "cancer," became a more common designation for the disease.

The word cancer has had a sinister connotation throughout history. This is understandable with a disease that might spread from a sore or lump to slowly and irrevocably produce a loss of weight and flesh, induce general weakness, lead to emaciation, and, finally, to death. To the fear occasioned by the obvious physical changes there was often added the uncertainty concerning the cause of the affliction. For centuries the word cancer was not used openly because of the mystery of its cause and an irrational stigma that was associated with its use. Today, on television and in newspapers and magazines the word cancer is used openly and its signs, symptoms, and course are frankly discussed.

Sometime during the realization that they may have a cancerous problem, patients and friends must have questions about the disease. What is this disease? Where did it come from? How long have we known about it? Why can't the doctors cure it, or prevent it, they have cured and prevented other diseases? I have led a decent life, why should this happen to me? Most of all: What is this disease?

What causes it? How does it cause such disastrous effects? The story of the search for some answers to these questions has been a long and intriguing one.

TUMOR, ULCER, NEOPLASM, AND CANCER

When many of the observations about cancer were first made in antiquity there was no understanding of the fundamental nature of the body, its anatomy, or its many functions. Diseases were vague entities that afflicted people and the words that were used to describe the physical effects of the disease were ambiguous. There were lumps or swellings, for instance in the breasts of women, some of which did no serious harm to the patient and may have persisted for years; they were called benign. Others grew and became ulcerating masses in the breast and overlying skin and eventually caused the death of the patient; these were called cancer. Early in antiquity "ulcers" of the skin, a loss of skin continuity, were recognized as being caused by injury, burns, and other agents. Most healed but a few did not and the latter spread widely and deeper into the skin, often causing disfigurement. The latter were also called cancers.

The only sure way that one could tell the difference between the innocuous ulcers or lumps and cancer was to follow the course of the disease. If the patient died with widespread disease, the lesion was cancerous; if the tumor did not spread and the patient lived for years, it was noncancerous.

A lump in the female breast or elsewhere was called a tumor by the Greeks (onkos, a swelling). From this came the term "oncologist," one who studies tumors. Later the Greek term, "oma," a tumor, was used as a suffix preceded by the organ of the body in which it occurred, e.g., osteoma (Greek: osteo, bone; oma, tumor), a bone tumor. Cancer could be a lump, and therefore a tumor, but many swellings or tumors were noncancerous, e.g., bleeding into an organ to produce a swelling, a hematoma (Greek: tumor of blood).

A tumor formed by the growth of new cells and tissue was called a neoplasm (Greek: new formation). Some neoplasms not only grew larger but they invaded adjacent tissues, spread to other organs of the body, and eventually caused the death of the patient if untreated. These tumors were called malignant (Latin: malicious, bad) neoplasms or cancers. The common cancer of the female breast was a malignant neoplasm.

There were some neoplasms that grew to a limited size, remained in place in the organ in which they arose, and did not invade adjacent tissues significantly or spread to other organs. They were called benign (Old French: benign; Latin: kind, gentle) neoplasms because they did not endanger the health of the patient. An example is the fibroadenoma of the female breast, a benign neoplasm.

Some benign neoplasms (an adenoma or polyp of the colon) change, over time, to malignant neoplasms (a cancer of the colon). For this reason they are removed surgically.

Both benign and malignant neoplasms are often called "tumor" (a swelling) in the everyday terminology of the physician, particularly when he does not know whether it is a benign or malignant.

PROGRESSION OF CANCER

The progression of cancers, in terms of their growth, varies greatly. The common basal cell cancer of the skin invades the skin slowly and rarely metastasizes; its behavior is essentially innocuous. At the other extreme, a cancer of the pancreatic ducts causes the death of most patients within months of diagnosis (2).

The organ in which the cancer arises is called the primary site of the cancer and the organ(s) to which the cancer cells spread is called the secondary site. At the secondary site the cancer cells grow into a colony which is called a "metastasis" (Greek: meta, change; stasis, place). The metastasis grows and makes a home for itself in an organ, most commonly the lungs, liver, or bone marrow. Primary and metastatic cancers absorb and rob the rest of the body of the sustenance and nutriments from the blood stream and cause a loss of weight and strength.

Most cancers, if untreated, invade the lymphatic vessels and adjacent lymph nodes draining the primary organ, or grow into the small veins of the primary organ and get into the bloodstream and spread to other organs. The lymphatic system also empties into the bloodstream. Cancer may spread by either or both systems.

Oncologists can give an average, statistically probable, figure for the length of survival of patients with a particular cancer but the survival of an individual patient may vary greatly from the average. The percentage of patients who are living 5 years after diagnosis of a cancer is called the 5-year survival rate; it is used as a rough indicator of prognosis and as a gauge of the effectiveness of different types of therapy.

If left untreated, most cancers eventually cause the death of the patient, unless death from another cause intervenes. Rarely, spontaneous disappearance of cancer has been reported (3,7) and very rarely a patient may live for years harboring a dormant cancer (4,7,7a). A dormant cancer may be activated, on occasion, to grow locally and metastasize (1,7).

PALEOPATHOLOGY AND CANCER

Was cancer present in ancient man, in prehistoric man, in some of his ape-man predecessors, in early mammals, or even in the earlier invertebrates, plants, or micro-organisms? If cancer appeared some time early in the evolutionary trail would there be any evidence of its presence in fossil remains?

The susceptibility of biologic tissues to the degradative effects of death and the results of burial or exposure to the elements for years usually preclude the preservation of any bodily remains except for bones and teeth. Organs such as heart, lungs, and kidneys and other soft tissues of the body are rarely preserved and then only under special circumstances.

The freezing of animals has resulted in a few mammalian specimens that were well preserved, such as the woolly mammoth whose flesh was eaten by sled dogs when thawed 30,000 years after it was frozen (20). The recently discovered Neolithic hunter found in the Alps was well preserved for about 4,000 years because of a combination of freezing and protection from the mechanical forces of disruption (12,13). Insects preserved in amber show a remarkable state of preservation over millions of years (10,11).

The study of pathologic lesions in animal or human remains of ancient times has been termed paleopathology (Greek: study of ancient disease). Evidence of disease has been found in fossil teeth of fish of the Permian period, about 25 million years ago (22). Dinosaur bones of the Mesozoic period, about 250 to 75 million years ago, have been examined for the presence of disease.

A few human remains preserved in acid soil, such as the "bog men" of Denmark, have been remarkably intact, so that even the half digested porridge of a last meal was recognizable (32). Artificial preservation of human remains was practiced by some cultures and is best illustrated by the Egyptian process of mummification (see below). It is only under such rare circumstances that human remains are available for examination centuries after death. Microscopic examination of prehistoric bone by histologic techniques has been performed in only a few fossils (8,17).

For the 2 to 3 billion years in which there is definite evidence of the existence of life on earth (25), the bones of large animals are the ones most frequently available. The reptilian era, represented by the well-known dinosaurs, occurred about 300 million years ago during the Carboniferous period; reptiles were the predominant life form from 230 to 70 million years ago. Bone "tumors" have been described in dinosaurs from the Mesozoic era (22) but they were probably the result of injuries, arthritis, or other noncancerous diseases.

"Cave bear tumors," from the Pleistocene epoch of about 600,000 years ago, have been found; these bone lesions were originally called sarcomas (cancers of connective tissue). Examination by pathologists revealed that the bone lesions were those of arthritis (31). Over 600 types of animals and plants from the late Pleistocene period (36,000 to 10,000 years ago) were preserved in the La Brea, California, tar pit (28,30); Moody found arthritis in the bones of many but no cancers (22).

The primates first appeared in the Paleocene epoch about 70 million years ago and the apes about 35 million years ago. The common ancestor of the hominids—the human family—was *Ramapithecus,* a small ape-like genus which appeared on the evolutionary scene about 12 million years ago. There followed a long void with an absence of fossil remains until the remains of three species of primates from about 3 to 4 million years ago were discovered in Africa. About 750,000 years ago, two of these species vanished and the third (fig. 1-1), *Homo erectus,* who walked upright, remained. The latter had a bone tumor that was originally called a "sarcoma," a cancer of bone (fig. 1-2) (9,19).

Homo erectus was called the Java man because his remains, a femur (thigh bone) and skull, were discovered on the left bank of the Solo River in central Java. They were estimated to be about 500,000 years old (9,19,25). The left femur (fig. 1-2) had a projecting growth of bone on its posterior aspect extending outward from a point where the

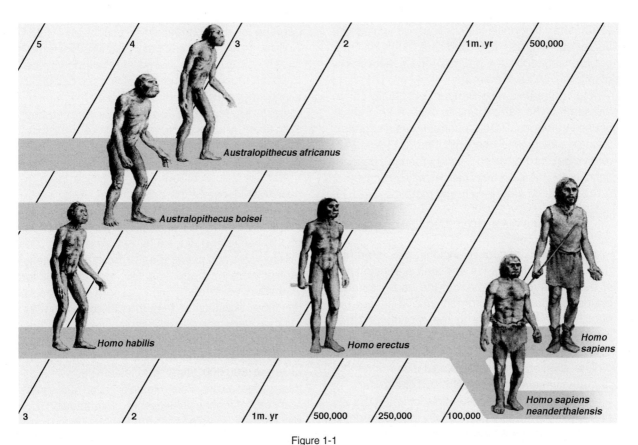

Figure 1-1
POSSIBLE SEQUENCE OF HOMO SAPIENS' ANCESTORS
A possible path of the evolution of man from the *Homo habilis* to *Homo sapiens. Homo erectus* was said to have a bone cancer.
(Modified from figure in reference 19.)

adductor muscle would have been inserted. Although called a bone sarcoma for years, the tumor probably was noncancerous and represented a calcification of muscle called myositis ossificans. This lesion occasionally occurs today following injury to, and hemorrhage into, muscle, which then becomes calcified (9,24). This bony muscle lesion may represent the oldest recognized example of primate pathology.

A small piece of a jawbone from a Neolithic man living about 500,000 years ago in the Stone Age was found in Kanam, Kenya. It contained a solid tumor, originally interpreted as a bone sarcoma (18). More recent study (29) of the tumor led to the diagnosis of a noncancerous bone callus of an infected fracture (9), although there is debate about this diagnosis (27).

A benign tumor in each of two femurs of Neolithic men has been described (16). A late Neolithic skull from the Pyrenees had "punched out" discrete holes

in bone, which may have been metastatic cancer from a nonskeletal primary, or a primary multiple myeloma of bone, a cancer of bone marrow (14). A tumor of the skull of a Dane of the Neolithic period has revealed osteolytic and destructive features of bone, possibly a cancer (9). The difficulty in differentiating a primary cancer of bone from a metastatic one, and these possibilities from artifacts, has been discussed (21,24,33).

The relative absence of primary and metastatic bone cancer in fossil remains has been striking. The scarcity may be related partially to the fact that ape-man and early man did not, on the average, live into the so-called cancer age—over 50 years of age—when most cancers of today occur.

A few cases with debatable evidence suggest the existence of rare benign and malignant bone tumors in late prehistoric man (16). Since organs composed of soft tissues—lungs, gastrointestinal

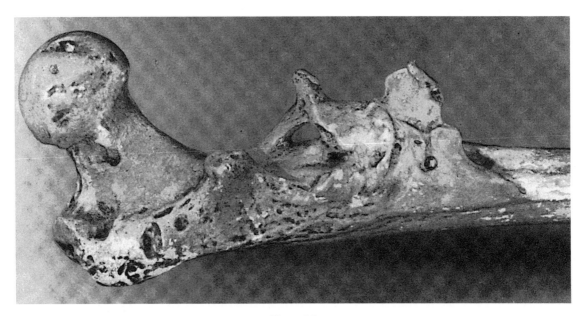

Figure 1-2
MYOSITIS OSSIFICANS, IN "JAVA MAN"
Hypertrophic bone lesion, probably caused by traumatic myositis ossificans, of the left femur of *Homo erectus (Pithecanthropus),* "Java man." Originally called a bone cancer, it probably was the result of calcification of injured muscle. Cast of the original specimen. (Fig. 96 from Ortner DJ, Putschar WG. Identification of pathological conditions in human skeletal remains. Smithsonian contributions to anthropology, No. 28. Washington, D.C.: Smithsonian Institution Press, 1981:84,85.)

tract, kidneys, or other organs—were rarely preserved and since most cancers today arise from soft tissues, it cannot be determined whether cancers of these organs existed in antiquity (Note 1). No cancer of soft tissues has, as yet, been satisfactorily identified in prehistoric remains.

REFERENCES

Cancer

1. Allen JC, Jaeschke WH. Recurrence of malignant melanoma in an orbit after 28 years. Arch Ophthalmol 1966;76:79–81.
2. Cubilla AL, Fitzgerald PJ. Tumors of the exocrine pancreas. Atlas of Tumor Pathology, 2nd Series, Fascicle 19. Washington, D.C.: Armed Forces Institute of Pathology, 1984.
3. Everson TC, Cole WH. Spontaneous regression of cancer. Philadelphia: WB Saunders, 1966.
4. Lowy AD Jr, Erickson ER. Spontaneous 19-year regression of oat cell carcinoma with scalene node metastasis. Cancer 1986;58:978–80.
5. Rather LJ. The genesis of cancer: a study in the history of ideas. Baltimore: Johns Hopkins Univ. Press, 1978:16.
6. Retsas S. On the antiquity of cancer; from Hippocrates to Galen. In: Palaeo-Oncology: the antiquity of cancer. London: Farrand Press, 1986:41–58.
7. Stewart F. Experiences in spontaneous regression of neoplastic disease in man. Texas Reports on Biology and Medicine 1952;10:239–53.
7a. Tchertkoff V, Hauser AD. Carcinoma of head of pancreas with spontaneous regression. NY State J Med 1974;74:1814–7.

NOTE 1: A recently developed technique, the polymerase chain amplification (PCA), multiplies small amounts of DNA up to a million or more times (23). This technique might be used to study DNA or RNA in an ancient body (12,13), in insects, or in cells that happened to be specially preserved (10,11).

As yet, there are no distinctive patterns in DNA recognized as diagnostic of cancer. If it were discovered that specific genetic changes are distinctive of cancer, it might be possible, under special considerations of preservation (15,23,26, 34), to document a cancer that had been present in prehistoric remains.

Paleopathology and Cancer

8. Blumberg JM, Kerley ER. A critical consideration of roentgenology and microscopy in paleontology. In: Jarcho S, ed. Human palaeopathology, New Haven: Yale University Press, 1966:150–70.

9. Brothwell D. The evidence for neoplasms. In: Brothwell D, Sandison AT, eds. Diseases in antiquity; a survey of the diseases, injuries, and surgery of early populations. Springfield, IL: Charles Thomas, 1967:320–45.

10. Cano RJ, Poinar HN, Roubik DW, Poinar GO. Enzymatic amplification and nucleotide sequencing of portions of the 18s rRNA gene of the bee Proplebeia dominicana (Apidae: Hymenoptera) isolated from 25-40 million year old Dominican amber. Medical Science Research 1992;20:619–22.

11. DeSalle R, Gatesy J, Wheeler W, Grimaldi D. DNA sequences from a fossil termite in oligo-miocene amber and their phylogenetic implications. Science 1992;257:1933.

12. Eijgenraam F, Anderson A. A window on life in the Bronze Age. The remains of a 4,000-year-old man may shed light on the racial structure and culture of early Europe. Science 1991;254:187–8.

13. Elmer-Dewitt P. The 4,000-year-old-man. Time, Oct. 7, 1991:48.

14. Fusté M. Antropologia de las poblaciones pirenaicas divante el periodo neo-eneolitico. Trab Inst Bernadino de Sahagún Antrop Y Etnologia 1955:14:109–55.

15. Herrmann B, Hummel S, eds. Ancient DNA: recovery and analysis of genetic material from paleontological, archeological, museum, medical, and forensic specimens. New York: Springer-Verlag, 1994.

16. Janssens P; Dequeecker I, trans. A. Paleopathology. Diseases and injuries of prehistoric man. London: J Baker, 1970.

17. Jarcho S. Human paleopathology; proceedings. New Haven: Yale University Press, 1966:162–3.

18. Lawrence JE. Appendix A. In: Leakey LS, ed. Stone Age races of Kenya. London: Oxford University, 1935:139.

19. Leakey RE, Lewin R. Origins. What new discoveries reveal about the emergence of our species and its possible future. New York: EP Dutton, 1977:32, 79–117, 132–6.

20. Mammuthus. New Encyclopedia Britannica. 15th ed. Micropaedia VI. Chicago: Encyclopedia Britannica, 1974:547.

21. Micozzi MS. Diseases in antiquity. Arch Path Lab Med 1991;115:838–44.

22. Moodie RL. Paleopathology: an introduction to the study of ancient evidences of disease. Urbana: Univ. Illinois Press, 1923:94, 128, 192–4, 221–42.

23. Mullis KB, Faloon F. In: Wu R, ed. Methods in enzymology. New York: Academic Press, 1987:335–50.

24. Ortner DJ, Putschar WG. Identification of pathological conditions in human skeletal remains. Smithsonian contributions to anthropology, No. 28. Washington, D.C.: Smithsonian Institution Press, 1981:84–5, 264–9.

25. Reader J. The rise of life. The first 3–5 billion years. New York: Knopf, 1986:27, 166–8.

26. Ross PE. Eloquent remains. Sci Am 1992;266:114–25.

27. Sandison AT. Kanam mandible's tumor [Letter]. Lancet 1975;1:279.

28. Stock C. Rancho La Brea: a record of Pleistocene life in California. Science series no. 37. Los Angeles: County Museum of Natural History, 1992.

29 Tobias PV. A re-examination of the kanam mandible. Actes du IVe Congrès Panafricain de Préhistoire et de l'Etude du Quaternaire. Tervuren, Belgium: Musée royal de l'Afrique Centrale. 1962:341–64.

30. Van Valkenburgh B, Hertel F. Tough times at La Brea: tooth breakage in large carnivores of the late Pleistocene. Science 1993;261:456–9.

31. Virchow R. Knochen vom Holenbaren mit krankhaften Veränderungen. Z Ethnol 1870;2:365.

32. Wells C. Bones, bodies and disease, evidence of disease and abnormality in early man. New York: Praeger, 1964:28.

33. Wells C. Pseudopathology. In: Brothwell D, Sandison AT, eds. Diseases in antiquity; a survey of the diseases, injuries, and surgery of early populations. Springfield, IL: Charles Thomas, 1967:5–9.

34. Zimmerman MR. An experimental study of mummification pertinent to the antiquity of cancer. Cancer 1977;40:1358–62.

Additional Pertinent References

Elerick DV. Human paleopathology and related subjects. An international bibliography. San Diego: San Diego Museum of Man, 1997.

Sandison AT. Pathologic changes in the skeletons of earlier populations due to acquired disease and difficulties in their interpretation. In: Brothwell DR, ed. The skeletal biology of earlier human populations. Oxford, Pergamon Press, 1968:205–43.

❊ ❊ ❊

2

THE SEARCH FOR CANCER AND ITS CAUSE IN ANCIENT CIVILIZATIONS

Was cancer recognized in the early river valley civilizations of Mesopotamia, Egypt, or India? Was it known in the early days of Chinese history? In a search of these and other ancient cultures do we find any evidence, definitive or suggestive, of the presence of cancer? If cancer were recognized as an entity by a civilization, what did the inhabitants believe caused it?

In the dawn of civilization ignorance of the world and superstition about its operation, as well as of man's own nature, must have led to constant consternation and fear of the unknown. Supernatural forces must have seemed to primitive man to be everywhere present and most powerful. Beset with such overpowering forces it is not surprising that human imagination gave rise to mythology, superstitions, demonology, and religions. Primitive man created supernatural forces, demons, gods, or spirits and he surrounded them with imaginary attributes to explain their supposed existence. Some appeared to give him protection, others caused him

harm. Many of the same diseases present today attacked him but early man had little understanding of them and no weapons with which to defend himself. Only an innate natural immunity protected him against disease and often that must have failed him in his fight for survival.

THE SUPERNATURAL— DEMONS, EVIL SPIRITS, AND GODS

Although they differed in a great many aspects, three civilizations, Mesopotamian, Egyptian, and Indian, had relatively similar beliefs in the supernatural as a cause(s) of disease.

Mesopotamia

In Mesopotamia, all misfortunes and mishaps were caused by demons (fig. 2-1) and evil spirits (fig. 2-2) (5,7). They existed everywhere and were always ready to attack, singly or in groups. The

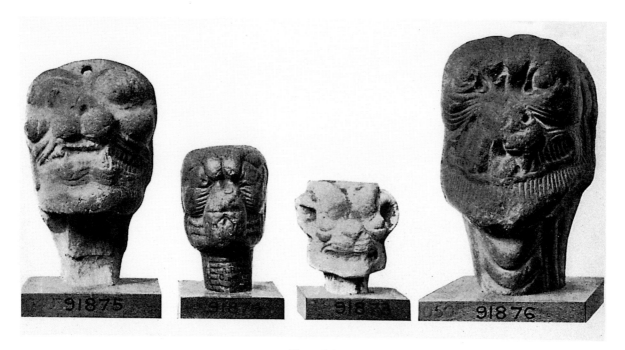

Figure 2-1
BABYLONIAN DEMONS
(Plate ii from Thompson RC. Devils and evil spirits of Babylonia. Vol 1. London: Luzac and Co., 1903:190.)

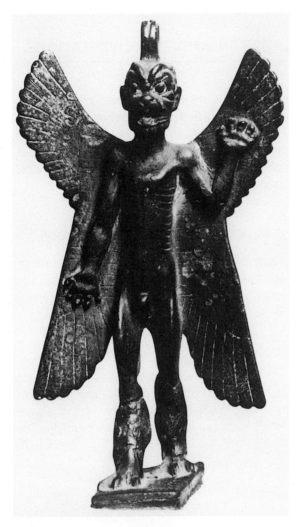

Figure 2-2
BABYLONIAN EVIL SPIRIT
Bronze figure of the dreaded sickness demon Pazuzu (c. 1000-500 BC). The Louvre, Paris.

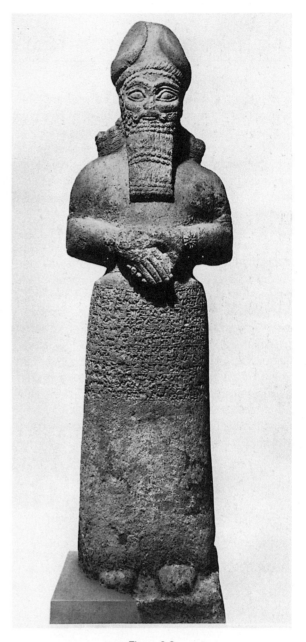

Figure 2-3
BENIGN GOD
A statue of an Assyrian god from the Nabu Temple at Nimrod (809-782 BC). (Courtesy of the British Museum, London.)

afflicting demons included disembodied human souls of the dead and ghosts; unhuman supernatural beings, fiends, and devils, differing from the gods by being of a lower order; and half-human, half-supernatural beings, born of human and ghostly parenthood, awful monsters (7).

The fear of demons was a large part of the life of the individual. Divination and astrology with their implication of a knowledge of the future were part of the magic employed to counteract the effects of demonic spirits (1,8).

There were gods who protected man (fig. 2-3) but they had to be invoked through the magic of the priesthood rituals and ceremonies. Anu, the great god of the heavens, was supreme over all. Good spirits might utilize magic and exorcism against demons and if these measures failed to protect, then as a last resort in Mesopotamia, the god Ea, the god of magic, was thought to alone possess the magic secrets that could conquer and repel the demons (5).

These beliefs were formed during the long evolution from the appearance of the cuneiform technique in about 4,200 BC (6) through the Sumerian period with the cities Ur, Erech, Lagash, and Kisk arising in the 3rd millennium BC (9,10).

In Lenormant's translations of Chaldean (Akkadian) cuneiform incantations there are words and phrases that suggest the possibility that cancer was recognized: "ulcers of a bad kind"; "ulcers which spread, malignant ulcers"; and "the nurse whose breast becomes ulcerated, the nurse who dies of the ulceration of her breast" (3). Did the translator use the word "malignant" as his own interpretation of the lesion and in light of the knowledge of his time (1879)? Did the original language indicate a significant difference in clinical behavior between an ulcer and a "malignant" ulcer? Was the "ulcer of the breast" an ulcer of the skin over the breast or a cancer of the breast causing an ulcer of the overlying skin? As Majno points out, there are many difficulties with the translation of Akkadian terms (2,4). These are questions that probably can't be answered.

There appeared to be no recognition of cancer as a distinctive disease in Mesopotamia.

Egypt

Egypt's category of agents causing disease covered a broader class of offenders than those in Mesopotamia. More specific causes were the result of curses or attacks from an enemy, a person with an evil eye, an animal or a reptile, a malevolent spirit of the dead, or even an inanimate substance. The spirit gained entrance to the body through the eyes, mouth, ears, or nose and spread throughout the body doing damage to various organs.

The power of the evil spirit was opposed by magic and the goal was to bring the evil force under the power of the individual. Magic was also important in the life after death (34).

The Egyptian religion taught that the death of the body was not the end of life, that there was an afterlife. Man was protected by many spiritual elements during life and at the death of the body, Ka, his primary soul, and Akh, his effective spirit which was to undertake the journey to the Next World, remained in the body. These and other spirits had to be maintained and food was placed in the tomb with the body for them. Preparation for the afterlife was achieved by an elaborate process of mummification (fig. 2-4) which

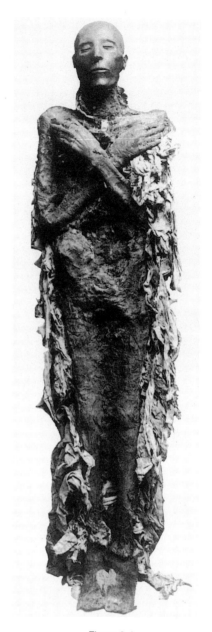

Figure 2-4
MUMMIFICATION
Pharaoh Sethos I; about 1300 BC. One of the well-preserved Egyptian mummies. (From Reeves N, Wilkinson RH. Complete valley of the kings. New York: Thames & Hudson, 1996:138.)

could preserve the body for centuries (16,23,29, 38). An estimated 30,000 mummified bodies have been found (33,38); a few have been examined by autopsy (29,33) and some by X ray (20,21) in the search for evidence of disease (12).

Mummification was accomplished by removing most viscera, desiccating the body for weeks in bags

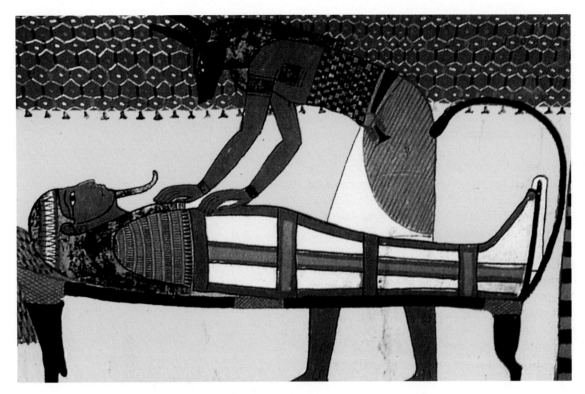

Figure 2-5
ANUBIS
The jackal-headed Anubis, god of the dead and patron saint of the embalmers. He was in charge of preparing the body for eternity.
(Fig. 233 from Siliottis A. Egypt. Splendors of an ancient civilization. New York: Thames & Hudson, 1996:233.)

of salt or in a concentrated solution of natron (sodium carbonate and other salts), and anointing the body with fragrant ointments and a paste of resins mixed with salt and soda fat. The body was then wrapped in bandages, enclosed in a series of overlapping coffins, and entombed in a hidden vault in a pyramid. Elaborate rituals accompanied the embalming process of the Pharaoh and the bodies of members of his court (fig. 2-5) (33); less involved procedures were used for lower ranking dignitaries and little attention was given to the remains of the lowest class, the fellahin. The latter received the cheapest and simplest burial—in the dry hot sands of the desert; ironically, such a burial sometimes preserved the body relatively well for centuries (23,33).

Some examples of neoplasia, benign and malignant, were recorded in Egypt. An important source of knowledge about disease in Egypt was contained in papyri—sheets of the papyrus plants used for recording events—and many have remained decipherable for centuries. The two most important were the Smith and Ebers papyri. In the Smith papyrus there was one case which involved a tumor—case #45, "Bulging Tumors of the Breast"—that has been considered to be a case of breast cancer (13). However, the tumors, in a man, consisted of swellings on the breast which extended beyond the breast and over the anterior portion of the chest wall. The lesions did not display the usual features of today's primary cancer of the breast: men with cancer of the breast today make up about 1 percent of the total number of cases of cancer of the breast in both men and women and in men, the cancer is usually confined to the nipple area but may extend into the breast and the lymph nodes of the contiguous axilla and metastasize (35). The tumors in the Egyptian man were probably caused by bilharziasis or tuberculosis. If the tumors were cancer, they were probably the result of a cancer elsewhere giving rise to metastases in the subcutaneous tissues of the chest.

In the Ebers papyrus there are suggestions of uterine and stomach cancer (17) but the evidence for these is not convincing.

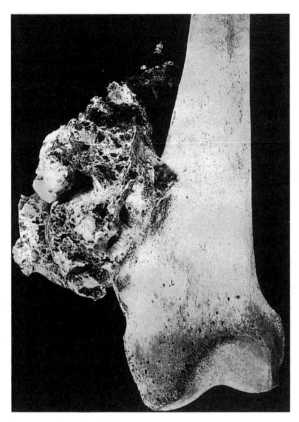

Figure 2-6
FEMUR TUMOR FROM A MUMMY
OF THE V DYNASTY (C. 2,500 BC)
Originally called an osteosarcoma (33), it is probably a
benign neoplasm of cartilage, an osteochondroma (15). (Fig. 64
from Smith GE, Dawson WR, MacVeagh L. Egyptian mummies.
London:Kegan Paul International,1991:144.)

G.E. Smith and W.E. Dawson, English Egyptologists, reported three bone sarcomas in mummies. In one case the tumor was in a femur and in two cases they occurred in head of the humerus of mummies of the V Dynasty of the Pyramid Age (about 2,700 BC) (33). The latter two cases were not described in detail or illustrated. The femur tumor (fig. 2-6) was probably an osteochondroma, a benign neoplasm of bone (15).

Cancer of the maxillo-alveolar region in a skull of an Egyptian of the III to V Dynasty (2,778 to 2,300 BC) was reported by Wells, an English pathologist (37). This probable carcinoma of the nasopharynx was associated with metastatic lesions of the skull. A tumor of cartilage in the right innominate bone of the pelvis was found in an adult female skeleton in the Rock Tombs, Lisht, Egypt (c. 1,800 BC) by M.A. Ruffer, an English pioneer paleopathologist (29). The tumor was a cartilaginous exostosis, a benign neoplasm (25). Ruffer and Willmore reported a tumor from about AD 250 Egypt in the right innominate bone of the pelvis, which was difficult to classify. It may have been an infection or an anomaly (25).

Two mummies had benign tumors of the covering of the brain, a meningioma that secondarily affected the skull (28). They were from the I and XX Dynasties. A genetic defect has been found recently in patients with meningioma and this raises the question of consanguinity being a factor in these neoplasms since it was prevalent in the Egyptian royalty (24).

Depictions of a prominent lower jaw (prognathism) of the Pharaoh Akhenaton (Amenophis IV), the heretic who substituted monotheism for the Egyptic polytheism, suggest the disease acromegaly (fig. 2-7) (25). This is a postpuberty enlargement of the hands, feet, and jaw as the result of a benign tumor of the pituitary gland (11,36). Other suggestions have been Fröhlich's syndrome and Marfan's syndrome, both non-neoplastic. The latter is more likely the correct diagnosis (14).

"Tumors of the god Chonsu," referred to in the Ebers' papyrus (28), are compatible with osteolytic lesions of metastatic cancer, multiple myeloma, a primary cancer of bone, or malignant lymphoma (25–27). However, one of three osteolytic lesions studied was believed not to be neoplastic (26,27).

Other tumors have been identified in mummies: a fibrous uterine cervical polyp (18), a possible ovarian tumor (19), a squamous papilloma of the skin (30), a calcified myoma of the uterus (31), and two cases of a syndrome that includes bone anomalies and a basal cell carcinoma of skin (32). A lipoma, a benign tumor of fat cells, was mentioned in the Ebers papyrus (22).

The definite evidence of neoplastic tumors in the Egyptians did not, apparently, lead to their recognition of cancer as an entity, even though mummification of bodies was practiced.

Costly Separation of Priests and Mummifiers. There was a dichotomy in Egyptian philosophy between the inhibition against dissection of the body and its preservation for life after death. This was resolved, symbolically, by having the initial incision of the abdomen of the dead person made by a designated person, the parischistes. After making this incision, the parischistes was chased away from the scene by a mock tirade against him so that the embalmers could then proceed with their task.

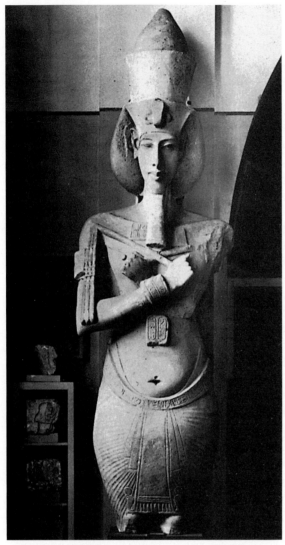

Figure 2-7
STATUE OF THE PHARAOH AKHNATON
A prominent lower jaw suggested the disease acromegaly, the result of a pituitary tumor. Frölich's syndrome was also suggested. (From Velikovski I. Oedipus and Akhnaton. Garden City, NY: Doubleday, 1960:91.)

Mummification was not an anatomic dissection (23,31,32). The low-caste embalmers were segregated from the priestly class physicians who were not involved in the mummification process; this prevented the physician from correlating the patient's signs and symptoms of disease with any changes present in the organs at embalming.

The internal organs of the body, except for the heart and sometimes the kidneys, originally were removed and stored in Canopic jars. Later in history they were restored to the body or placed between the legs. The soft tissues of the mummies have not been generally available for microscopic study, although Ruffer was able to study some (29).

Long, a pathologist, commented ruefully about the mummification process (22):

"... some three quarters of a billion human bodies with all the ills to which the flesh is heir, passed under the hands of Egyptian embalmers. A large proportion of these were opened in the process and countless thousands of diseased hearts, shrunken, abscessed and tuberculous lungs, cirrhotic livers, enlarged and atrophic spleens, infected kidneys and bowels, hardened arteries and clotted veins, in gigantic solemn procession must have been seen, handled and sealed in jars or thrown away ..."

by the uneducated, uninterested workers during the Egyptian period. A correlation between clinical signs and symptoms of disease and anatomic findings at autopsy was not firmly established until the 18th century when an Italian clinician-pathologist made the connection and an understanding of disease processes began (see chapter 7).

Despite the presence of cancerous tumors and the widespread use of mummification, the Egyptians apparently did not recognize cancer as a disease entity.

SIN IN A PREVIOUS LIFE— A CAUSE OF DISEASE?

India

The belief of the Mesopotamian and Egyptian cultures that supernatural forces, demons, and devil spirits caused diseases was part of the Indian philosophy as well. Sin was also an important cause of disease, possibly sin in an earlier life cycle, a reflection of the Indian philosophy of repetitive cycles of existence. Evil men and the caprice of a malevolent god were also thought to influence disease. Kali (fig. 2-8), the goddess of disease, death, and destruction, was feared (40,45,46).

India's health scriptures were the four Vedas, sacred books written in Sanskrit, which may date back to the 2nd millennium BC (45,46). A system of medicine, the Ãyurveda (the knowledge of life), was believed to have been received from Brahma by Dhanvantari who became the god of Indian medicine.

The supernatural attacks by the demons and evil forces focused on the three normal humors (fluids)

During the golden age of Indian medicine (the Brahmanistic period from 800 BC to AD 1000 [45]) two treatises were accepted as the basis of much of Ãyurvedic medicine: 1) The Susruta Samhitã, a compilation by Susruta of surgical procedures, which also contained medical treatment for diseases (44); and 2) The Caraka Samhitã (39,41), a medical treatise compiled by Caraka, a physician. Susruta was the royal physician to Kaniska (42), king of Gandhara, who reigned from 120 to AD 162 (41). The Caraka Samhitã is dated from about the 1st century AD.

Susruta, in mentioning over 1,100 diseases, described tumors, called Gulmas, which occurred inside the body, some in the ovary and uterus. Their cause was not known. The cause of incurable skin tumors was known, however. They were the product of the actions of the doshas, individually or in concert (44). Anatomy was not investigated extensively because the physicians were Brahmins and contact with body wounds, injuries, or death was degrading. The prohibition against cutting into a human body which was sacred in death was circumvented by a method described in the Susruta Samhitã. For examination, the body was placed in a basket and sunk in a pool of water for 7 days. On the removal of the body, tissue would be macerated and could be separated with a stick without cutting into the body. By this means some anatomy—mostly that of bones, ligaments, and joints—was learned (44).

The supernatural constantly intervened in daily life. Majno states that even with an operation as simple as piercing the earlobes for earrings, in order to receive protection from the "evil influences of malignant stars and spirits," the operation had to be postponed until the proper month of the year and until the right lunar and astral combinations occurred. Daily life was full of Beings, good and bad, that could not be neglected. There was a yaksha, a ghost, ". . . in every tree" (fig. 2-9) (40).

Prayer and invocations to the gods were the primary methods of treatment. Magic spells were directed against the demons of disease or the wicked men who were the instigators of witchcraft. Vishnu, a protector of good against evil, was one of the most powerful gods (fig. 2-10).

In addition to the Gulmas mentioned by Susruta (44), Rây and Gupta listed 149 diseases and 103 pathologic conditions mentioned in the Susruta Samhitã (41): tumors of the nose; neck of the bladder; rectal or urinary passage tumors; and a

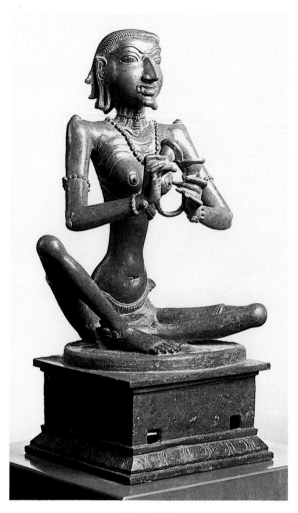

Figure 2-8
KALI, GODDESS OF EVIL
Copper statue of Kali, a goddess of evil, associated with disease, death, and destruction. The Nelson-Atkins Museum of Art, Kansas City, Missouri.

of the body. These humors (doshas), in varying proportions, acted with the blood. They were capricious and easily deranged, and when in disequilibrium caused disease. The doshas were *Vater* (Váyu), wind; *Pitta* (Pittam), bile; and *Kapha* (Kapham), phlegm; one dosha usually predominated. The blood, Rakta, became upset every time the three humors became unbalanced. Health depended on the normal equilibrium of these three substances in the blood; disequilibrium caused pathologic changes. The belief that three substances affected life also occurred in Greek medicine (see below) suggesting communication between the civilizations.

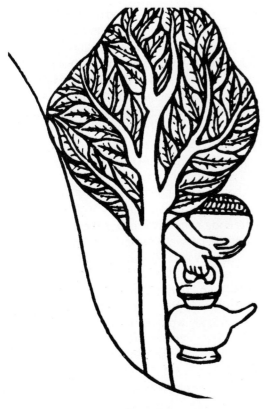

Figure 2-9
A GHOST, A YAKSHA, IN A TREE
Symbolic of the ubiquitous presence of non-human ghosts in Indian life. The Indian Museum, Calcutta, India.

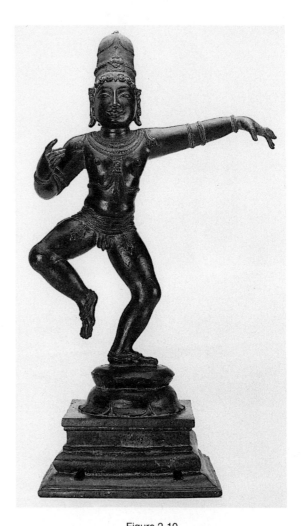

Figure 2-10
COPPER STATUE OF VISHNU,
A PROTECTOR GOD WHO WARDED OFF EVIL
Vishnu appears as Krishna, one of his incarnations. The Nelson-Atkins Museum of Art, Kansas City, Missouri.

chain of tumors around the neck were noted. Also described were vaginal tumors and skin tumors.

J.N. Susraiya, of the Surgery Department of the Tata Memorial Hospital, Bombay, India, translated the Sanskrit of the Susruta Samhitā and suggested that various cancers could be identified in the treatise by retrospective evaluation of the historical clinical record (43). Such retrospective diagnoses are questionable because of the vagaries of the descriptions of the illnesses and the clinical similarities in appearance between many neoplasms and infections. One of the tumors described by Susruta had the appearance of being malignant (43).

Under the heading of etiology and pathology of cancer there is Suraiya's statement: "Three disturbed humours of the body, Vata, Pitta and Kapha interacting with blood, flesh and fat produce the swelling." Blunt injury was considered to be a cause of muscle cancer and overindulgence in eating meat was believed to be another cause of cancer (43).

Whether many of the tumors cited by Susruta, Caraka, or Suraiya were cancers cannot be definitively decided since no modern methods of cancer diagnosis were extant. Some descriptions are not coercive, some are suggestive and others describe tumors that appear to have been cancers. Of the latter, the most likely were those of the oropharynx (43). Today there is a relatively high incidence of oropharyngeal cancer in regions of the old Indian empire.

By the beginning of the Christian Era, it appears that cancer was recognized in India as a definite disease entity. It was believed to have been caused by supernatural forces or the evil exploits of wicked men acting through the doshas.

THE CHINESE COSMOGONY

"ABSOLUTE NOTHING," CHAOS, WU CHI: REPRESENTED BY ○
which evolved of itself the
"GREAT ABSOLUTE" or "GREAT ULTIMATE" or
"GREAT LIMIT" or *T'AI CHI* "PRIMORDIAL MATTER" Represented by ●
This congealed by Revolving, by Unions and Disunions and Formed
the *LIANG I*, or, VITAL ESSENCES
OF THE UNIVERSE: TWO GREAT PRINCIPLES OF THE COSMIC BREATH, OR
CH'I
these are the
YANG I, AND *YIN I*,

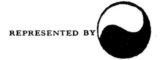

REPRESENTED BY

THE GREAT POSITIVE AND NEGATIVE PRINCIPLES OF THE DUALISM OF CHINESE COSMOGONY.
Their ceaseless permutations produced the four *Hsiang*

SSŬ HSIANG

T'AI YANG	THE GREATER POSITIVE, THE SUN.
T'AI YIN	THE GREATER NEGATIVE, THE MOON.
SHAO YANG	THE LESSER POSITIVE, THE FIXED STARS.
SHAO YIN	THE LESSER NEGATIVE, THE FIVE PLANETS.

In their productions and decay, unions and disunions, there was followed an inscrutable and inevitable law in strict accord with mathematical principles. The law of these changes is the
Li or Tao and the fixed form the *SU*

Figure 2-11
THE CHINESE COSMOGONY
The concept of Yin and Yang and the Tao. (Table 1 from Morse WR. Chinese medicine. Clio Medica, XI. New York: Paul B. Hoeber, 1934:4.)

MAN'S LACK OF HARMONY WITH THE UNIVERSE

China

In contrast to Mesopotamian, Egyptian, and Indian cultures, spirits and demons did not play as significant a role in causing disease in Chinese medicine (52). Man himself was responsible for much of the blame (54).

An ancient Chinese Taoist myth stated that a god, P'an Khu, chiseled out the universe after the separation of primeval chaos into two forces: Yang, the female (negative) and Yin, the male (positive). In women the Yang force predominated and in men the Yin was dominant but both forces were present in each sex to some degree. Yin and Yang circulated throughout the body by way of 12 channels or ducts (52).

Man, who was created with the universe, owed his life and health to his harmony with natural forces. If the relationship was upset, disease and death might result. It was up to man to comply with Tao, the way, a method of harmonizing this world and beyond by shaping earthly conduct to comply with the demands of the other world. One also had

to keep the proper balance of Yin with Yang (fig. 2-11) (52,54). An excess of Yin or Yang, or obstruction to the flow of blood or pneuma (air), gave rise to disease. Man's lack of balance between these and other forces, and a disharmony between the organs of the body, the planets, the seasons, and the colors and sounds corresponding with each organ, caused disease.

The concept of disease localized entirely to one area or organ of the body, prevalent in the modern Western World, did not exist in traditional Chinese medicine (54); disease affected the entire body. Most of man's ailments were caused by a dyscrasia (Greek: bad mixing) of the five elements, a lack of balance between Yin and Yang brought about by the weather or by an infringement against the Tao (54). Less frequently, disease could also arise from internal or external causes, such as demons (fig. 2-12) (50).

Written Chinese medical records began early in the second millennium BC, possibly preceded by oral recitation (50,56). The classic texts include: the *Shu Ching (Classic of History)* and the *Shih Ching (Book of Songs),* written not long after 1000 BC; *The Nei Ching, The Yellow Emperor's Classic of Internal*

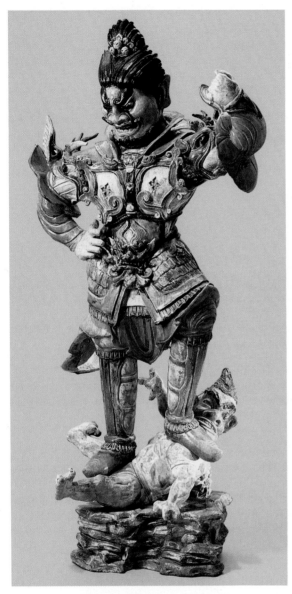

Figure 2-12
PROTECTOR WARRIOR KING

The guardian (King Lokapala), protector of one of four quarters of the Buddhist heaven, is represented as a ferocious warrior destroying a demon. Tang dynasty, AD 700-750. The Nelson-Atkins Museum of Art, Kansas City, Missouri.

Medicine, attributed to Huang Ti, the "Yellow Emperor" (54); and the *Shih Chi, Records of the Historian.*

The Yellow Emperor's Classic, an important exposition of medical philosophy, was written in the form of a dialogue between Huang Ti and his Prime Minister, Chi Po. The Emperor asks questions pertaining to health; the Prime Minister answers, generally espousing a philosophic or medical maxim (54). The book is dated as the first century BC (50, 54). Veith states that it is difficult to determine with any degree of certainty the actual date of the composition of the Yellow Emperor's Classic of Internal Medicine (54). Ascribing the date of writing to the time of the Emperor's life was in keeping with Chinese custom that an important work be ascribed to an ancient emperor.

According to Gwei-Djen Lu, a physician, and Joseph Needham, the British eminent historian of Chinese science, many diseases present today existed in China in 1500 BC (50). They believed, along with Bridgeman, that early Chinese medicine was on a par with, and paralleled, that of Grecian medicine (47,50,51). Some of the diagnoses made by Lu and Needham are debatable: a patient who was a police chief was said to be ". . . too far gone to recover . . ." from "bladder cancer accompanied by intestinal obstruction due to heavy ascaris infestation (chia)." These retrospective diagnoses, which include the patient's general health and three specific diseases, bladder cancer, intestinal obstruction, and the parasitic ascaris infection, require considerable imagination (50). In order to make a diagnosis of bladder cancer today, an experienced oncologist, even in the presence of hematuria, would want a cystoscopic examination of the urinary bladder and a biopsy of any tumor present.

As yet, no large number of body remains have been unearthed in China, as were the mummies of Egypt. In 1974 in Changsha, Hunan, Chinese archaeologists discovered in a tomb the well-preserved remains of the wife of a feudal marquis and an abundance of treasures from the Han period. The "Han lady," as she has been called, was estimated to have died soon after 168 BC (48,49,51–54). The tomb was one of three found in the area; the second tomb was that of her husband and the third was believed to be that of her son.

The lady was dressed in 20 elaborate garments and surrounded by many articles including silk clothing, furniture, toiletries, bamboo food containers, medicinal herbs, wooden figurines to ward off evil spirits, musical instruments, burial money, and various other articles. The tomb of the son contained over 1,000 articles including lacquers, clothing, provisions, a crossbow, and musical instruments. Texts on bamboo, wood, and silk included two medical treatises with breathing exercises (53) and recipes for treating 52 types of ailments (49).

Painted banners and coffins portrayed the soul's journey to the netherworld, the paradise of the immortals. The tombs contained many art treasures of the Han period (206 BC to AD 220) (53).

A recent autopsy of the lady revealed that her left coronary artery was almost totally blocked by atherosclerosis and a cardiologist believed that she died of a heart attack (54). There was no evidence of cancer.

Wong and Wu stated that a patient with cancer of the stomach was reported during the Han dynasty. However, no description of the cancer was given (56).

It would appear from the records available today that cancer was not recognized as an entity in the ancient Chinese repertory of diseases. There is no significant evidence available, at present, to substantiate a diagnosis of cancer in ancient China.

MORE SIN—MONOTHEISM AND JEHOVAH: THE BIBLE AND TALMUD

Ancient Hebrew medical tradition was a reflection of Mesopotamian influences. Disease was believed to be caused by supernatural forces, the demons and spirits of the Assyro-Babylonian cultures. Later came influences from Egypt and Greece (59,60).

The major belief that distinguished Hebrew tradition was monotheism and with this philosophy came the concept of Jehovah, God (58). Health was given to and taken from man by God and any bodily ailment was an affliction for a previous violation of a religious ordinance (60). Since disease was the result of sin, prayer and repentance were necessary for healing or to prevent recurrence (59,60).

Physical and mental health were interdependent and cleanliness of the body was inextricably tied to the purity of the soul. The primary mission of medicine was that of social hygiene. Many diseases were mentioned in the Bible such as plagues, infections, epidemics, and leprosy (59). Galenism (see chapter 3) later became the basis of Talmudic medicine (60,61,63), but the humoral theory is rarely mentioned (60).

Concerning the occurrence of neoplasms during the Biblical period, Preuss stated that ". . . the only body tissue that is ordinarily classified as a tumor is the *shuma,* or mole." There was no mention of the relationship of the mole (nevus) to melanoma, a cancer that may develop in a mole. The occurrence of moles in families and the presence of the hairy mole were noted (60). Preuss mentioned other lesions that are more difficult to identify (60).

After Titus destroyed the temple in Jerusalem he experienced headaches for 7 years and at his autopsy a tumor was said to have been found in his brain. One might speculate that a meningioma (a benign tumor of the covering of the brain) would have given such symptoms, have a relatively long course, and be consistent with the autopsy findings (60). King Jehoram died after 2 years of bowel disease and Preuss suggested the possibility of a rectal carcinoma; other commentators believed the disease was more likely was a noncancerous infection (60).

Steinfeld and McDuff found in the Talmud a report of what probably was a dermoid cyst of the vagina (62). A woman was aborting objects that appeared to be hairs. A physician stated that the woman had a wart in her internal organs from which the hairs grew and these were aborted through the vagina. Dermoid tumors are benign developmental malfunctions that contain skin elements including appendages such as hair.

There appears to be no recognition of cancer as a discrete disease entity in the Bible or Talmud.

CANCER IN THE AMERICAS

Neoplastic tumors of bone have been found in Peruvian, Chilean, and American Indian pre-Columbian skeletal remains (fig. 2-13) (64,65,68). With some of these there is the problem of proper dating.

Urteaga and Pack have described diffuse osteolytic lesions which contained a black pigment, assumed to be melanin, in the bones of nine pre-Columbian Inca Indians of Peru (fig. 2-14) (70). They believed that the lesions were the earliest evidence of metastatic melanoma (a malignant tumor, primarily of skin). Some of the associated remains were 2,400 years old, as determined by radiocarbon (^{14}C) dating.

Remains of an adult female Indian found in the Indian Knoll Site, Kentucky, United States, showed diffuse lytic lesions of bone throughout the skeleton. The case is believed to be metastatic carcinoma and the dating of the bones varies widely, but one date thought probably accurate is 800 to AD 1700 (67). The lesion has also been interpreted as a multiple myeloma (67,69). Osteolytic lesions present a problem in diagnosis between cases of multiple myeloma and metastatic cancer (66,67,71).

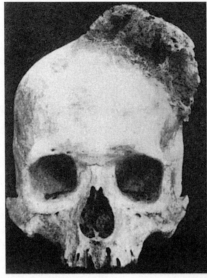
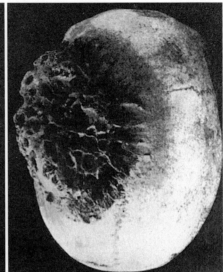

Figure 2-13
HYPEROSTOSIS–SKULL

Bone tumor in skull involving the left parietal and frontal bones (left panel) of a Peruvian male Indian, estimated to be about 60 years old (65). The tumor is probably a hyperostosis (increased growth) of skull bone (right panel), secondary to the pressure of a meningioma, a benign tumor arising in the underlying covering of the brain. (Plate XXXIX from MacCurdy GG. Human skeletal remains from the highlands of Peru. Am J Phys Anthropol 1923;6:218–329.)

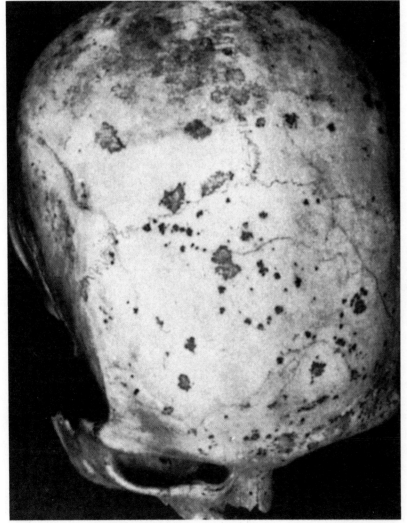

Figure 2-14
EARLY METASTATIC MELANOMA

Multiple osteolytic lesions with associated black pigment, assumed to be melanin, in the skull of a pre-Columbian Inca Indian (70). Radiocarbon (^{14}C) dating of materials associated with the skull were estimated to be 2,400 years old. This is believed to be the earliest recorded melanoma, a cancer most commonly arising in the skin. (Fig. 2A from Urteaga OB, Pack GT. On the antiquity of melanoma. Cancer 1966;19:607–10.)

Bone lesions, representing both benign and malignant neoplasms, have been reported in the remains of Indians in United States and South America, Canadians, and Eskimos. Critical analyses and interpretation of these and other ancient American remains have been published (66,67,71).

REFERENCES

Mesopotamia

1. Jayne WA. The healing gods of ancient civilizations. New Hyde Park, NY: University Books, 1962:89–128.
2. Labat R. Geschwulst, Geschwür, Hautkrankheiten. In: Eberling E, Meissuer B, eds. Reallexikon der Assyriologie, vol III. Berlin: W de Gruyter & Co, 1964:231–3.
3. Lenormant F. Chaldean magic and sorcery. Its origin and development. English translation. London: Bagster, 1878:4–5.
4. Majno G. The healing hand: man and wound in the ancient world. Cambridge, MA: Harvard Univ. Press, 1975:38, 430.
5. Saggs HW. The greatness that was Babylon: a sketch of the ancient civilization of the Tigris-Euphrates Valley. New York: Hawthorne Books, 1962:459–71.
6. Sigerist HE. A history of medicine. Primitive and archaic medicine, vol 1. New York: Oxford Univ. Press, 1951:375–497.
7. Thompson RC. The devils and evil spirits of Babylonia. London: Luzac & Co, 1903.
8. Thorndike L. A history of magic and experimental science, vol 1. New York: Macmillan, 1923:1–35.
9. Woolley CL. The Sumerians. Oxford: Clarendon Press, 1929.
10. Woolley CL. Ur of the Chaldees: a record of seven years of excavation. New York: W.W. Norton, 1965.

Egypt

11. Aldred C, Sandison AT. The Pharaoh Akhenaton: a problem in Egyptology and pathology. Bull Hist Med 1962;36:293–316.
12. Boulos FS. Oncology in Egyptian papyri. In: Restas S, ed. Paleo-oncology, 1986:35–40.
13. Breasted JH. The Edwin Smith surgical papyrus, published in facsimile and hieroglyphic transliteration with translation and commentary in two volumes. Chicago: Univ. Chicago Press, 1930.
14. Brier B. The murder of Tutankhamen: a true story. New York: GP Putnam's Sons, 1998.
15. Brothwell D. Evidence for neoplasms. In: Brothwell D, Sandison AT, eds. Diseases in antiquity. A survey of the diseases, injuries and surgery of early populations. Springfield, IL: Charles Thomas, 1967:323–4.
16. Dawson WR. The beginnings; Egypt and Assyria. Clio Medica. New York: B Hoeber Inc, 1930:31–8.
17. Ebbell B. The papyrus Ebers: the greatest Egyptian document. Copenhagen: Levin and Monksgaard, 1937.
18. Egypt. Survey department. The archaeological survey of Nubia, vol 2. Cairo: National Printing Department, 1908:29.
19. Granville AB. An essay on Egyptian mummies: with observation of the art of embalming among the ancient Egyptians. Philos Trans Royal Soc London 1825;115:269–316.
20. Gray PH. A radiographic skeletal survey of ancient Egyptian mummies. In: Gaillard PJ, van den Hooff A, Steendiejk P, eds. 4th European symposium on calcified tissues. Excerpta Med Int Congr Ser No 120, Amsterdam: Excerpta Medica 966:35–8.
21. Harris JE, Weeks KR. X-raying the Pharaohs. New York: Scribner, 1973.
22. Long ER. A history of pathology. Baltimore: Williams & Wilkins, 1928:516.
23. Majno G. The healing hand. Man and wound in the ancient world. Cambridge, MA: Harvard Univ. Press, 1975:130–9.
24. Mark J. Chromosomal abnormalities and their specificity in human neoplasms: an assessment of recent observations by banding techniques. Adv Cancer Res 1977:24:165–222.
25. Ortner DJ, Putschar WG. Identification of pathologic conditions in human skeletal remains. Washington, D.C.: Smithsonian Institution Press, 1981:264–9, 289–398.
26. Pahl WM. Pathologic findings on a head of a mummy from Dynastic Egypt. Anthropologia Contemporanea 1980;3:27–33.
27. Pahl WM. La tomographmographie par ordinateur appliquée aux momies égyptiennes. Bulletin et Mémoires de la Société d'Anthropologie de Paris (Serie XIII), 1981:343–56.
28. Rowling JT. Pathologic changes in mummies. Proc Roy Soc Med 1961:54:409–15.
29. Ruffer MA. The paleopathology of ancient Egypt. In: Moodie RL, ed. Studies in paleopathology of Egypt. Chicago: Univ. Chicago Press, 1921.
30. Sandison AT. Squamous papilloma of the skin, possibly a solar keratosis, of a woman possibly of late dynastic period. In: Brothwell D, Sandison AT, eds. Diseases in antiquity. A survey of the diseases, injuries and surgery of early populations. Springfield, IL: Charles Thomas, 1967:454–5.
31. Sandison AT, Wells C. Diseases of the reproductive system, In: Brothwell D, Sandison AT, eds. Diseases in antiquity. A survey of the diseases, injuries and surgery of early populations. Springfield, IL: Charles Thomas, 1967:511–3.
32. Satinoff MI, Wells C. Multiple basal cell naevus syndrome found in ancient Egypt. Med Hist 1969;13:294–7.
33. Smith GE, Dawson WR. Egyptian mummies. London: G. Allen & Unwin, 1924.
34. Thorndike L. A history of magic and experimental science. During the first thirteen centuries of our era, vol 1. New York: Columbia University Press, 1923:7–14.
35. Treves N, Holleb AI. Cancer of the male breast, a report of 146 cases. Cancer 1955;8:1239–50.
36. Velikovsky I. Oedipus and Akhnaton: myth and history. Garden City, NY: Doubleday, 1960.
37. Wells C. Ancient Egyptian pathology. J Laryngol Otol 1963;77:261–5.
38. White JE. Ancient Egypt. Its culture and history, New York: Dover, 1970:20–4.

India

39. Caraka; Karviratna AC, transl. Caraka Samhita. Calcutta, India: Sri Satguru, 1896–1912.
40. Majno G. The healing hand: man and wound in the ancient world, Cambridge, MA: Harvard Univ. Press 1975:261–312.
41. Rây P, Gupta. Caraka Samhit. A scientific synopsis. New Dehli: National Institutes of Sciences of India, 1965:38–85, 99–111, 143.
42. Smith V. History of India, from the earliest times to the end of 1911. Oxford: Clarendon Press, 1920:130–7.

43. Suraiya JN. Medicine in ancient India with special reference to cancer. Ind J Cancer 1973;10:391–402.
44. Suruta Samhit; Bhishagratna KL, trans-ed. 3 vols. Varanasi, India: Chowkhamba Sanskrit Series Office, 1998: 172, 246–264.
45. Underwood EA. India. Medical history. Encyclopedia Britannica, 15th ed., Macropaedia, Chicago: Encyclopedia Britannica, 1974;11:823–4.
46. Zimmer HR, Edelstein L, eds. Hindu medicine. Baltimore: Johns Hopkins Univ. Press, 1948:178–83.

China

47. Bridgman RF. La Médecine dans la Chine Antique. Mélanges Chinois et Bouddhiques, vol 10. Brussels, Instit. belge des hautes etudes chinoises, 1955.
48. Hall AJ. A lady from China's past. Nat Geogr 1974;145:661–81.
49. Harper DJ. The Wu-Shih-Erh Ping Fang: translation and prolegomena. Ph.D. dissertation, Univ Ca, Berkeley, Ann Arbor: Univ. Microfilms International, 1982:75–83.
50. Lu GD, Needham J. Records of diseases in ancient China. In: Brothwell D, Sandison AI, eds. Diseases in antiquity. Springfield, IL: Charles Thomas 1967:222–5, 230–7.
51. Majno G. The healing hand: man and wound in the ancient world, Cambridge, MA: Harvard Univ. Press 1975:230–2, 255–7.
52. Morse WR. Chinese medicine. Clio Medica, XI, New York: Paul B. Hoeber, 1934:1–38, 45–9.

53. Pirazzoli-t'Serstevens M. Life in this world and the next: the Mawangdui tombs. In: The Han civilization of China (trans. J. Seligman), Oxford: Phaidon Press, 1982:41–60, 207–8.
54. Time-Life Books, eds. Lost civilizations. China's buried kingdoms. Alexandria, VA: Time-Life Books, 1993:148–9.
55. Veith I; Huang Ti Nei Ching Su Wên, trans. Yellow emperor's classic of internal medicine. Birmingham, AL: The Classics of Medicine Library, 1988:4–24, 49–58.
56. Wong KC, Wu LT. History of Chinese medicine: being a chronicle of medical happenings in China from ancient times to the present period. Tientsin, China: Tientsin Press, 1932:31, 45.
57. Yang WS. The Chinese language. Sci Am 1973;228:51–60.

Bible and Talmud

58. Cahill T. The gifts of the Jews: how a tribe of desert nomads changed the way everyone thinks and feels. New York: Doubleday, 1998.
59. Neuburger M; Playfair E, trans. History of medicine. London: Henry Frowde: Hodder & Stoughton, 1910:38–42, 318–22.
60. Preuss J; Rosner F, ed. Julius Preuss' biblical and talmudic medicine. New York: Sanhedrin Press, 1978:6, 142, 183, 200–6, 262–3, 317, 350.

61. Snowman J. A short history of talmudic medicine. New York: Hermon Press, 1974:7–11.
62. Steinfeld AD, McDuff HC. An ancient report of a dermoid cyst of the vagina. Surg Gynecol Obstet 1980;150:95–6.
63. Sussman M. Diseases in the Bible and the Talmud. In: Brothwell DJ, Sandison AT, eds. Diseases in antiquity. A survey of the diseases, injuries and surgery of early populations. Springfield, IL: Charles Thomas, 1967:209–21.

The Americas

64. Allison MJ, Gerszten E, Dalton HP. Paleopathology in pre-Columbian Americans. Lab Invest 1974:30:407–8.
65. MacCurdy GG. Human skeletal remains from the highlands of Peru. Am J Phys Anthropol 1923:6:218–329.
66. Micozzi MS. Disease in antiquity. The case of cancer. Arch Pathol Lab Med 1991;115:838–44.
67. Ortner DJ, Putschar WG. Identification of pathological conditions in human skeletal remains. Smithsonian contributions to anthropology, no. 28, Washington, D.C.: Smithsonian Institution Press, 1981:265–9, 365–98.

68. Ritchie WA, Warren SL. The occurrence of multiple bony lesions suggesting myeloma in the skeleton of a pre-Columbian Indian. Am J Roentgenol 1932;28:622–8.
69. Steinbock RT. Paleopathological diagnosis and interpretation: bone diseases in ancient human populations. Springfield, IL: C.C. Thomas, 1976.
70. Urteaga O, Pack GT. On the antiquity of melanoma. Cancer 1966;19:607–10.
71. Wells C. Pseudopathology. In: Brothwell D, Sandison AT, eds. Diseases in antiquity. A survey of the diseases, injuries and surgery of early populations. Springfield, IL: Charles Thomas, 1967:5–9.

Additional Pertinent References

Mesopotamia

Civil M. Prescriptions médicales summériennes. Revue d'Assyriol 1960;54:59–72.

Kramer SN. The Sumerians. Their history, culture, and character. Chicago: Univ. of Chicago Press, 1963:93–9.

Labat R. Traité Akkadien de Diagnostics et Prognostics Médicaux. 1: Transcription et Traduction. Collect. de Trav de l'Acad. Internat. d'Hist. des Sci., no. 7, Paris, 1951.

Layard AH. Nineveh and its remains: with an account of a visit to the Chaldar Christians of Kurdistan and the Yezidis, as devil worshippers and an inquiry into the ancient Assyrians. 2 vols. New York: D. Appleton, 1854.

Majno G. The healing hand: man and wound in the ancient world. Cambridge, MA: Harvard University Press, 1975:29–68.

Oppenheim AL. Ancient mesopotamia: portrait of a dead civilization. Chicago: Univ. Chicago Press, 1964.

Pritchard JB. The code of Hammurabi. In: Ancient near eastern texts relating to the old testament. Princeton: Princeton Univ. Press, 1950:163–80.

Strommenger E, Hirmer M; Haglund SC, trans. 5000 years of the art of Mesopotamia. New York: Abrams, 1964.

Thompson RC. Assyrian medical texts. Proc Roy Soc Med. 17: Sect Hist Med. 1923–4;1–34, 19:29–78.

White W Jr. An Assyrian physician's vade mecum. Clio Medica 1969;4:159–71.

Egypt

Dawson WB. Egypt's place in medical history. In: Underwood EA, ed. Science medicine and history. Essays on the evolution of scientific thought and medical practices, vol 1. London: Oxford Univ. Press, 1953:47–60.

Dawson WR. The Egyptian medical papyri. In: Brothwell D, Sandison AT. Diseases in antiquity. Springfield, IL: Charles Thomas, 1967.

El-Gazayerli MM, Abdel-Aziz AS. On bilharziasis and male breast cancer in Egypt: a preliminary report and review of the literature. Br J Cancer 1963;17:566–71.

Erman A. Zaubersprüche für Mutter und Kind. Aus den Papyrus 3027 des Berliner Museums. Berlin, Der Königl: Academie der Wissenschaften, 1901.

Estes JW. The medical skills of ancient Egypt. Science history publications, USA. Canton, MA: Watson Pub Intl, 1989.

Ghalioungui P. Malignancy in ancient Egypt. In: Retsas S, ed. Paleo-oncology, 1986:27–33.

Hurry JB. Imhotep: the Egyptian god of medicine. London: Oxford Press. 1926:22–5.

Jonckheere F. Le Papyrus Medical Chester Beatty. Brussels: de la Fond. Egyptol. Reine Elizabeth, No. 2. 1947.

Ortner DJ, Putschar WG. Identification of pathologic conditions in human skeletal remains. Washington, D.C.: Smithsonian Institution Press, 1981:378–9.

Pickard C, Callen JP, Blumenreich M. Metastatic carcinoma of the breast, an unusual presentation mimicking cutaneous vasculitis. Cancer 1987;59:1184–6.

Rather LJ. The genesis of cancer: a study in the history of ideas. Baltimore: Johns Hopkins Univ. Press, 1978.

Retsas S. Paleo-oncology. The antiquity of cancer. London: Farrand Press, 1986.

Sandison AT. The first recorded case of inflammatory mastitis: Queen Atossa of Persia and the physician Democedes. Med Hist 1959;3:317–22.

Sigerist HE. A history of medicine. Primitive and archaic medicine, vol 1. New York: Oxford Univ. Press, 1951:297–373

Strouhal E. Tumours in the remains of ancient Egyptians. Am J Phys Anthropol 1976;45:613–20.

Todd TW. Egyptian medicine, a critical study of recent claims. Am Anthrop 1921;23:460–70.

White JM. Everyday life in ancient Egypt. New York: Dorset Press, 1963.

India

Castiglioni A; Krumbhaar EB, trans.-ed. A history of medicine. New York: Jason Aronson, 1975:90–4.

Filliozat J. La doctrine classique de la médicenne indienne, ses origines et ses paralleles Grecs. Paris: Imprimerie Nationale, 1949:199–215.

Needham J. Science and civilisation in China, Cambridge: Cambridge Univ. Press, 1965;1:191–248.

Neuburger M; Playfair E, trans. History of medicine. London: Henry Frowde: Hodder & Stoughton, 1910:47.

Sigerist HE. A history of medicine. II. Early Greek, Hindu and Persian medicine. New York, Oxford Univ. Press, 1961:161.

Zimmer HR. Hindu medicine. Baltimore: Johns Hopkins Univ. Press, 1948:184.

China

Harper D. Chinese demonography of the third century B.C. Harvard J Asiatic Studies 1985:45:459–8.

❋ ❋ ❋

3
THE BEGINNING OF SCIENCE

The pre-Socratic period of Greek history from about 600 BC until shortly before 400 BC is usually regarded as the beginning of science. Thales of Miletus (fl. 585 BC), the founder of the Ionian school of natural philosophy and science, believed that all matter was composed of a single element, water (5). Eventually the philosophers of the Ionian school added fire, air, and earth to water as the essential ingredients of matter. Pythagoras (525 BC) placed great importance on the mathematical aspect of matter and life (2).

THE ATOMIC HYPOTHESIS

Various Greek philosophers had attempted to define matter as being formed from small particles (3). Leucippus of Miletus (fl. 430 BC) postulated that matter was composed of atoms, homogeneous indivisible hard units which existed in the void of space. Space was the sum total of those parts of the whole world which at any given moment was not occupied by the atoms. The variety of phenomena in the world was explained by the atoms being of different shape, arrangement, and position, and their ability to form different compounds, combinations of atoms. Atoms in motion were constantly forming compounds as they jostled and collided with each other. Even in compounds there was in each atom a constant state of atomic vibration (1). Richard Feynman, the late Nobel physicist, describes the atomic hypothesis as: ". . . all things are made of atoms—little particles that move around in perpetual motion, attracting each other when they are a little distance apart, but repelling when being squeezed into one another" (4).

Democritus (460–457 BC) (fig. 3-1), a pupil of Leucippus, came to Aldera, Thrace, and founded the Atomistic School there. He agreed with Leucippus but made the theory more definite and systematic, and he added to it. The material universe was infinite and eternal, nothing could be added to it or subtracted from it. "Necessity" foreordained all things that happened or could happen. Religion was banished from consideration in favor of a physical world (1).

Atomism had an uneven course in the history of physical science over the centuries after the speculative reasoning of Leucippus and Democritus (5, 7). It flourished in Greece from about 430 to 280 BC. Much later, with the advances in physics and chemistry in the 17th and 18th centuries, atomism again became an important hypothesis. In 1803, John Dalton, an English physicist, published a definitive work which stated that each chemical element was composed of identical atoms, hard and permanent, of fixed characteristic mass. Compounds were combinations of different elements in simple numerical proportions (6). Advances in the basic sciences led to the current atomic theory (4).

THE DAWN OF RATIONAL MEDICINE

In Greece, medicine began in myth with the healing god, Apollo. His son, Aesculapius, was born of the unfaithful Coronis. When Apollo learned from his talking raven of his wife's proclivities he

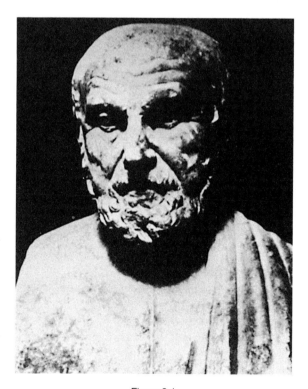

Figure 3-1
DEMOCRITUS
Democritus was co-founder of the atomic theory of matter. Roman copy of Greek sculpture. Museo Capitolino, Rome.

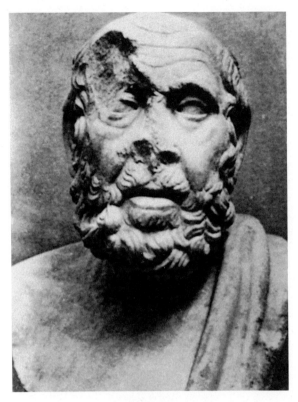

Figure 3-2
HIPPOCRATES

This Greek bust found near Ostia in 1940 is believed to be a true representation of Hippocrates. Probably a Roman copy of a Greek original. (Courtesy of the Museo della via Ostiense, Rome) (9).

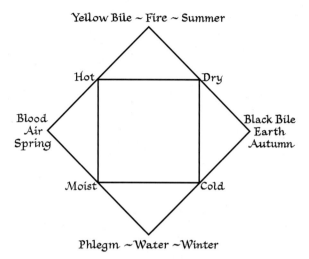

Figure 3-3
HUMORAL DOCTRINE

Greek composite schematic representation of the four elements, the four humors, the four seasons, and the four qualities that determined health and disease. (Modified from fig. 3 from Peart WS. Humors and hormones. Harvey Lecture Series 1977-78;73:262.)

shot an arrow into her breast. Before Apollo carried her to the funeral pyre he opened her abdomen and womb and delivered his son by a pre-Caesar "caesarean" section. Aesculapius evolved into the Grecian god of medicine and his reputation grew with the passage of time. Soon a cult was organized and temples to Aesculapius were erected; in these shrines the sick were treated (24).

Early in Greek history it was believed that the gods sent disease upon mankind for various reasons: offenses against the gods, impiety, vows not kept, lack of sacrifices to the gods, and the innate wickedness of the human heart. The deities caused pestilence and disease to descend upon the hapless Greeks. Later, in the 5th century BC Greek medicine was influenced by the earlier Ionian philosophy and a school of medical thought arose that was rational and secular. The Greeks adopted the Ionian belief in the existence of a natural law that governed the universe, one that could be discovered by observa-

tion and rational deduction. The coupling of the Greek love of intellectual manipulation of ideas and the development of various schools of philosophy, plus experience in the practice of medicine, evolved into a doctrine of medical thought and practice ascribed to a Greek physician, Hippocrates.

The Corpus Hippocraticum

In the 5th century BC, Hippocrates (460–335), a physician of Athens (fig. 3-2), published a compendium of medicine later called the *Corpus Hippocraticum*. It was a collection of medical treatises written at different time periods (9,18–22,24). There is debate as to which treatises were written by Hippocrates and which were written before or after his life (18,28). The corpus has been regarded as the bible of medicine. Hippocrates also formulated a code of ethics for the medical profession, the Hippocratic Oath, which physicians have sworn to obey, with some modifications, to this day.

The Humoral Doctrine

One of the most important concepts in the history of medicine was a hypothesis that eventually hardened into a doctrine. It was first proposed by Hippocrates (18,19) and later modified by Galen in

The Beginning of Science

the 2nd century AD (fig. 3-3) (17,24,32). The Humoral Doctrine was a combination of the contributions of these two leaders in medicine and is more easily understood if considered, arbitrarily, as a single concept. Galen admired Hippocrates (32) and ascribed the original hypothesis to him (30).

The Humoral Doctrine was based on the belief that four fluids of the body, called humors, controlled human health and disease (fig. 3-3) (24,26, 29). An excess of one humor gave rise to the personality and behavior of the individual (33). The four fluids—blood, phlegm, black bile, and yellow bile—regulated health and disease. If the humors were in proper proportion throughout the body there existed a crasis (Greek: krasis, a mingling) which gave health to the individual.

An excess of the blood humor described someone who was of a sanguine temperament, healthy and cheerful; excessive phlegm produced a personality with a cold temperament, caused by this clammy humor; a choleric temperament arose from an excess of yellow bile which produced a bitter or prejudiced personality; and a melancholy or gloomy temperament was caused by a predominance of black bile. The latter was predisposed to develop cancer because of the excess of black bile (15,33). A disproportionate increase or decrease of one of the humors led to disease. Other factors were important, such as the qualities of the humors and the seasons of the year. This hypothesis was consistent with the Greek ideal of moderation, a proper balance between competing elements (29,32).

Clarissimus (Claudius) Galen (AD 129–201)

Galen (fig. 3-4) is one of the most prominent and debatable figures in the history of medicine. He was a prolific author and his prolixity was proverbial; his output ran to over 20 volumes (32). Although born in and retired to Pergamos, Asia Minor, Galen spent much of his life in Rome in the court of Emperor Marcus Aurelius Antoninus where he was physician to the latter's son Commodus. His approach to medical problems generally was a rational one and based on practical experience.

The concept of the humoral doctrine is thought by some to have arisen from the occurrence of two common health complaints in ancient Greece: chest diseases, leading to the prominence of phlegm (mucus) and malaria with its association with hemorrhage (blood) which sometimes accom-

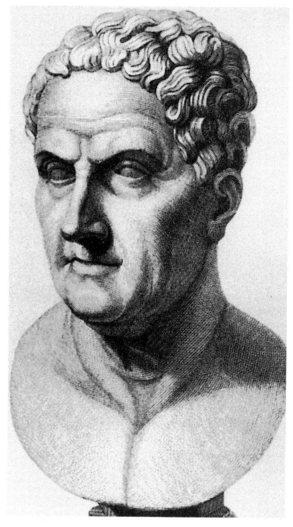

Figure 3-4
CLAUDIUS GALEN
Greek bust believed to be that of Claudius Galen, one of the most influential leaders in medicine. He was a co-founder of the Humoral Doctrine that lasted almost 2,000 years. (Courtesy of the British Library, London.)

panied the malarial fevers. Yellow and black bile may have been suggested by the vomit of recurrent malaria (20). Surprisingly, there is practically no information in the treatise entitled "Humors." The treatise is called, ". . . a scrap-book of the crudest sort . . ." by Jones (20).

Galen added the theory of the Pneumatists to the Hippocratic version of the humoral concept, i.e., that pneuma, which carried the vital forces, was an important component of life (24,30).

Mechanism of Disease Formation

Health was not only the "presentation" of the humors in the right amounts to the organs of the body but, in addition, there had to be a proper "adhesion" of the humor to the organ. When a proper amount of the right kind of fluid reached an organ it adhered to it and was utilized (forerunner of the receptor theory?). An excess of bile in the blood gave rise to jaundice in the tissues because the excess black bile failed to adhere to the spleen and the latter could not remove it from the blood (30). When black bile was in excess in an organ it caused cancer (30).

Secularization of Disease

One of the great contributions of the Greeks to the epidemiology of diseases was the offering of a rational explanation of the afflictions (9,13). Hippocrates indelibly indicated this freedom from the belief in the supernatural as a cause of disease when he discussed epilepsy. The disease had been called the Sacred Disease because it was thought to be caused by the gods. Hippocrates' statement is definitive: "It is thus with regard to the disease called Sacred: it appears to me to be nowise more divine nor more sacred than other diseases, but has a natural cause from which it originates like other afflictions" (18).

The Humoral Doctrine and Cancer

The diagnosis of a tumor in Hippocratic times was limited to an examination by sight, smell, and touch. A clear-cut distinction between inflammations, such as tuberculosis and other infections, and cancer was not possible until the advent of bacteriology and pathology in the latter half of the 19th century.

Hippocrates' book on cancer, *On Carcinosis,* has been lost but Pournaropoulus is quoted as having found 12 references to cancer by Hippocrates in the *Corpus Hippocraticum* (29). Cancers of the breast, uterus, pharynx, nose, and internal organs were mentioned. The general symptoms associated with cancer of internal organs were listed. Their treatment was not advocated. Most cancers were said to be associated with old age.

Galen's Contributions to Cancer

Galen believed that melancholic women had more cancer than women of sanguine tempera-ment because black bile predominated more frequently in melancholic persons. Black bile thickened and accumulated mainly in the face, lips, and breast (29). Because black bile was corrosive when it attacked the skin, it produced an ulcer. A flux of black bile mixed with blood gave rise to a kind of hard inflammation called scirrhous (Greek: hard, fibrous), one form of which was related to, or was capable of being converted into, cancer. Menstrual suppression and hemorrhoids were believed to be carcinogenic because they prevented black bile from being evacuated (34).

Galen classified tumors (swellings) into three groups and this scheme was followed until after the Renaissance, 1,200 years later (34): *Tumores secundum naturam* (tumors secondary to nature), physiological normal swellings, e.g., breast at puberty and the pregnant uterus; *Tumores supra naturam* (tumors above nature), productive and reparative processes following injury, e.g., callus formation around a fractured bone; *Tumores praeter naturam* (tumors contrary to nature), benign and malignant neoplasms (the group also included inflammatory lesions, localized edema, gangrene, cysts, and other lesions which Galen could not differentiate from neoplasms).

Some of Galen's words (29) are notable: "carcinoma is a tumor malignant and indurated, ulcerated or non-ulcerated. It is named after the animal cancer [crab]."

Galen believed that female breast cancer was the most common form of cancer, with a high incidence after the menopause. He also referred to cancers of the male and female genitalia, palate, intestine, and anus (29). He believed that cancers discovered early in their course could be cured but that once the cancer had attained a considerable size no one could cure it without surgery. Galen advised the excision of the affected cancerous part "without leaving a single root . . ." (29). The Greeks described many organs in which cancer was said to have originated (Table 3-1) (30).

Early in his career Galen made substantial achievements in anatomy, embryology, experimental pathology, and in studies of the movement of the blood (23,26,32). He studied the flow of urine from the kidneys and the effects that followed cutting of the spinal cord at different levels in animals. The recurrent laryngeal nerve of a pig was cut and that caused the pig to stop its squealing. This experiment was repeated in other animals and

Table 3-1

ANATOMIC SITES INVOLVED BY CANCER AS RECORDED BY ANCIENT GREEK MEDICAL WRITERS*

Sites	Authors
Head	Aetius
Eyes	Paulus Aeginita, et al.
Eyelids	Rufus
Lip	Rufus
Ear	Rufus
Nose	Hippocrates, et al.
Neck	Rufus
Axilla	Rufus
Chest	Hippocrates
Thorax	Aetius
Thenar	Rufus
Back	Aetius
Groin	Aetius
Anus	Galen et Rufus
Pubes	Rufus
Genitalia, male and female	Galen et Rufus
Glans penis and prepuce	Oribasius
Uterus	Hippocrates, Galen, et al.
Breast(s)	Hippocrates, Galen, et al.
Glands	Paulus Aegineta
Mouth	Philumenus
Palate	Galen
Tonsils	Philumenus
Pharynx	Hippocrates
Intestines, large and small	Galen, et al.

*Listing of the anatomic sites where cancer was said by Retsas to have been recognized by ancient Greek medical writers. (Modified from Table III from reference 29.)

again the voice disappeared, demonstrating the importance of the nervous system in the control of speech. Long, a pathologist and historian, thought highly of Galen's achievements (23). Later in life Galen became a mystic who believed in the power of divination and dreams (30). Because of Galen's renown it became almost sacrilegious in the subsequent centuries to deny or even to question any of his statements. The rigid adherence to his principles prevented significant advances in medical science for hundreds of years and resulted in Galen becoming stigmatized for his disciples' blind adherence to his doctrines.

The Greeks left few skeletal remains, in comparison to the number of mummies preserved by the Egyptians. They usually buried or burned their dead, although some were exposed to the elements or to animals outside the city limits for destruction.

The Alexandrian Center

After the contributions of the Greeks to oncology it might have been expected that the great scientific center in Alexandria, Egypt, would have extended these initial advances. With the death of Alexander the Great in 323 BC his general, Ptolemy I Soter of Macedonia and the latter's son, Ptolemy II Philadelphus, established the famous museum and library at Alexandria, Egypt. The library contained hundreds of thousands of papyri and vellum scrolls (26,31).

With its museums, library, and medical school, Alexandria became the world center of science and medicine. It remained dominant well into the Roman hegemony and advances were made, particularly in mathematical, mechanical, and astronomical fields (10,11). Its library contained the *Corpus Hippocraticum* and great intellects from many parts of the world gathered there. The study of botany, numerology, and the physical sciences was encouraged. Dissection of the human body was pursued and human anatomy was the medical subject in which progress was made. There was an attempt to organize and subsidize science with state support.

Two anatomists emerged from the center: Herophilus (before 300 BC) and Erasistratus (310–250 BC). They described and named many of the body's organs (28). Herophilus was one of the first to search for the cause of disease in the dissection of the human body. Erasistratus studied the physiology of many organs, including the brain.

Alexandrian science gradually lost its intellectual vigor and in 48 BC most of the library was destroyed. Unfortunately, the writings of the Alexandrian physicians were lost; Celsus and others such as Galen were sources of information about some aspects of the medical studies at the center.

Aristotle

Aristotle (384–322 BC), the Greek philosopher, did not contribute directly to oncology but his fundamental contributions to biology were important. He contributed extensively to comparative anatomy, embryology, and zoology (8). His remarks on human anatomy were limited and fanciful but his dissection of animals fostered the study of anatomy. He spoke in generalities of disease and health in man (12) and described some diseases of animals. Aristotle's observations of natural phenomena and his organization and classification of biologic forms of life were important pioneer contributions.

Aristotle's concept of a fixed pattern of the various forms of life and the separate creation of these different classes was later overthrown by the Darwinian theory of evolution (14). Nevertheless, Darwin praised him highly for his contributions. Aristotle's teleologic concepts and approach to biologic problems have found disfavor with modern scientists (27).

During the Hippocratic period there appears to have been a higher incidence of cancer in the Greeks than the Egyptians. The Greeks were better clinicians and they had a more rational approach to disease and possibly they lived to an older age, but the higher incidence of cancer in the Greeks appears to be greater than could be accounted for by more accurate recognition of the disease.

Was there an increase in dietary or environmental carcinogens during the period? Or was there an increase of cosmic ray radiation from outer space which may have caused mutations in the Grecian genes? One extraterrestrial source of radiation, a binary star, Cygnus X-3, at the edge of the Milky Way, temporarily, in 1972, increased its radiation of high energy gamma rays by a factor of 1,000 (25). Recently, gamma ray bursts of very high intensity have been recorded by the space instruments of the astrophysicists (16). The bursts' energy is estimated to be between 100,000 and 1 million electron volts (the photons of optical light from the sun have energies of a few electron volts). One burst of unknown cause was found recently in the Orion constellation; among the possible causes is the collapse of a binary neutron-star system, or a neutron star, an ordinary star, or a white dwarf, colliding with a black hole. Up to 1,000 bursts a year might occur in the sky (16). It will be important to learn more about these and similar blasts of radiation because of their potential carcinogenic effects. Are they a cause of some of the mutations now known to be present in many genes?

Cancer was recognized and recorded probably for the first time in history as a distinct disease of humans by the Greeks, at least by 400 BC, possibly earlier. In addition, they proposed a rational hypothesis that suggested that black bile was its cause. This suggestion became a doctrine that was accepted for almost 2,000 years.

REFERENCES

Beginning of Science

1. Bailey C. The Greek atomists and epicurus. Oxford: Clarendon Press, 1928:74–108, 109–214, 215–534.
2. Clagett M. Greek science: origins and methods. In: Greek science in antiquity. 2nd ed. Princeton Jct, NJ: Scholar's Bookshelf, 1988:33–48.
3. Crombie AC. Medieval and early modern sciences, vol I, 2nd ed. Cambridge, MA: Harvard Univ. Press, 1963:28–9.
4. Feynman RP. Six easy pieces: essentials of physics explained by its most brillant teacher. Reading, MA: Helix Books, 1995:4.
5. Lloyd GE. Early Greek science: Thales to Aristotle. New York: Norton, 1970:1345–9.
6. Moore FJ. Dalton and the atomic theory. In: A history of chemistry. New York: McGraw-Hill, 1918.
7. Whyte LL. Essay on atomism: from Democritus to 1960. New York: T Nelson, 1961.

Greek Medicine

8. Aristotle; Barnes J, ed. The complete works of Aristotle. Revised Oxford translation. Princeton: Princeton Univ. Press, 1984.
9. Barrow MV. Portraits of Hippocrates. Med Hist 1972:16:85–88.
10. Bernal JD. Science in history. The emergence of science, London: Watts, 1954:198–223.
11. Bernand A. Alexandrie la Grande. Paris: Arthaud, 1966.
12. Byers JM. From Hippocrates to Virchow. Reflections on human disease. Chicago: ASCP Press, 1988:31–3.
13. Castiglioni A; Krumbhaar EB, trans. A history of medicine. New York: A.A. Knopf, 1969:148–78.

14. Darwin C. On the origin of species. A facsimile of the first edition. New York: NY Univ. Press, 1988.
15. Fahraeus R. The suspension-stability of the blood. Acta Med Scand 1921;LV:1–228.
16. Fishman GJ, Hartmen DH. Gamma-ray bursts. New observations illuminate the most powerful explosions in the universe. Sci Am 1997;277:46–51.
17. Galen; Kühn GC, ed. Clavdii Galeni Opera Omnia. Lipsiae: Off Libr C Cnoblochii, 1821–1833.
18. Hippocrates; Adams F, trans. The genuine works of Hippocrates. Birmingham, AL: Classics of Medicine Library, 1985:Section 1:3–130, 843.
19. Hippocrates; Chadwick J, Mann WN, trans. The medical works of Hippocrates, vol 4. Springfield, IL: Charles Thomas, 1950:204.
20. Hippocrates; Jones WH, trans. General introduction. London: Heinemann, 1923:ix–lxix, xlvi–lii.
21. Hippocrates; Jones WH, Withington BT, trans., vols 1–4. Cambridge, MA: Harvard Univ. Press, 1959–1962.
22. Hippocrates; Littré E, trans. Oeuvres complètes d'Hippocrate. Paris: JB Bailliere, 1839–61.
23. Long ER. A history of pathology. Baltimore: Williams & Wilkins, 1928:26–37.
24. Lund FB. Greek medicine. Clio medica, vol 18, New York: PB Hoeber, 1936:27–47, 67–71, 95–126, 201–205.
25. MacKeown PK, Weekes TC. Cosmic rays from Cygnus X-3. Sci Amer 1985;253:60–9.
26. Majno G. The healing hand: man and wound in the ancient world. Cambridge, MA: Harvard Univ. Press, 1975:313–338, 395–419.
27. Medawar PB, Medawar JS. Aristotle to zoos: a philosophical dictionary of biology. Cambridge, MA: Harvard Univ. Press, 1983:26–9.
28. Neuburger M; Playfair E, trans. History of medicine, vol. 1. London, H. Frowde, 1910:12–60, 69–87.
29. Retsas S. On the antiquity of cancer; from Hippocrates to Galen. In: Retsas S, ed. Paleo-oncology. The antiquity of cancer. London: Farrand Press, 1986:43–9.
30. Sarton GG. Galen of Pergamon. Lawrence: Univ. Kansas Press, 1954:15–17, 27–41, 49–53, 59–60.
31. Sarton GG. A history of science. Cambridge, MA: Harvard Univ. Press, 1959.
32. Temkin O. Galenism, rise and decline of a medical philosophy. Ithaca, NY: Cornell Univ. Press, 1973:15–8, 18, 101–4, 153–8.
33. Thorndike L. A history of magic and experimental science, vol 1. The first thirteen centuries of our era. New York: Columbia Univ. Press, 1923:127, 157–62.
34. Wolff J. The science of cancerous disease from earliest times to the present times. Ayoub B, trans. Science History Publications, Canton, MA: Watson Publishing, 1989:9–10.

Additional Pertinent References

Beginning of Science

Neuburger M; Playfair E, trans. History of medicine, vol 1. London: H. Frowde, 1910:201–11.

Nutton V. Roman medicine, 250 B.C. to A.D. 200. In: Conra LI, Nutton V, Porter R, Wear A, eds. The Western medical tradition. 800 B.C. to A.D. 1800 by members of the academic unit, the Wellcome Institute for the History of Medicine. Cambridge: Cambridge Univ. Press, 1995:39–69.

Greek Medicine

Bowra CM. The Greek experience. New York: New American Library, 1957;177–98.

Clagett M. Greek science. Origins and methods. In: Greek science in antiquity. 2nd ed. Princeton Jct., New Jersey: A Scholar's Bookshelf, 1988:33–48.

Fleming D. Galen on the motions of the blood in the heart and lungs. Isis 1955;46:14–21.

Galen. On the usefulness of parts of the body. May MT, trans. Ithaca, NY: Cornell Univ. Press, 1968:47–61.

Harvey W. Exercitatio anatomica de motu cordis et sanguinis in animalbus. Leake CC, trans. Springfield, IL: Charles Thomas. 1941.

Lloyd GE. Early Greek science: Thales to Aristotle, New York: WW Norton, 1970:13.

Rather LJ. The genesis of cancer: a study in the history of ideas. Baltimore: Johns Hopkins University Press, 1978.

Reedy J. Galen on cancer and related diseases. Clio Medica, 1970;10:227–38.

Temkin O. Greek medicine as science and craft. Isis. 1953;44:213–25.

✳ ✳ ✳

4

THE ONCOLOGICALLY SOMNOLENT CENTURIES (AD 200–1500)

After the disintegration of the Greek and Roman cultures and the invasion of the barbarians, medicine went into a long eclipse. With the rise of Christianity there was also a parallel rise of Galenism. There seemed to be little conflict of principles between them. Illness was often viewed as a consequence of man's innate sinful nature and he obviously needed help, spiritual or otherwise, in the battle against disease. Christianity thrived eventually and Galenism persisted for centuries. Increasing numbers of shrines of the Christian saints and martyrs arose and patients visited them in the hope of a miraculous cure through supernatural intercession (23).

SCRIBES AND THE PRESERVATION OF KNOWLEDGE

The preservation of Greco-Roman medical knowledge occupied the monks of the monasteries and hospitals (10,12) and later the Arabian scholars who translated the Greek medical treatises into Arabic (24). The conquest of the Eastern Empire by the Mohammedan invaders in the 7th century AD cut off Greek culture from Western Christianity for centuries. By the 10th century, the writings of Aristotle, Hippocrates, Galen, and other Greeks had been translated into Arabic, and with the spread of Arab-Islam culture, Greek medical knowledge was preserved and spread throughout the Arab-Islam world (15). Significant contributions were made by the Arab-Islamic culture to medicine, e.g., the works of Rhazes (865–925) (27) and Avicenna (980–1037) (2).

In oncology, cancers of the stomach and esophagus were described by Avenzoar (1113–1162) at Cordova (27).

ANGLO-SAXON MEDICINE

Anglo-Saxon medicine is usually dated from the introduction of Christianity into England by Augustine in AD 597 to the Norman Conquest, AD 1066 (25). This was a time of almost continuous warfare, devastation, and epidemics of famine and disease. Anglo-Saxon medicine was primitive and probably indicative of the low level of much of the medicine practiced throughout England and possibly Europe

(29). Disease, in the pre-Norman Conquest period, was thought to have been produced by venoms; "flying venom" and "livid venom" were among the nine venoms that caused specific diseases. A great worm, a wind, and the elf-shot (mischievous hidden elfs shooting arrows at passersby) also were responsible for afflictions (29).

The primary sources of medical knowledge were the manuals, leech-books and vernacular texts for the "leeches," as the practitioners of medicine were called (4,5,7,13,14,25). The leeches passed on their crude craft from father to son and practiced medicine only as a side issue to earning their livelihood (fig. 4-1). Singer did not believe that there was any element of rationality or learning from experience evident in the practice of medicine (29). Cameron claimed, however, that Anglo-Saxon medicine was on a par, admittedly at a low level, with that practiced by Mediterranean contemporaries who inherited directly Greco-Roman views of medicine (fig. 4-2) (11).

With the Norman Conquest came ecclesiastics, who treated patients as well as performing their

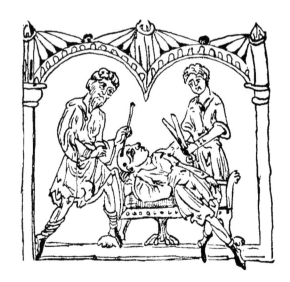

Figure 4-1
NON-TONSURED PHYSICIANS ("LEECHES"),
EARLY ANGLO-SAXON TIMES
(Fig. 1 from Singer CJ. Early English magic and medicine. Proc. British Academy. IX:3,4. London: Oxford Press, 1919–1920:344.)

"Five Leaf, Cinquefoil (Potentilla reptans) III

9. If thou will blind a cancer, or prevent its discharging, then take fiveleaf, the wort, seethe it in wine, and in an old barrow pigs grease without salt; mix all together, work to a plaister, and then lay it on the wound; then it will soon heal.

(From Apuleius)

XIII

5. For cancer, the head of a mad dog burnt to ashes and spread on, healeth the cancer wounds.

(From the Medicina de Quadrupedibus of Sextus Placitus)

Figure 4-2
ANGLO-SAXON PRESCRIPTIONS FOR CANCER
Anglo-Saxon prescriptions, probably of Greek origin. (Items 1:89 and 1:371 from Cockayne TO. Leechdoms, wortcunning and starcraft of early England. 3 vols. London: Holland Press, 1864–1866; revised edition, 1961.)

spiritual duties. Military surgeons also arrived with the Normans. By the 13th century, Oxford and Cambridge were teaching medicine to a few students (12,27). The Anglo-Norman practitioner, Gilbertus Anglicus (c. 1180–1250), wrote the *Compendium Medicinae*, which contained most of the medical knowledge of the day (1).

EARLY OXFORD SCIENCE

During the 13th century there was considerable intellectual ferment instigated by two figures at Oxford University. Robert Grosseteste (1175–1253), Chancellor of Oxford, began to employ inductive reasoning in problems of physics and optics, emphasizing experimental and mathematical methods (16,22). Roger Bacon (1214–1294), the Oxford friar and mystic, called Doctor Mirabilis because of a da Vinci-like array of inventions, espoused the inductive reasoning process, emphasizing observation and experimentation in physics and optics (3,16, 22). The use of inductive reasoning in the 13th century by these two Oxford luminaries was believed by Crombie (16) to be the beginning of a revolution in science that occurred earlier than the generally accepted view that modern science began in the late 16th or early 17th centuries (9).

THE RISE OF THE UNIVERSITIES

The pioneer medical school of Salerno, Italy, was founded in the 11th century. Salerno introduced Arabic medicine into Western Europe, thereby introducing Greek ideas which had been translated from the Arabic into Latin. Salerno had been famous as a center of medical practice for

centuries before its facilities were formalized into a medical school (24). The development of the universities began in the 13th and 14th centuries; medical schools were activated in Bologna and Padua in Italy, Montpellier and Paris in France, and Oxford and Cambridge in England. Surgery became prominent and led to an increased interest in human anatomy. From 1200 to the end of the Middle Ages about 80 universities were founded in Europe (27). Their influence on medical science was great, but medicine had also been practiced earlier in communities (24).

ANATOMY, AUTOPSIES, AND CANCER

One of the most important steps in the study of disease was the beginning of the study of anatomy, mostly in the universities, particularly at Bologna (8,27). The dissection of the human body was important in the training of surgeons, medical students, and artists, but only rarely were such autopsies performed because of antagonism to the opening of the human body after death. Forensic questions occasionally required an autopsy and in the academic world of Europe a few dissections were performed in the 12th and 13th centuries. Joseph Needham, the great scholar of Chinese science, states that anatomic dissection was practiced in China by Pien Chhio, attested to at the time of Wang Mang (AD 9), and continued a little later into the San Kuo period (c. AD 240), after which it vanished until the late middle ages (23).

Two folios were found in the Bodleian Library of Oxford which contained eight illustrations inserted loosely in an unrelated treatise on gynecology from the late 13th century. The folios portrayed the illness, death, and autopsy of a young lady. The illustrations

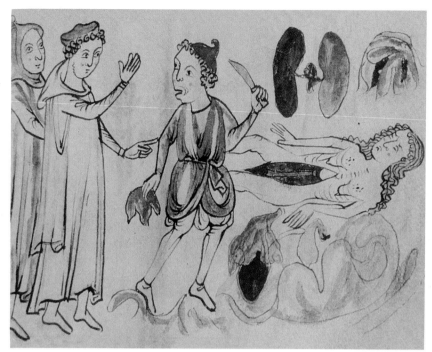

Figure 4-3
AN EARLY AUTOPSY
Representation of an autopsy performed about AD 1290 on a young woman. (Ashmolean manuscript 399, folio 34. The Bodleian Library, Oxford University.)

were estimated by Bober to be from AD 1270–1290. The depiction of the autopsy has given rise to speculation as to the illness causing the death (fig. 4-3) (21,30,32). Singer suggested that the prosector represents a low surgeon who was interrupted in his nefarious task (30). It has also been suggested that what the prosector was holding was not a liver but was a mandrake plant that the patient had placed in her vagina to abort her pregnancy and this was the cause of her death (32). It is more likely that the object being held by the prosector was the liver which often had been represented in antiquity as being trilobed. The suggestion has been made that a septic infection of the uterus occurred (32). If the liver were much smaller than usual, as it appears to be, it would suggest that the cause of death was an acute infectious hepatitis. The relatively gigantic kidneys seem to illustrate the anatomic inexperience of the artist, plus the possibility that they were relatively large. If so, a nephrosis could be considered a possible cause of death.

The cause of the disease is uncertain but the depiction of an autopsy indicates that attention was being paid to changes in the organs that might indicate the cause of death. A fresco on the wall of a catacomb in Rome may have depicted an autopsy in the 4th century AD, but there is doubt as to this interpretation (26).

The first recorded public human dissection, an executed criminal, was performed in AD 1315 by Mondino dei Luzzi in Bologna. In 1316 he published a textbook of anatomy, *Anatomia,* based on his dissections of a few human bodies. The book passed through at least 40 editions and was used until the end of the 16th century (see fig. 5-6) (17).

Antonio Benivieni (c. 1443–1502), an independently minded physician in Florence, did not adhere to the Humoral Doctrine. After his death, his relatives published his notes about some of his patients. The book recorded the postmortem examinations of 15 of Benivieni's patients, performed or observed by him (6,28). The autopsies were undertaken in an attempt to determine the site of the disease and to explain the signs and symptoms which occurred during life.

One patient was a relative of Benivieni who had vomited all food, gradually wasted away and died. Upon dissection of the body Benivieni found a thickening of the wall of the stomach which obstructed the passage of food from the distal portion of the stomach into the duodenum. This probably was a carcinoma of the pyloric end of the stomach. Another case revealed a cancer of the colon.

This alert practicing physician focused attention on the possibility that the cause of disease might be revealed by a postmortem examination (fig. 4-4) (20).

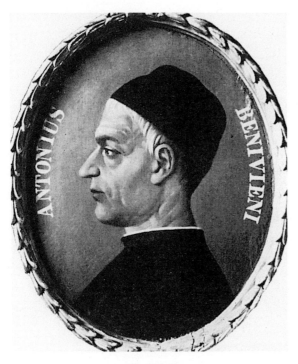

Figure 4-4
ANTONIO BENIVIENI
A medical practitioner in Florence, who autopsied some of his patients in order to find the cause of their death. (Frontispiece from Benivieni A; Singer C, trans. De abditis nonnullis ac mirandis morborum et sanationum causis. Springfield, IL: C.C. Thomas, 1954.)

CANCER IN THE RENAISSANCE

During the 14th and 15th centuries much attention in medicine was preoccupied with compilations, commentaries, glossaries, concordances, and consilia (collections of clinical cases). The questioning of concepts, medical as well as religious, was not generally encouraged, accepted, or rewarded by the political and religious establishments in the early Middle Ages. In the words of Garrison, "The scholiast and the dialectician ruled supreme until more advanced spirits became rank sophists, or skeptics, thus preparing the ground for the true Revival of Learning" (18). There still were adherents of Galenism in the 16th century (19).

Whereas the natural scientists of the 12th and 13th centuries were involved in the study of light and many static phenomena, the basic scientists of the 16th and 17th centuries more often studied motion. In the process they reformed cosmology, overturned the doctrine of geocentricity, and invented a new mathematics, calculus. Involved in these activities were such scientific giants of the Renaissance as Copernicus, Kepler, Galileo, Newton, Francis Bacon, Déscartes, and many others of similar stature (9).

The general state of medicine in the 16th and 17th centuries throughout Europe may be inferred from conditions present in England during that period. Wear has described the social conditions and geographic environment affecting health and disease, and pointed out the difficulty in getting accurate figures for such a fundamental fact as the cause of death (31). "Searchers of the dead," usually old women of the parish, certified deaths based on the symptoms of the deceased as recalled by friends or family. Causes of death such as "old age," "bloody flux," and, "struck suddenly," were reported. In England, in 1665, 68,596 deaths were listed as caused by the plague; consumption (tuberculosis) gave rise to 4,808 deaths; French pox (syphilis) killed 86 people; and cancer, gangrene, and fistula combined caused 56 deaths (31). The incidence of stroke, heart attack, and cancer could not be accurately assessed from such bills of mortality although the predominance of infectious diseases is obvious.

Illness during the 16th and 17th centuries was frequently considered to have been sent by God for one's sins or as a trial of one's faith. The faithful prayed to the saints or to God, and made pilgrimages to shrines where it was believed that miracles might occur.

Oncology slumbered on, undisturbed, with only the unheeded voice of Benivieni and a few other investigators who indicated that examination of the human body might reveal the anatomic cause of some deaths.

REFERENCES

1. Anglicus Gilbertus. Compendium medicinae. London, 1510.
2. Avicenna; Cameron O, trans. A treatise on the canon of medicine of Avicenna. London: Luzac and Co, 1930.
3. Bacon R. In: Little AG, ed. Roger Bacon essays, contributed by various writers on the commemoration of the seventh centenary of his birth. Oxford: Clarendon Press, 1914
4. Bald's Leechbook. (British Museum Royal Manuscript 12D xvii.) In: Wright CE, ed. Early English manuscripts in facsimile, vol 5. Copenhagen: Rosenkilde & Bagger, 1955.
5. Bede; Thompson AH, ed. Bede, his life, times and writings: essays in commemoration of the twelfth century of his death. Oxford: Clarendon Press, 1935:596–612.
6. Benivieni A; Singer C, trans. De abditis nonnullis ac mirandis morborum et sanationum causis. Springfield IL: Charles C. Thomas, 1954.
7. Bonser W. The medical background of Anglo-Saxon England: a study in history, psychology and folklore. London: The Wellcome Historical Medical Library, 1963:12–33.
8. Bullough VL. Medieval Bologna and the development of medical education. Bull Hist Med 1958:32:201–15.
9. Butterfield H. The origin of modern science 1300–1800. London: G Bell, 1951:48–82.
10. Cahill T. How the Irish saved civilization: the untold story of Ireland's heroic role from the fall of Rome to the rise of medieval Europe. New York: NA Talese/Doubleday, 1995.
11. Cameron ML. Anglo-Saxon medicine. Cambridge: Cambridge Univ. Press, 1993:185–6.
12. Castiglioni A; Krumbhaar EB, ed. A history of medicine. New York: J. Aronson, 1975:292–9, 339.
13. Cockayne TO. Leechdoms, wortcunning and starcraft of early England. 3 vols. London: Longman, Roberts & Green, 1864–1866.
14. Colgrave B. Bede's miracle stories. In: Thompson AH, ed. Bede, his life, times and writings: essays in commemoration of the twelfth century of his death. Oxford: Clarendon Press, 1935:201–2.
15. Conrad LI. The Arab-Islamic medical tradition. In: Conrad LI, Wellcome Institute for the History of Medicine, eds. The western medical tradition: 800 BC to 1800 AD. Cambridge: Cambridge Univ. Press, 1995:89–138.
16. Crombie A. Medieval and early modern science, vols I,II. Cambridge, MA: Harvard Univ. Press, 1963:I:102–6; II:11–24.
17. de Vigevano G, ed. Mondino dei Luzzi 1326 Anatomia. Geneva: Slatkine Reprints, 1977.
18. Garrison FH. An introduction to the history of medicine with medical chronology suggestions for study and bibliographic data, 4th ed. Philadelphia: WB Saunders, 1929:166.
19. Ingrassia GF. De tumoribus praeter naturam (1553). Quoted by Shimkin M. Contrary to nature. Washington D.C.: Government Printing Office, 1977:51,52.
20. King LS. A history of the autopsy. A review. Am J Pathol 1973;73:514–44.
21. MacKinney LC, Bober H. A thirteenth-century medical case history in miniatures. Speculum. A journal of medieval studies. 1960;35:251–9.
22. Marrone SP. William of Auvergne and Robert Grosseteste: new ideas of truth in the early thirteenth century. Princeton NJ: Princeton Univ. Press, 1983:3–24, 25–292.
23. Needham J. 1965. Science and civilization in China. Cambridge, MA: Harvard Univ. Press, 1965:150–1.
24. Nutton V. Medicine in late antiquity and the early middle ages. In: Conrad LI, The Wellcome Institute for the History of Medicine, eds. The western medical tradition: 800 BC to 1800 AD. Cambridge: Cambridge Univ. Press, 1995:71–87, 139–205.
25. Payne JF. English medicine in Anglo-Saxon times. Oxford: Clarendon Press, 1904:1–94.
26. Proskaur C. The significance to medical history of the newly discovered fourth century Roman fresco. Bull NY Acad Med 1958;34:672–86.
27. Riesman D. The story of medicine in the middle ages. New York: PB Hoeber, 1935:52–60, 165–72.
28. Shimkin MB. Morbid anatomy begins: Benivieni. In: Shimkin MB, ed. Contrary to nature. Washington D.C.: Government Printing Office, 1977:49–50.
29. Singer C. Early English magic and medicine. Proceedings of the British Academy. London: Oxford Univ. Press, 1920:17, 34.
30. Singer C. Thirteenth century miniatures illustrating medical practice. Proc Royal Soc Med 1915;9:29–41.
31. Wear A. Medicine in early modern Europe 1500–1700. In: Conrad LI, The Wellcome Institute for the History of Medicine, eds. The Western medical tradition: 800 BC–1800 AD. Cambridge: Cambridge Univ. Press, 1995:207–361.
32. Weedon FR, Heusner AP. A clinical-pathological conference from the middle ages. Bull Sch Med Univ NC 1960;8:14–20.

Additional Pertinent References

Crombie AC. Medical and early modern science, vol I. Cambridge, MA: Harvard Univ. Press, 1963:225.

Grattan JH, Singer C. Anglo-Saxon magic and medicine: illustrated specially from the semi-pagan text "Lacnunga," London: Oxford Press, 1952:92.

Riddle JM. Dioscoridies on pharmacy and medicine. Austin: Univ. Texas Press, 1985.

Thompson P. The disease that we call cancer. In: Campbell S, Hall B, Klausner P, ed. Health disease and healing in medieval cultures. New York: St. Martin's Press, 1992:1–11.

✳ ✳ ✳

5

THE REVOLT AGAINST THE HUMORAL DOCTRINE

Until the 16th century the Humoral Doctrine continued to hold sway in medicine. One of the early major personalities who doubted its validity and preached against it was an itinerant practitioner of medicine who may or may not have attended a medical school or university. The peripatetic skeptic had the impressive name of Theophrastus Philipus Aureolus Bombastus von Hohenheim, usually shortened to Paracelsus (fig. 5-1) (7,8).

PARACELSUS (1493–1541)

Paracelsus grew up in the mountains of Switzerland, the son of a practicing physician who was the impoverished scion of a noble family of Swabia. He obtained extensive knowledge of the traditional medicine of the time and impressed all with his learning and capability.

Paracelsus rebelled against ancient medical traditions, denounced academic faculties of medicine, and railed against the local practicing physicians everywhere he traveled to such a degree that he often had to leave a town shortly after arrival. He not only questioned Galenism but advised the burning of the books of medical authorities, including Galen and Avicenna (3).

Paracelsus believed in a chemical approach to disease, yet he could not rise above the superstitions of the time. He taught that the stars and constellations affected the fate of man, including his health, by transmitting poisons from the stars to mankind. The essence of disease was a morbid seed which became implanted in an organ of the body (8).

According to Paracelsus three chemical substances represented various aspects of man: mercury, the spirit; sulfur, the soul; and salt, the body

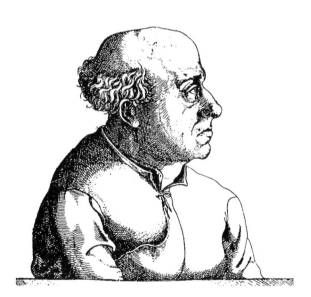

Figure 5-1
PARACELSUS
The revolutionary figure who disparaged Galenism and suggested a chemical approach to disease, including cancer. (Fig. 4 from Pagel W. Paracelsus: an introduction to philosophical medicine in the era of the Renaissance, 2nd ed. Basel: Karger, 1982:29.)

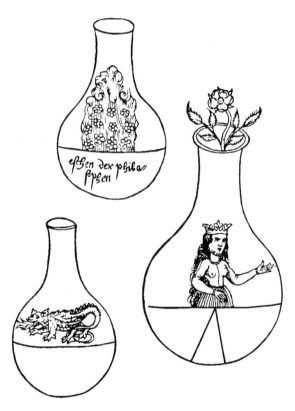

Figure 5-2
CHEMICAL ASPECTS OF MAN
Representation of the three important chemicals, mercury, sulfur, and salt, of Paracelsus' Tria Prima. (Fig. 29 from Pagel W. Paracelsus: an introduction to philosophical medicine in the era of the Renaissance, 2nd ed. Basel: Karger, 1982:268.)

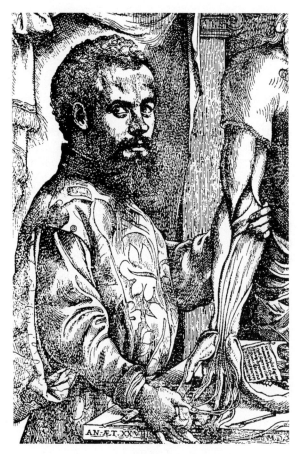

Figure 5-3
VESALIUS
Vesalius, the anatomist, dissecting an arm. (Frontispiece from O'Malley CD. Andreas Vesalius of Brussels, 1514–1564. Berkeley and Los Angeles: Univ California Press, 1964.)

(fig. 5-2). But these three chemicals could also produce disease (8).

Concerning cancer Paracelsus stated, "When you see Cancer, say there is Calcothar" [the salt of vitriol]. Vitriol represented the sulfur salts of metals which after distillation left a residue called "fixed vitriol" (8). Erysipelas and cancer differed by their chemical constitutions, i.e., erysipelas was caused by vitriol and cancer was produced by calcothar, the melancholy dregs, or the residue of vitriol. Cancer was also thought to be correlated with the deposit of arsenic in the world, therefore it could be cured by arsenic since, in Paracelsus' philosophy, the disease and its remedy were attuned to each other as a lock and key (8).

Although he contributed little directly to the advance of oncology, Paracelsus instigated an overall skepticism about ancient medical dogmas and helped to destroy the rigid worship of the tradition and authoritarianism of the Humoral Doctrine. He has justifiably been called the Martin Luther of medicine (10).

ANDREAS VESALIUS (1514–1564)

In contrast to Paracelsus, Vesalius was a studious anatomist who originally believed in the Humoral Doctrine and Galenistic teachings (fig. 5-3). He was a humanist who wrote in Ciceronian Latin (2). Born in Brussels in 1514, Vesalius at the age of 15 years went first to the University of Louvain and then to medical school in Paris. There he was exposed to the Greek doctrines that had been recently translated from Arabic to Latin. In 1537 he enrolled in the medical school at Padua. A brilliant student, he was appointed to the chair of anatomy and surgery the day after he received his medical degree.

Anatomy was taught by the professor sitting in a high chair reading from Galen while a lowly barber-surgeon did the dissection. A third person, the ostensor, pointed out with a stick the object of the exercise. Vesalius dispensed with the barber-surgeon and ostensor, doing the autopsy and lectures himself, quoting Galen (fig. 5-4). Soon Vesalius began to notice from his autopsies that there were omissions and errors in Galen's anatomic studies and found a large number of mistakes in Galen's writings. For instance, there was no *rete mirabilis* in the human brain as Galen taught; it was confined to the ungulates that Galen autopsied (fig. 5-5).

In a short period of 2 1/2 years, Vesalius wrote and published in 1543 his classic book on human anatomy, translated by O'Malley as *Seven Books on the Structure of the Human Body* and is generally called, the *Fabrica* (6). This masterpiece was remarkable not only for its superb drawings, probably by an artist from the Titian school, but for the detailed dissections and the accuracy of his findings (figs. 5-6, 5-7). The Fabrica is regarded as the fundamental study upon which modern anatomy rests and as a model blending of science, art, and topography.

Vesalius' effect on the study of anatomy and medicine was monumental. All of medicine eventually benefited from his solid contributions to the knowledge of the anatomy of the human body and his questioning of Galenism and the Humoral Doctrine (6).

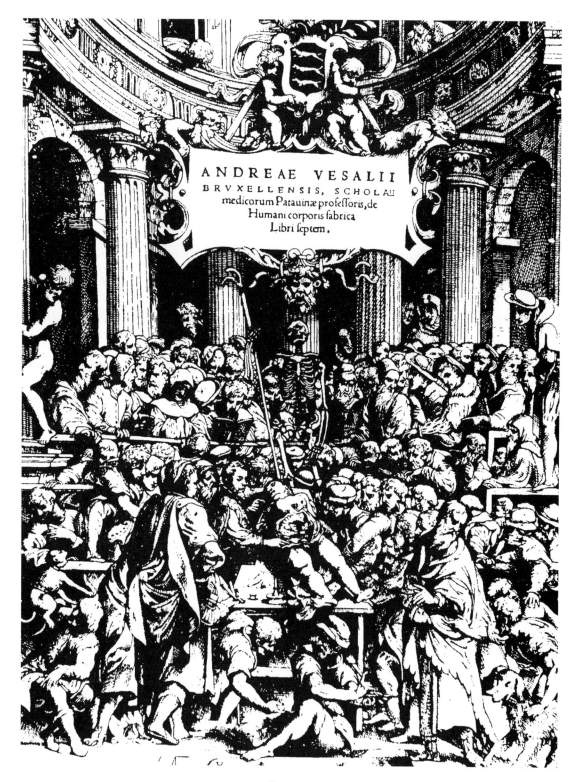

Figure 5-4

VESALIUS DEMONSTRATING ANATOMY

Vesalius doing his own dissections and lecturing while assistants who, prior to Vesalius, did the dissection are confined to a space beneath the autopsy table sharpening knives. (Plate 25 from O'Malley CD. Andreas Vesalius of Brussels, 1514–1564. Berkeley and Los Angeles: Univ California Press, 1964.)

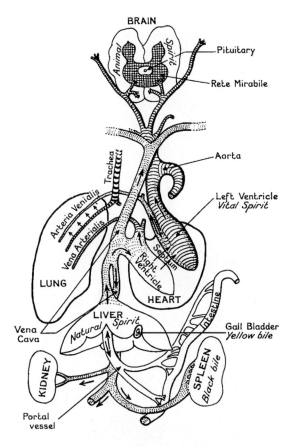

Figure 5-5

DIAGRAM OF GALEN'S PHYSIOLOGY

Rete mirabile at the base of the brain was thought by Galen to be present in humans because he found it in ungulates (hoofed animals). Vital spirits were believed to be transformed into animal spirits there. Vesalius found no such organ in humans. (Plate XIX from Crombie AC. Medieval and early modern science. vol. 1. Cambridge, MA: Harvard Univ. Press, 1963.)

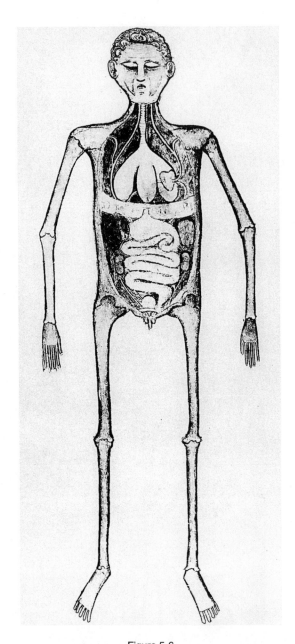

Figure 5-6

HUMAN ANATOMY IN THE FOURTEENTH CENTURY

(Figure from Wickersheimer E. Anatomies de Mondino dei Luzzi et de Guido de Vigevano, 1316. Geneva: Slatkine Reprints, 1977.) (Compare with figure 5-7.)

Prior to Vesalius, Leonardo da Vinci (1452–1519), the great artist and imaginative inventor of the Renaissance, stated that he had performed 30 autopsies in studies of human anatomy. His notebook sketches of various parts of the human body revealed not only his artistic ability but a realistic detailed study of human anatomy. At his death in 1519 the manuscripts were passed to Francesco Melzi and his son but neither published them. Some became available only in 1587. The notebooks were then dispensed to collectors and museums over the next century. Vesalius did not mention Leonardo and presumably the latter's work was not known to him (4).

Michelangelo (1475–1564), another giant of the Renaissance, also dissected human bodies made available to him in the hospital Chiesa di Santo Spirito in Florence. However, his interest was essentially artistic, i.e., to obtain a knowledge of the surface modeling of the body in rest and in motion. The muscles were studied for this purpose (4).

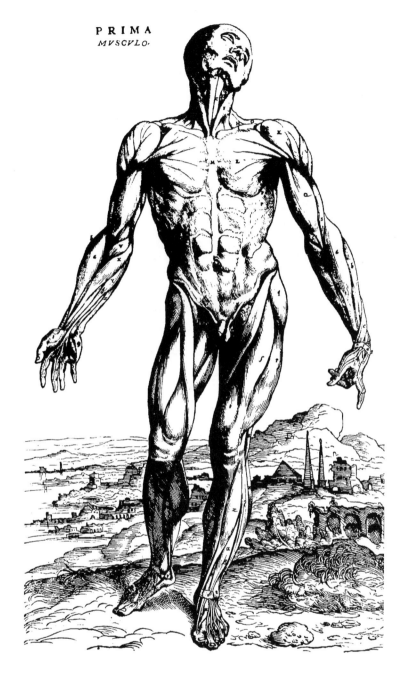

PRIMA
MVSCVLO·

Figure 5-7
MUSCLES OF THE HUMAN BODY,
BY VESALIUS

An accurate portrayal of musculature,
an artistic representation including land-
scape. (Plate 30 from O'Malley CD. Andreas Vesalius of Brussels, 1514–1564.
Berkeley and Los Angeles: Univ. California
Press, 1964:44.)

CLAUDE DESHAIS-GENDRON (1630–1750) THE SOLIDITY OF CANCER

It was more than a century after Vesalius'
Fabrica before the Humoral Doctrine was again
seriously questioned. Deshais-Gendron, a French
surgeon, physician to the brother of Louis XIV, the
"Sun King," challenged the Humoral Doctrine in a
book published in 1700 (1). He contradicted the

concept that cancer consisted of a fluid, the black
bile of the ancients (5,9).

On the basis of his dissection of tumors, Gendron
stated that ". . . cancers were composed of solid
structural substance of degenerate character that
derived from transformation of nervous, glandular
and vascular parts and were inherently capable of
continued destructive growth" (1); cancers were
hard and of ". . . an uniform Nature, very like a

tender Horn, penetrated with blood vessels" (1). Deshais-Gendron's finding of the solid nature of cancer led to his further belief that cancer was a localized resectable entity. It could be cured if completely resected, otherwise it was incurable (1).

After the studies of Paracelsus, Vesalius, and Deshais-Gendron, it would seem that the demise of the Humoral Doctrine was at hand. Yet this did not occur for another 150 years.

REFERENCES

1. Deshais-Gendron C; Taylor J, trans. Enquiries into the nature, knowledge and cures of cancer. London: J Taylor, 1701:5–6, 26–7, 74.
2. Edelstein L. Andreas Vesalius the humanist. In: Tempkin O, ed.; Tempkin CL, trans. Ancient medicine. Selected papers of Ludwig Edelstein. Baltimore: Johns Hopkins Univ. Press 1967:444–54.
3. Grabman JP. Theophrastus Paracelsus. J Hist Med All Sci 1974;29:228–9.
4. McMurrich JP. Leonardo da Vinci, the anatomist (1452–1579). Baltimore: Williams & Wilkins, 1930.
5. Mustacchi P, Shimkin MB. Gendron's enquiries into the nature, knowledge and cure of cancers. Cancer 1956; 9:645–7.
6. O'Malley CD. Andreas Vesalius of Brussels, 1514–1564. Berkeley and Los Angeles: Univ. California Press, 1964.
7. Pachter HM. The story of Paracelsus, magic into science. New York: Henry Schuman, 1951
8. Pagel W. Paracelsus: an introduction to philosophical medicine in the era of the Renaissance, 2nd ed. Basel: Karger, 1982:82–9, 130, 140-141, 146, 147, 367.
9. Rather LJ. The genesis of cancer: a study in the history of ideas. Baltimore: Johns Hopkins Univ. Press, 1978:35–9.
10. Sigerist HE. Four treatises of Theophrastus von Hohenheim called Paracelsus. Baltimore: Johns Hopkins Univ. Press, 1941:8, 12.

Additional Pertinent References

Crombie AC. Medieval and early modern science, 2 vols. Cambridge, MA: Harvard Univ. Press, 1963.

✳ ✳ ✳

6

SPIRITS, SEEDS, POISONS, BLOOD, AND LYMPH STASIS

Although cancer had been recognized as a disease entity in the 16th through the 18th centuries, it did not appear to have been a major cause of concern as were infectious diseases. The Humoral Doctrine, however, was being challenged by other hypotheses explaining the cause of disease during this period.

THE ARCHEUS

Jean Baptiste Van Helmont (1577–1644) (fig. 6-1), a follower of Paracelsus, was a Flemish Capuchin friar, physician, biochemist, and founder of the iatrochemical (Greek: iatro, physician) school. He had an extensive background in the chemistry of his day and an interest in ferments (enzymes), and he performed experiments in chemistry and physiology.

Van Helmont was antagonistic to the Greek Humoral Doctrine and believed in vitalism, a doctrine which proclaimed that human life could not be described in only physical or chemical terms. He believed there was a spiritual, nonmaterial essence in life that separated it from material substances.

Von Helmont believed that in all matter there was an indwelling seed which shared the nature of spirit and matter. The seed contained information that determined the future. In each seed there was an *archeus,* a sensitive soul controlling the body through the means of minor archei scattered throughout the body. Life was regulated by the chief spirit, the archeus, who functioned through ferments (enzymes) in the blood (6). Infection was caused by the invasion of foreign archei (7). The emotional outbursts of a patient might misdirect the archeus so that it sent its ferment to the wrong place. If a woman's breast was injured, the archaeus, furious at the insult, produced a tumor (8).

Cancer was differentiated from other diseases. Cancer was not an imbalance of humors but was the reaction of the archeus to a virulent "light" in tissue which infuriated it to produce a cancer. The "light" was an immaterial force (6).

As with many of his contemporaries, Van Helmont combined a mixture of a belief in spirits with a beginning chemical approach to disease (6). He may have suggested the first clinical trial of a remedy by matching a group of patients given the remedy against a control group of patients not exposed to it (10).

ANIMISM, CIRCULATORY STASIS, AND CANCER SEEDS

Georg Ernst Stahl (1660–1734), a professor of medicine at Halle and Berlin, was a member of the iatrochemical school. He considered most diseases to be the result of stasis (Greek: standing still, stagnation) of the blood in the vascular system (2–4).

Stahl was a dynamist who declared that Animism (nature) represented the unity of the entire body and soul. The soul animated the body, directed its functions, and was in charge of reasoning, intelligence, and voluntary action. The anima protected the

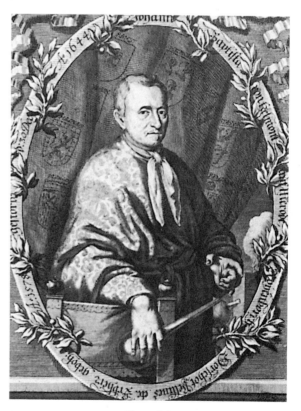

Figure 6-1
JEAN BAPTISTE VAN HELMONT
J.B. Van Helmont of Brussels, friar, physician, and biochemist. Founder of the iatrochemical school. (From Pagel W. John Baptista van Helmont. Cambridge: Cambridge Univ. Press, 1982:18.)

organism from the deterioration to which it tended, and against putrefaction which occurred in the absence of anima. Anima provoked the organism to movement; when the vital movements of life were altered disease supervened.

The activity of nature was expressed through the circulatory system. Stasis of the circulation of the blood led to its thickening; unfavorable reactions resulted in a block in circulation which gave rise to disease; and bile was trapped in solid parts of the body, broke down, and in the ensuing inflammation could become a cancer. The blockage could lead to a scirrhus, a hard tumor incapable of being completely resolved, or it could degenerate into a corrosive and putrid form that caused cancer (9,11).

Stahl resorted to "ferments" and "seeds" to explain the recurrence of cancer after surgical removal of the breast. The true seeds, or roots of the cancer, sat within one's blocked blood vessels. If left behind after surgery the seed, a ferment, could disseminate into minute branches of the vasculature and be the source of a recurrence of the cancer. The cancer ferment, or seed, could reproduce itself and thereby give rise to recurrence (9).

Stahl was involved in the biochemical controversy involving combustion and he proposed the hypothetical substance phlogiston (1).

As with Van Helmont, there was an odd combination in Stahl of beginning chemical and physical sciences, with an emphasis on circulatory stasis and an overriding of mystical substances, the seeds, which caused the cancer.

LYMPH STASIS AND CANCER

Frederick Hoffmann (1660–1742), a professor of medicine at Halle and a member of the iatromechanical school, thought that all processes of the body were regulated by the reaction of atomic particles and that blockage of these movements was the cause of disease (2,3,5). "When the pores and openings are injured and distorted, the humors not only stagnate, but become corrupt, as evidenced by stromas, excrescences, scirrhuses and cancerous ulcers" (5). Hoffmann emphasized that excessive or overly tenacious lymph might retard lymph flow and give rise to its stagnation, a change towards an acid condition leading to suppuration (formation of pus), or result in a hard tumor, a scirrhus. If a scirrhus was formed, under the action of corrosive matter the end result was a cancer (5,9).

King stated that Hoffmann's approach to medicine was dependent on rationalism, inference, and assertion without any need for concrete evidence to bolster his hypotheses (6).

The variety of concepts proposed for the cause of cancer during the 16th to early in 18th centuries indicates that the Humoral Doctrine was losing adherents. However, the opposing hypotheses, with their combinations of spirits and seeds and/or the interference with blood or lymph flow, did not gain lasting support.

No significant advance in concepts concerning carcinogenesis appears to have been made during these centuries.

REFERENCES

1. Butterfield H. The history of science origins and results of the scientific revolution: a symposium. London: Cohen and West, 1951:177–82.
2. Castiglioni A; Krumbhaar EB, trans. A history of medicine. New York: Knopf and J Aronson 1975:582–5.
3. Garrison FH. An introduction to the history of medicine, 4th ed. Philadelphia: WB Saunders, 1929:312–4.
4. Haigh E. Xavier Bichat and the medical theory of the eighteenth century. London: Wellcome Institute for the History of Medicine, 1984:26–8.
5. Hoffmann F; King LS, trans. Fundamenta medicinae. New York: Elsevier, 1971:96.
6. King LS. The road to medical enlightenment. London: MacDonald, New York: Elsevier, 1970:37–62, 181–204.
7. Pagel W. Jean Baptista Van Helmont: reformer of science and medicine. New York: Cambridge Univ. Press, 1982.
8. Pagel W. Van Helmont's concept of disease–to be or not to be? The influence of Paracelsus. Bull Hist Med 1972;46:419–54.
9. Rather L. The genesis of cancer. Baltimore: Johns Hopkins Univ. Press, 1978:32–5..
10. Van Helmont JB; Chandler J, trans. Oriatrike or physik refined. Cited by Debus AG. In: The chemical dream of the Renaissance. Cambridge: Heffer 1968:27.
11. Wolff J. The science of cancerous disease. From earliest times to the present, vol 1. Canton, MA: Science History Publications, 1989:598–9.

7

THE ORGAN—THE SITE OF THE ORIGIN OF CANCER

From the 16th through the 18th centuries, as more autopsies were performed, many diseases were reported to be associated with changes in an organ of the body (1) (Notes 1,2). Cancers were described as present in the stomach, bladder, uterus, ovary, brain, rectum, bone, and a genital organ of either sex (1,3,5,6). The concept that cancer was a disease of the humors of the body began to lose credence.

GIOVANNI BATTISTA MORGAGNI (1682–1771)

In 1761 a book that correlated the clinical signs and symptoms of diseases with their effects on the body, as demonstrated at autopsy, was published (10). Its author, Morgagni (fig. 7-1), was a pioneer figure in pathology, often called the father of gross pathologic anatomy. He held the chair of anatomy at Padua, was a practicing physician, pathologist, and popular teacher, an intimate of famous figures of his day, and a recipient of scientific honors from many countries in Europe (7,9,10,13).

Morgagni's fame arose from his book *De Sedibus et Causis Morborum* (The Seats and Causes of Disease), a report of about 700 autopsies, most of which he or his friends had performed. The book recorded observations made by Morgagni over a 50-year period (10). Characteristic of Morgagni's report was a succinct clinical history of the patient, with signs and symptoms of the disease, often including colorful pertinent data, correlated with an accurate description of the pathologic changes found in the organs of the body at autopsy. Many of the patients had been treated or seen in consultation by Morgagni in his clinical medical practice (9,10).

In his book, Morgagni described various diseases: infections such as lobar pneumonia, cirrhosis of the liver, kidney diseases, defects of the blood vascular system, and many others. He described the gross appearance of cancers of the mouth, stomach, rectum, pancreas, adrenal gland, prostate, ovary, and esophagus (10). He noted the enlarged lymph nodes in the axilla of a patient with breast cancer and other enlarged lymph nodes associated with the nearby presence of a cancer, but apparently he did not recognize the process of metastasis (7).

The following case history indicates Morgagni's correlation of pertinent clinical history and his accurate findings at autopsy:

"A man of about fifty-four years of age, had begun, five or six months before, to become somewhat emaciated, in his whole body, when in the beginning of the month of August, of the year 1689, a troublesome vomiting came on, of a fluid which resembl'd water, tinctured with soot. And the same kind of fluid was discharged by stool, sometimes, when the vomiting was upon the patient, and sometimes, when it was absent, but this discharge was not constant. In the meanwhile, scarcely any pain was perceiv'd in the region of the stomach. But the physician having prescribed salt

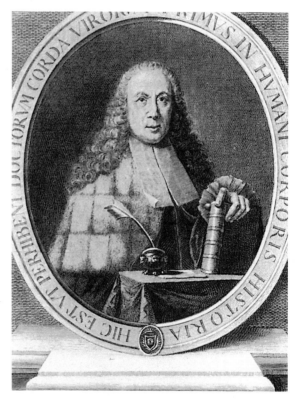

Figure 7-1
GIOVANNI BATTISTA MORGAGNI
Morgagni was an Italian clinician-pathologist of Padua who focused attention on the individual organ as the site of disease and correlated clinical signs and symptoms with the changes in organs at autopsy (10). (From Shimkin MB. Contrary to nature. Washington D.C.: U.S. Department of Health, Education, and Welfare, 1977:74.)

of wormwood, it created such uneasiness in the stomach that it was never given afterwards. At length the vomiting being very violent, with a discharge of the same matter and the pulse growing, by degrees, very languid, death took place of life on the thirteenth of November."

Morgagni's autopsy description of the stomach follows:

In the stomach towards the pylorus [distal end of the stomach where it enters the duodenum], was an ulcerated cancerous tumor, and this seemed to be made up of a congeries of glands, which, being pressed, discharged a kind of humor, like the male semen [probably the mucin of a mucous adenocarcinoma]. And the stomach contain'd three pints of a matter, almost of the same nature with that, which was thrown up by vomiting. Betwixt the stomach and the spleen were two glandular bodies, of the bigness of a bean, and in their color, and substance, not much unlike that tumor which I have described in the stomach. These were the appearances in the belly." Letter XXX, Articles 1, 2, pp. 43, 44 (10).

Morgagni's account is a classic story of carcinoma of the stomach in a patient who had advanced, untreated disease. The age and sex of the patient, the general emaciation, the progressively severe vomiting, and the ultimate death are typical of untreated stomach cancer. The black (soot-like) vomitus and stool represented the bleeding caused by the cancer, altered in color by the gastric and intestinal contents. The "two glandular bodies" between the stomach and the spleen were probably lymph nodes containing metastatic cancer.

Throughout recent history autopsy has played an important role in clarifying the presence and spread of cancer (4,11,14) (Note 2). It still is a significant factor in verifying the presence of cancer and judging the effects of various types of treatment. It may reveal side effects of therapy on organs and cells of the body and other diseases present in the patient (4,7,11,14) (Notes 3,4).

Morgagni's study showed that cancer was a discrete solid entity of neoplastic tissue involving a single organ. This contradicted the Humoral Doctrine with its concept of a derangement of the fluids of the body by black bile.

Morgagni described the anatomic findings of the cancer in organs and correlated these with the clinical signs and symptoms. This was a monumental step forward in furthering clinical medicine, gross pathologic anatomy, and oncology.

DISTINCTION BETWEEN BENIGN AND MALIGNANT TUMORS

In 1643, an important distinction between benign and malignant tumors was attempted by an Italian professor of surgery and anatomy in Naples, Marco Aurelio Severino (1580–1656) (fig. 7-2). Severino described differences between tumors of

---

Note 1: Théophile Bonet (1620–1689), a physician trained at Bologna, collected the written records of over 3,000 autopsies in a book called *The Sepulchretum*. All autopsies were performed in the 16th to 17th centuries (1). The cases were not critically analyzed but they indicate that at that time it was slowly being realized that one might learn much about the cause of disease by a postmortem examination of the human body.

Note 2: In 1586, Marcello Donato, an Italian surgeon, discovered a cancer of the rectum at autopsy of an elderly man who was severely constipated. Donato exhorted his fellow physicians to obtain autopsies on their patients. His comments are still valid today: *"Let those who interdict the opening of bodies well understand their errors. When the cause of a disease is obscure, in opposing the dissection of a corpse which must soon become the food of worms, they do no good to the inanimate mass, and they cause a grave damage to the rest of mankind, for they prevent the physicians from acquiring a knowledge which may afford the means of a great relief eventually to individuals attacked by a similar disease. No less blame is applicable to those physicians who, from laziness love better to remain in the darkness of ignorance than to scrutinize laboriously the truth, not reflecting that by such conduct they render themselves culpable toward God, themselves and society at large."* (3)

Note 3: A more recent reiteration of the value of autopsies is that of the late Sigmund Wilens of the autopsy service at New York City's Bellevue Hospital: *"The old adage that, 'Dead men tell no tales,' does not hold true as far as the medical profession is concerned. Dead men have for centuries been telling doctors the story of how they got sick and why they died, and the doctors have made use of this information very effectively in the treatment of other sick people. The story can be unfolded only by anatomical dissection . . . . The public owes to the dissectors of the dead a debt that it has seldom recognized or acknowledged"* (14).

Note 4: Recently an issue of the Archives of Pathology and Laboratory Medicine was devoted to the subject of autopsies (13). A study from a large teaching medical center showed that there was a discordance between the clinical and autopsy diagnoses of malignant neoplasms: of the 250 malignant neoplasms diagnosed at autopsy 111 (44 percent) were not diagnosed or misdiagnosed clinically. Fifty-four percent of the patients with undiagnosed or wrongly diagnosed malignant neoplasms had local invasion of the tumor or distant metastases (2).

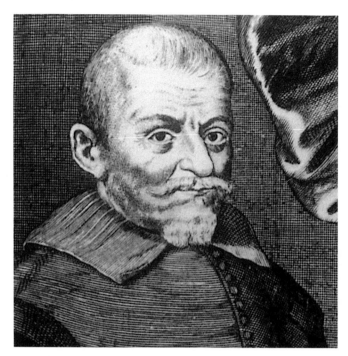

Figure 7-2
MARCO AURELIO SEVERINO
Severino was a professor of surgery and anatomy in Naples who stated that some breast lesions fixed to the chest wall were malignant; other tumors that were freely movable were benign. This was an early attempt to separate benign and malignant lesions of the breast by clinical signs. (From Shimkin MB. Contrary to nature. Washington D.C.: U.S. Department of Health, Education, and Welfare, 1977:68.)

the female breast, separating them into four categories: tumors of glands and stroma, and scirrhous and cancerous tumors. Tumors of glands and stroma did not adhere to underlying flesh, did not occupy the entire breast, were movable, and could be pulled in different directions. These he believed were not cancerous and did not seriously affect the life of the patient. The scirrhous and cancerous tumors were fixed to the underlying chest wall and spread to other organs. They were malignant (8,12).

Severino's separation of benign from malignant tumors based on the correlation of their physical characteristics and behavior was an important landmark dividing the generic term, "tumor" or "neoplasia" into two clinical categories—benign and malignant neoplasms. Although the criteria are not valid in early stage cases seen most often today, nevertheless, Severino's observations were a start towards the separation of benign and malignant neoplasms.

REFERENCES

1. Bonet T. Sepulchretum; sive anatomica practica ex cadaveribus morbo denatis propanens historias et observationes onmium pene humani corporis efectuum. Genevae Sumptilous Leonardi Chouex, 1679.
2. Burton EC, Troxclair DA, Newman WP III. Autopsy diagnoses of malignant neoplasms: how often are clinical diagnoses incorrect? JAMA 1998;280:1245–8.
3. Donato M. de historia medica mirabilis libri sex. Book 4, chapt. 10. Frankfort Gregor/Horst, 1713.
4. Hill RB, Anderson RE. The autopsy: medical practice and public policy. Boston: Butterworth, 1988.
5. King LS, Meehan MC. A history of the autopsy. A review. Am J Pathol 1973;73:514–44.
6. Long ER. History of pathology. Baltimore: Williams & Wilkins, 1928.
7. Long ER. A history of pathology. New York: Dover Publications, 1965:63–75.
8. McLendon WW, ed. College of American Pathologists Conference 29: restructuring autopsy practice for health care reform. Arch Pathol Lab Med 1996;120:693–781.
9. Morgagni G; Jarcho S, trans. The clinical consultations of Giambattista Morgagni. Boston: Countway Library of Medicine, 1984.
10. Morgagni JB; Alexander B, trans. The seats and causes of diseases. Birmingham AL: The classics of medicine library, 1983.
11. Severinus MA. De recondita abscessicum natura, Libri viii. 2nd ed. Francofurti: Impensis Joamis Beyeri, 1643.
12. Shimkin MB. Contrary to nature. Washington, D.C.: Department of Health Education and Welfare, 1977:67–8.
13. Shimkin MB. Gross pathology emerges: Morgagni. In: Contrary to nature. Washington, D.C.: Dept Health Education Welfare, 1977:73–4.
14. Wilens S. My friends the doctors. New York: Atheneum, 1961.

8

THE INDIVIDUAL TISSUE—THE SITE OF ORIGIN OF CANCER

After Morgagni's studies focused attention on the organ as the site of the formation of cancer, the next major advance came from the work of a brilliant French surgeon-pathologist, Marie Francois-Xavier Bichat (1771–1802) (fig. 8-1). Bichat was assistant to Pierre-Joseph Desault, Chief Surgeon of the Hôtel-Dieu in Paris in 1794. At the end of the 18th century, Bichat, after performing about 600 autopsies, wrote that the functioning units of the body consisted of 21 individual membrane (tissue) components (2,3,5,6).

MULTIPLE TISSUES IN EACH ORGAN

In his Traité des Membranes (2,5), Bichat described new categories of units of the body which he called membranes, but are now called tissues. Different combinations of tissues made up the individual organs. Organs had different proportions of the various tissues. Before Bichat it was believed that organs were composed of globules or a hypothetical fiber as the ultimate constituent of tissues (see chapter 10). Blood and fluids were not tissues, according to Bichat, because they lacked vital properties. Rather pointed out that most of Bichat's 21 tissues could be included in the present day categories of epithelium, connective tissue, muscle, and nerve (8).

Bichat was correct: organs of the body are composed of different types of tissue. For example, the stomach contains epithelial mucosa (the inner secreting part), the muscular layers, vascular channels, and the supporting connective tissue. Bichat did not use the microscope. He believed that microscopic instruments at the time were "... a species of agents from which physiology and anatomy, do not seem to me, besides ever to have derived any great assistance, because when we view an object obscurely, everyone sees in his own way, and according as he is affected" (5). The defective lenses of the compound microscope with their chromatic and spherical aberrations were not corrected until the 1820s, after Bichat's death. Instead he used the knife, the naked eye, and a few simple chemical reagents as tools to dissect the organs and identify the tissues (4).

Bichat believed that each tissue exercised the vital properties of irritability and contractility, independent of the body as a whole or of the organ in which the tissue was located. In each individual tissue was the essence of life, whereas previously, a generalized vital principle, a nonmaterial force in the body as a whole, was thought to represent life (8). He realized that disease, while occurring in an organ, afflicted a specific tissue of the organ. The tissues differed from each other in composition and vital properties, therefore each tissue differed in its diseases because diseases were alterations of vital properties. Most diseases were localized to a specific tissue in an organ, except for inflammatory lesions and cancer which could afflict all tissues (5).

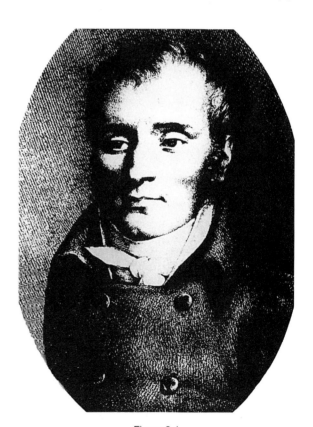

Figure 8-1
MARIE FRANCOIS-XAVIER BICHAT

Bichat was a brilliant French pathologist who stated that organs were composed of different tissues; one of the latter might be the site of disease (5). (From Shimkin MB. Contrary to nature. Washington D.C.: U.S. Department of Health, Education, and Welfare, 1977:65.)

All tumors arose from the *tissu cellulaire* (connective tissue), Bichat believed, even tumors of epithelial, muscular, tendinous, or cartilaginous character. The characteristic matter of the tumor was deposited later in the base of the tumor after its origin in the connective tissue of the involved organ, a hypothesis that states that all tumors arise from the connective tissues and the stroma of the body (3).

Bichat's concept of the tissue as the site of disease was a correct one because most diseases, including cancer, do arise in a specific tissue of an organ. Cancer of the stomach is most commonly an adenocarcinoma of the lining layer of the stomach, the mucosa, and it only secondarily affects the muscular or connective tissue components. The muscular tissue of the stomach may, independent of the mucosa, give rise to a muscle tumor: a leiomyoma (Greek: smooth muscle tumor), a benign tumor, or a leiomyosarcoma (Greek: smooth muscle flesh-like cancer), a malignant tumor.

Bichat was mistaken in the belief that the connective tissue of organs was the source of all cancers. Most cancers arise in the epithelial tissues although a much smaller number—the sarcomas—do arise in connective tissues.

Bichat's major contribution to oncology was that of indicating that a distinctive tissue of an organ was the site of origin of disease, including cancer. This was a more specific localization than Morgagni's identification of the organ as the primary site of cancer.

Where previous investigators regard all organs as wholly detached and entirely independent, Bichat realized that there were tissue elements that made up part of most organs and that cancer was built up in the same manner. In his mind cancer was adventitious tissue (7).

Bichat was a prodigious worker who became afflicted with tuberculosis and died at the age of 31 years, possibly from an infection received while performing an autopsy (1,4).

REFERENCES

1. Bayle AL, Thillaye AJ. Biographie médicale par order chronologique, d'apres Daniel Leclerc, Eloy, etc. Mis dans un nouvel ordre, revue et completee par Bayle et Thillaye. Amsterdam: Boekhandel & Antiquariaat, BM Israel (reprint), 1967:867–71.
2. Bichat X. Traité des membranes en général et de diverses membranes en particulier. Nouvelle édition augmentée d'une notice historique sur la vie et les ouvrages de l'auteur. Par M. Husson. Paris: Méquignon-Marvis, 1816.
3. Bichat X; Hayward G, trans. General anatomy applied to physiology and medicine, vol 1. Boston: Richardson & Lord, 1922:140–64.
4. Bichat X; Husson M, Coffin JG, trans. An historical notice of the life and writings of Marie Fr. Xavier Bichat. A new edition. Enlarged by an historical notice of the life and writings of the author. Boston MA: Cummings and Hilliard, 1813. Birmingham AL: Classics of Medicine Library (reprint), 1987:2–19.
5. Bichat X; Husson M, Coffin JG, trans. Treatise of the membranes. In general and on different membranes in particular. In: A new edition. Enlarged by an historical notice of the life and writings of the author. Boston: Cummings and Hilliard, 1813. Birmingham, AL: Classics of Medicine Library (reprint), 1987:40–2.
6. Haigh E. Xavier Bichat and the medical theory of the eighteenth century. London: Wellcome Institute for the History of Medicine, 1984.
7. Oberling C. The riddle of cancer. New Haven: Yale Univ. Press, 1944.
8. Rather LJ. The genesis of cancer. A study in the history of ideas Baltimore: Johns Hopkins Univ. Press, 1978:55–6.

9

THE BLASTOMA—THE ORIGIN OF LIFE

Blood has always had a mystical quality, particularly in some ancient cultures where it was associated with superstition and religious practices. Severe blood loss from wounds of the battlefield or from accidents was often a prelude to death and this added to its importance and mystique. The thought must have occurred to many individuals that the blood contained some vital life-giving element.

The Humoral Doctrine emphasized the importance of the proper equilibrium of the humors in blood and the importance of blood itself. The practice of expelling noxious substances by blood-letting was a result of this belief.

BLASTOMA

The word "blastoma" (Greek: sprout) was said to have appeared in the Hippocratic corpus and in Galen's writings in reference to the plastic exudate of eruptive lesions on the skin (13). Later it was extended to indicate the generative source of all tissues. Schwann, a proponent of the Cell Theory (see chapter 10), used the term blastoma and later changed it to "cytoblastoma," meaning that cells arose from the blastoma exuded from the blood (12,13) and from these cells evolved the tissues of the body. Earlier, William Harvey, the discoverer of the circulation of the blood, had believed in the primacy of the blood as the source of all tissues when he noted that the first sign of life in a hen's egg was the appearance of blood, followed later by the pulsation of the blood. He concluded that all subsequent living tissues were derived from the blood (4).

COAGULATING LYMPH AND THE BLASTOMA

One of the most popular hypotheses concerning the cause of cancer in the late 18th and early 19th centuries was that of John Hunter (1728–1793), a British teacher of pathologic anatomy and a practicing surgeon, often called the father of experimental pathology and surgery (fig. 9-1). Born near Glasgow, Scotland, he joined his brother William in London in 1748 where they founded a famous museum that was used for the clinical teaching of physicians and surgeons. John Hunter elevated surgery to a branch of scientific inquiry with his

experimental approach, made contributions to the practical techniques of surgery, and wrote books on surgery and venereal diseases (7). There is even a question as to whether Hunter infected himself with pus from gonorrheal exudate in the study of venereal diseases or whether he did the experiment on a patient (6,10,11,16) (Note 1).

Hunter believed that "coagulating lymph" was a major substrate for the development of cancer. The "lymph" of his hypothesis was a component of the circulating blood, a fluid substance that would coagulate outside the blood. It was later named fibrin. When the coagulated lymph formed a solid substance in the interstices of tissues, a blastoma was

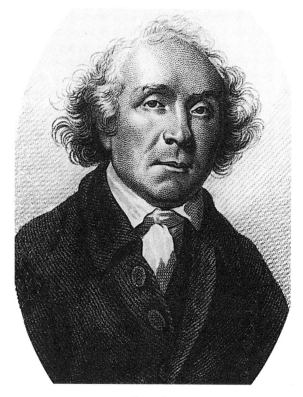

Figure 9-1
JOHN HUNTER

Portrait of John Hunter, noted English surgeon and experimentalist, who believed that cancer was formed from the "coagulable lymph" of the blood. (From Shimkin MB. Contrary to nature. Washington D.C.: U.S. Department of Health, Education, and Welfare, 1977:85.)

created and from it arose cells, organs, and tissues. Even the embryo and tissues of the adult body were formed from it. The blastoma nourished the organs and cells of the body throughout life. The fibrin of the blood was the vital substance of the blastoma.

Hunter's concept is illustrated by two quotations: 1) "To conceive that blood is endowed with life, while circulating, is perhaps carrying the imagination as far as it well can go, but difficulty arises merely from its being fluid, the mind not being accustomed to the idea of the living fluid."; and, 2) "When all the circumstances attending this fluid [blood] are fully considered, the idea that it has life within itself may not be so difficult to comprehend; and indeed, when once considered, I do not see how it is possible we should think it to be otherwise, when we consider that every part is formed from the blood, that we grow out of it..." (7).

The coagulating lymph concept was based on Hunter's observation that when blood was at rest, it separated out into red cell particles, serum, and coagulable lymph. The latter was called "coagulating lymph" because it could coagulate by itself (7). Restitution of damaged tissue, repair and maintenance of the solid parts of the body, as well as inflammation and cancer evolved from the coagulating lymph.

Hunter believed that during a perverted, unhealthy inflammatory response the active coagulating lymph became contaminated by an agent from the air, a "cancerous poison," and the combination gave rise to cancer. The cancerous poison was not further identified (12).

He also believed that hereditary predisposition was a factor in the causation of some cancers but he had not yet ascertained its importance. Age was a factor in that more cases occurred in the 40- to 60-year age group. The susceptibility of the organ was also a consideration, e.g., the breasts and uterus in women and the testicles in males were the "most disposed to cancer." Hunter thought that climate might also be a possible modulating influence (2,9).

Because of Hunter's prominence and contributions to surgery and medicine, his hypothesis of coagulating lymph and a cancerous poison replaced the black bile etiology of the Humoral Doctrine. His was the dominant hypothesis concerning the cause of cancer in the first half of the 19th century.

In 1824, Julius Vogel, a pathologist at the University of Giessen, described the blastoma as an amorphous substance, similar and probably identical to coagulated fibrin, with the sometimes inclusion of modified protein or fat. Both normal and abnormal cells and tissues could arise from the amorphous formative substance, or from a cytoblastoma, derived from the blood. The cells were transformed from the cytoblastoma into normal or abnormal tissues, including cancer. A solid cancerous cytoblastoma could then arise and lead to many types of cancers (12,15).

Paul Broca, a French pathologist, stated in 1852 that there were as many blastomas as tissues, as well as a traumatic or inflammatory blastoma and a cancerous blastoma (1). J.F. Heller, a physiological chemist in Schuh's laboratory in Vienna, analyzed the blood of cancer patients and reported that it contained an increase of fibrin three or four times that normally present (14). F. Führer classified the chemical end products of tumors into albuminous, cartilaginous, and glutinous blastomas. Nitric acid supposedly differentiated blastomas rich in albumin, from which cancers developed, by the different color produced by the action of the acid on the blastoma. Other types of blastoma stained differently. He believed that the blood and its derivatives were the germinal sources of cancer (3).

NOTE 1: To resolve the problem of whether gonorrhea and syphilis were caused by the same agent but manifested different signs and symptoms, it has been reported that Hunter dipped a lancet into the gonorrheal discharge of a patient and introduced by puncture the pus into the foreskin and head of his own penis (11).

When this procedure was followed by the clinical signs of a syphilitic infection, Hunter concluded (wrongly) that the two diseases, gonorrhea and syphilis, although clinically different from each other, were caused by the same agent. Presumably, the pus contained not only the bacterium causing gonorrhea but also the spirochete of syphilis. After waiting for the signs of syphilis to appear, the penile lesions were cauterized and the syphilis was treated with mercury.

Qvist has raised the question whether Hunter experimented upon himself or performed the experiment on one of his patients (11). Weimersherch and Richter have found evidence recently that Hunter claimed to have performed the experiment on himself (16). It has also been debated whether Hunter developed syphilis and that this caused central nervous system signs and symptoms in his later life (6,10).

COAGULABLE LYMPH, SEROUS MEMBRANES, AND CANCER

In 1836, Thomas Hodgkin, a pathologist at Guy's Hospital in London, published the hypothesis that cancer arose from Hunter's coagulable lymph and the serous membranes formed from a blastoma. The serous membranes gave rise to cysts, as well as to areas of solid tumor. New cysts arose within the original cysts from the serous membranes and the process continued until a solid cancer was formed from the compound layers of successive serous membranes of the cysts and solid tumor. The corrected compound microscope was not used, although Hodgkin had such an instrument, and only dissection and visual examination of the tumors were performed. Hodgkin took the serous and mucinous tumors of the ovary as models for his hypothesis (5).

Pathology was only one of the interests of Hodgkin who was involved in many social and political matters, such as the abolition of slavery, as well as in medical and scientific societies (8).

It was eventually realized that the blastoma concept was too simplistic; it ignored the complexity of tissues and organs and their widely diverse functions. Soon a new world of substructure, unrecognizable to the naked eye, would be revealed through the advent of the corrected compound microscope with its new vista of different tissues, cells, subcellular organelles, bacteria, and parasites. This necessitated a complete reorientation of the approach to the cancer problem—a look at the subvisible world.

REFRENCES

1. Broca P. Anatomie pathologique du cancer. Mem de l'Acad Nat de Med 1852;16:453–820.
2. Dobson J. John Hunter's views on cancer. Am Roy Coll Surg Engl 1959;25:176–81.
3. Führer F. Umrisse und Bemerkungen zur pathologischen Anatomie der Geschwülste. Deutsche Klinik 1852:222–4.
4. Harvey W; Willis R, trans. The works of William Harvey. New York: Johnson Reprint, 1965:237–8.
5. Hodgkin T. Lectures on morbid anatomy of the mucous and serous membranes. London: Sherwood, Gilbert & Piper, 1836.
6. Hunter IJ. Syphilis in the illness of John Hunter. J Hist Med 1953;8:249–62.
7. Hunter J. A treatise on venereal disease. In: Palmer JF, ed. The works of John Hunter F.R.S. London: Longman Rees Osme Braun Green and Longman, 1835:229–31, 1837:17, 104–5.
8. Kass A, Kass E. Perfecting the world: the life and times of Thomas Hodgkin. New York: Harcourt Brace & Jovanovich, 1988.
9. Otley D. The life of John Hunter F.R.S. In: Lectures on the principles of surgery by John Hunter with notes by J.F. Palmer, vols. 3, 4. Philadelphia: Haswell Borrington and Haswell, 1839: 3:2, 376–89; 4:618–31.
10. Power DA. Hunterian oration. John Hunter as a man. Lancet 1925;1:369–76.
11. Qvist G. John Hunter's alleged syphilis. Am Roy Coll Surg Engl 1977;59:206–9.
12. Rather LJ. The genesis of cancer: a study in the history of ideas. Baltimore: Johns Hopkins Univ. Press, 1978:41–5, 95–9, 118–24.
13. Rather LJ, Rather P, Freirichs JB. Johannes Müller and the nineteenth century origins of tumor cell theory 50 (note 84). Canton, MA: Science History Publications, 1986.
14. Schuh F. Ueber die Erkentniss der Pseudoplasma. Wien Seidel, 1851.
15. Vogel J; Day GE, trans. The pathological anatomy of the human body. Philadelphia: Lea & Blanchard, 1847:265–78.
16. Weimerskirch PJ, Richter GW. Hunter and venereal disease. Lancet 1979;1:503–4.

PART I I

THE CELL—

THE RENAISSANCE OF ONCOLOGY

(19TH CENTURY)

10

THROUGH A LOOKING GLASS SEEN CLEARLY—
THE COMPOUND MICROSCOPE

If there was a Renaissance in the field of oncology analogous to the explosion of creative energy in the humanities and arts of the 16th and 17th centuries it probably was the comparable outburst of knowledge and concepts that illuminated the biological and medical sciences of the 19th century.

The increasing number of autopsies performed in the 17th and 18th centuries had shown that cancer could be found in many organs and tissues of the body. But were the cancers of one organ or tissue the same or different from those of another organ or tissue? Was there a common unit in all these cancers? What was the relationship of cancer to normal tissue? Before these and many other questions could be answered fundamental technical problems had to be solved.

Although there are some characteristics of cancers of different organs that had been discovered by the naked eye, such as tumors that were cystic or contained recognizable substances such as fat, cartilage, or bone, in many cases the changes in physical appearance were not distinctive enough to make a definitive diagnosis separating some inflammatory or other noncancerous pathologic processes from cancer. Some infectious diseases, particularly tuberculosis, often resembled cancer clinically, and, rarely, even during the gross pathologic examination of the tissue at autopsy. There were no definitive criteria by which one could decide the matter, even the death of the patient was not evidence of cancer because there were many noncancerous causes of death.

There evolved in the 17th century the use of a convex glass lens that furnished a magnified image of part of an object. This device was called a simple microscope because it used only one glass lens. The microscope revolutionized biology and medicine because it did for the human eye what the telescope did for astronomy—it opened a new universe (7).

THE SIMPLE MICROSCOPE

Antoni Van Leeuwenhoek (1632–1723) (fig. 10-1), a citizen of Delft, used the simple microscope most effectively and described a new world of subvisible organisms and structures (15). He made his own microscopes by grinding lenses out of very small circular pieces of thin ordinary glass (7,15). The overall dimensions of the plates holding the lens was less than 2 inches in length, about 1 inch in width, and just over a millimeter (1/25 of an inch) in thickness (fig. 10-2).

Leeuwenhoek had no formal training in science yet his observations were accurate and his descriptions of what he saw were clearly expressed (15) (Note 1). He described free-living protozoa and bacteria ("the little animals") (fig. 10-3). The subvisible structure of biological objects including striated muscle, blood corpuscles, hair, teeth, and spermatozoa

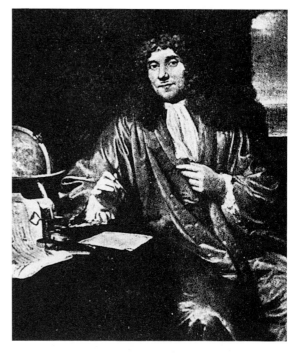

Figure 10-1
ANTONI VAN LEEUWENHOEK

Antoni Van Leeuwenhoek of Delft who with a simple home-made microscope opened up a new world of subvisible biological structures and organisms (7). Portrait by Johannes Verkolje. (Plate XI from Dobell C. Antoni van Leeuwenhoek and his "little animals"; being some account of the father of protozoology and bacteriology and his multifarious discoveries in the disciplines. New York: Russell & Russell, 1958:49.)

Figure 10-2
LEEUWENHOEK'S
SIMPLE MICROSCOPE

A drawing of the two halves of the microscope (left) and the whole microscope (right). The side view drawing (right) shows the bolted halves (15) with the lens at L. The pointed metallic rod upon which the specimen was impaled could be moved up or down to bring the specimen within the line of sight of the lens. (Left: Fig. 3.4 from Bradbury S. Microscope. The evolution of the microscope. Oxford: Pergamon Press, 1967:78. Right: Plate XXXI from Dobell C. Antoni van Leeuwenhoek and his "little animals"; being some account of the father of protozoology and bacteriology and his multifarious discoveries in the disciplines. New York: Russell & Russell, 1958:328.)

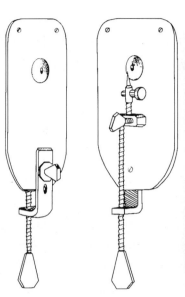

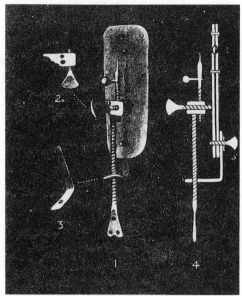

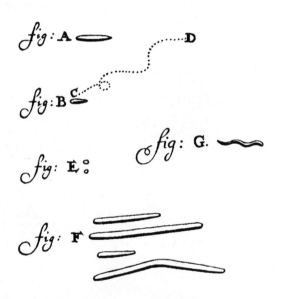

Figure 10-3
BACTERIA FROM THE HUMAN MOUTH, DEPICTED BY LEEUWENHOEK

(Plate XXIV from Dobell C. Antoni van Leeuwenhoek and his "little animals"; being some account of the father of protozoology and bacteriology and his multifarious discoveries in the disciplines. New York: Russell & Russell, 1958:239.)

LEEUWENHOEK'S FIGURES OF BACTERIA FROM THE HUMAN MOUTH
(Letter 39, 17 Sept. 1683)
Enlarged (× 1½) from the engravings published in *Arc. Nat. Det.*, 1695.

Fig. A, a motile *Bacillus*.
Fig. B, *Selenomonas sputigena*.   C . . . . D, the path of its motion.
Fig. E, Micrococci.
Fig. F, *Leptothrix buccalis*.
Fig. G, A spirochæte—probably "*Spirochaeta buccalis*," the largest form found in this situation.

Note 1: In 1673, Leeuwenhoek came to the notice of the scientific world as the result of a letter he sent to the Royal Society in London. The letter told of his observations through a simple microscope of the sting, mouth parts, and eye of the bee and louse. The Fellows of the Royal Society were pleased with the letter that was translated from Dutch and published it in the Society's Philosophical Transactions. They invited Leeuwenhoek to send more observations and he sent them 190 letters over a period of 50 years. In 1680, he was made a Fellow of the Royal Society (15).

was examined. Also studied was the life cycle of ants, aphids, and mussels, as well as the structure of plants. The achievements of this amateur scientist using a homemade simple microscope are astounding.

THE COMPOUND MICROSCOPE

At the end of the 16th century many instrument makers, particularly in Holland, were making telescopes. The environment was conducive to the invention of optical instruments (7). It was found feasible to increase the magnification of the simple microscope by using a second lens to magnify the image given by a first lens, thereby adding to the ultimate magnification. Credit is usually given to the spectacle-makers Hans Janssen and his son Zacharis of Holland for the invention of the compound microscope (about 1590–1609) (7). It was much easier to use the compound microscope than the simple microscope but it had defects (Note 2).

THE MICROSCOPE AND THE CELL

Robert Hooke (1635-1703), an English physicist, designed a compound microscope and examined many objects with it. He examined a thin section of cork and described what he saw as a "cell" (27). Hooke often receives credit for the discovery of the cell, although this claim is debatable (7). What he saw were the walls of the plant cell; his microscope had a magnifying power of about 30 times.

Correction of Chromatic and Spherical Aberrations

At the end of the 18th century, a defect in the compound microscope gave rise to a major problem—overlying color fringes in the microscopic image, called "chromatic aberration." It was caused by the different degrees of refraction to which the component colors of white light were subjected. Green light was refracted more than red light so that there was an overlap of color fringes which caused the blurring of the image and confusion in the mind of the observer (7).

Another defect of the compound microscope that decreased resolution was "spherical aberration." This occurred when rays of light passing through the peripheral parts of the lens were bent more strongly toward the central axis than those rays which passed through the lens nearer to its optical axis (7).

In the 1730s, the barrister Chester More Hall, an amateur optician and astronomer, found that flint glass differed but little in refractive power from the ordinary crown glass used for the lens of a telescope, but its dispersive power (the breaking up white light into its constituent color components) was more than double that of crown glass (7). Using Hall's discovery, Joseph Jackson Lister fitted together lenses that corrected both types of aberration (7,30).

In 1827, Lister, a wine merchant, physicist by avocation, and father of the surgeon Lord Lister, together with Thomas Hodgkin, one of the "Great" physicians at Guys Hospital, London, published a paper using his lenses. They described the microscopy of blood, muscle fibers, nerve fibers, and the fibers of cellular tissue (26). In contrast to the findings of previous microscopists (32,38), they saw no globules in any of the tissues examined; these observations destroyed the theory of the globular nature of biological matter (32). They believed that the fundamental unit was a fiber, as suggested by the Greeks. The electron microscope later showed that the ultrastructure of biological matter was more complicated.

Optical firms soon incorporated the corrected lenses in their microscopes. Microscopes made in England, Vienna, and Berlin earned a good reputation for their resolving power, which from about 1840 could resolve about one micron (1/25,000th of an inch), a marked increase over earlier instruments and a boon to the biological sciences (fig. 10-4). With these microscopes individual cells and cell contents could be visualized. Later in the 19th century, Ernst Abbé of the Zeiss firm in Jena, Germany, made many major contributions to the further development of microscopy (7). A whole new outlook on the structure of cells and biological organisms was provided by these advances in microscopy.

Note 2: The simple microscope was more effective and gave better resolution than the compound microscope available during Leeuwenhoek's lifetime because it distorted the image less. Because he had to hold his microscope close to his eye, Leeuwenhoek saw light rays close to the central axis of the rays where chromatic and spherical aberrations were minimal. In the uncorrected lenses of the compound microscope, more of the peripheral rays were viewed and their distortion of the image by chromatic and spherical aberrations was greater than with the simple microscope, even though higher magnification could be achieved with the former (7).

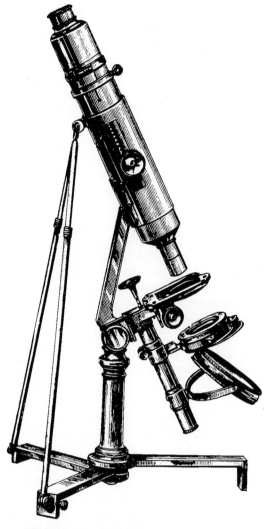

Figure 10-4
EARLY ACHROMATIC COMPOUND MICROSCOPE
An achromatic microscope from 1826 which was commissioned by J.J. Lister. (Fig. 5.14 from Bradbury S. Microscope. The evolution of the microscope. Oxford: Pergamon Press, 1967:196.)

TISSUE PROCESSING

When insects were used as specimens for the simple microscopes of the 17th and 18th centuries, none of the details of inner structure were visible because light cannot penetrate tissue to any appreciable extent. Very thin slices (sections), preferably 10 microns (1/2500 of an inch) or less in thickness, had to be cut so that visible light could penetrate the tissue and be visualized through the microscope.

In order to cut very thin sections of soft biological tissue, the latter would have to be hardened and kept rigid. In addition, the process of decay, which occurs when tissue is removed from the body or an organism dies, had to be stopped. A "fixative," a means whereby the degradative action of enzymes present in the tissues was stopped and the tissue hardened, was required. Among the substances used to preserve and harden tissues were: freezing (37,39,55), alcohol (12), acids (6,31), and formalin fixation (3).

Alcohol had been employed occasionally in the past for preserving bodies. The body of the British admiral, Lord Nelson, was "fixed" in a cask of brandy for its return to England after the battle of Trafalgar (12). Alcohol dehydrates and fixes tissue but it distorts its fine structure, limiting its use for microscopic studies. Formalin has been used probably more than any other fixative of tissue; it is part of many embalming solutions and distorts tissue only slightly, permitting light microscopic studies.

The Microtome

After the biological specimen was hardened, it had to be cut into very thin slices of tissue (sections) of about 5 microns (1/500th of an inch) or less in thickness. To obtain this thinness requires a mechanical slicing device called a microtome. John Hill, an English investigator of the structure of wood, invented a microtome in 1770 that he claimed could cut thin slices of wood (1/2000 of an inch) for microscopic examination (25). Between 1830 and 1870 many different types of microtomes were described (6, 57) and further advances were made. Today, microtomes are finely machined instruments that can cut sections of tissue a few microns in thickness. A microtome can be operated in a refrigerated device so that a piece of tissue, suspected of being cancerous, can be frozen, sliced, stained, and examined under the microscope—the "frozen section"—in a few minutes. A surgeon may thereby receive from the pathologist during surgery a report as to whether the tissue is benign or malignant.

Imbedding of Tissue

A major advance in the cutting of thin sections occurred when Edwin Klebs (1834–1913), a peripatetic German pathologist-bacteriologist, immersed fixed dehydrated tissues in molten paraffin which diffused throughout the tissue. When the paraffin preparation cooled and hardened at room temperature, it formed a solid block containing the tissue, which was held rigid enough so that very thin sections could be cut by the microtome with little distortion (28).

Staining of Tissue Sections

The sliced paraffin-imbedded tissue was placed on a glass slide, the paraffin dissolved out, and the tissue stained. Because unstained tissue did not have enough contrast between its components to reveal the structure of the tissue or cells when viewed through the light microscope, the tissue was stained with different dyes; this allowed intracellular structures to be distinguished from each other. The nucleus of a cell could be easily distinguished from the cytoplasm because it stained differently (23). A commonly used dye, hematoxylin, colors the nucleus of a cell blue to black but has little effect on the cytoplasm (5). S. Ramon y Cahal, the Spanish neuropathologist, used silver salts to study the cells of the central nervous system (9). Hundreds of stains for the differential staining of cellular structures have been described (9,14, 29,37,47,54). Some identify specific biochemical compounds, but most do not have that specificity.

An important indicator of the presence of deoxyribonucleic acid (DNA) in the cell nucleus was the Feulgen reaction, introduced in 1924 by R. Feulgen and H. Rossenbeck, German investigators (19). This was widely used for decades by cytologists in cancer research because of its differential staining of the chromatin and the chromosomes of the nucleus of the cell. A different group of stains was introduced by Paul Ehrlich who used aniline dyes to identify different types of blood cells in health and disease (16). These were important in the delineation of the cancers of the blood cells, the leukemias.

What appears, in retrospect, to be a sequence of relatively minor advances in microscopic and histologic techniques added up to a major improvement in the ability of investigators to examine the new subvisible world of structure, cells, and organisms. Previously unrecognized cell organelles, bacteria, and parasites could now be seen and examined. They could be correlated with normal structures and functions, or disease processes. These discoveries impacted on the fields of biology, embryology, bacteriology, immunology, pathology, medicine, and eventually, oncology in the latter half of the 19th century.

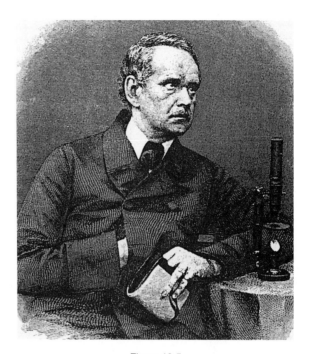

Figure 10-5
MATTHIAS JACOB SCHLEIDEN,
PROPONENT OF THE CELL THEORY
(Frontispiece from Mabius M. Matthias Jacob Schleiden. Zu seinem 100 gerbur totage. Leipzig: W. Engelmann, 1904.)

THE CELL THEORY

One of the most important concepts in biology and medicine had among its proponents two graduate students who met in 1834 in a Berlin café. Matthias Jacob Schleiden (1804–1881), a botanist and one-time student of law at Heidelberg, developed his hobby of botany into a full time graduate pursuit (fig. 10-5). He met Theodore Schwann (1810–1882), a graduate in medicine at Bonn and a psychologist (fig. 10-6). They were students in the laboratory of Johannes Müller, chairman of the Department of Anatomy and Physiology at the Friedrich Wilhelm University in Berlin.

Schleiden told Schwann about his microscopic discoveries (48). In all plants that he had examined, he had seen two common structural units (fig. 10-7): a cell, previously described by Robert Hooke (27), and a nucleus within the cell, reported earlier by Robert Brown (2,8). Schwann decided to look at animal tissues to see if they contained the same units that Schleiden had seen in plant tissue. In the notochord and cartilaginous tissue of amphibian larvae, Schwann found the same two units: cells and nuclei within cells (fig. 10-8) (50–52).

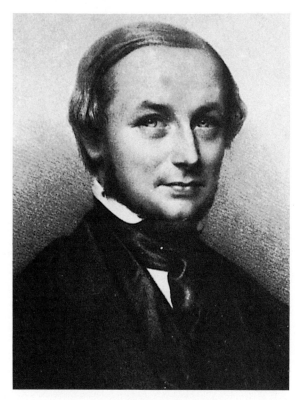

Figure 10-6
THEODORE SCHWANN

Theodore Schwann who, with Schleiden, propagated the Cell Theory. (Plate 26 from Florkin M, Stotz RH. A history of biochemistry. Amsterdam: Elsevier, 1972:135.)

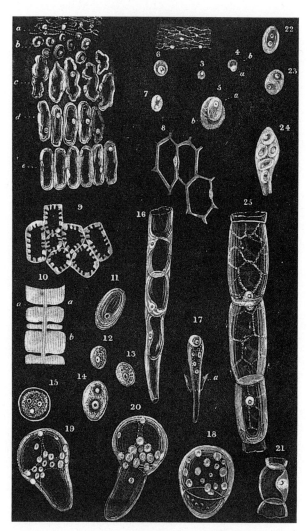

Figure 10-7
SCHLEIDEN'S PLATE ILLUSTRATING
NUCLEI IN PLANT CELLS

The "watch glass" model is present on cytoblasts 4, 5, 6, and 7. (Plate 1 from Schleiden MJ. Contributions to phytogenesis. In: Schwann T; Smith H, trans. Microscopic researches into the accordance in the structure and growth of animals and plants. London: Sydenham Society, 1847:264.)

In 1838, Schleiden wrote that in the formation of new cells, nuclei arose from granules in the cytoplasm of the mother cell. A new nucleus became the nucleus for a daughter cell, and became surrounded by material in the mother cell cytoplasm. As soon as the new cell had reached full size, it appeared as a fine transparent vesicle rising up from the surface of the original cell with the new cell lying on the original cell, like the glass on the face of a watch—the "watch glass" model. Schleiden emphasized that the new cell arose from within the mother cell, thereby preserving continuity of successive generations of cells (48).

Schwann initially stated that he was able to trace the origin of animal cells to the same type of "watch glass" model that Schleiden described in plant cells (50–52). Later, Schleiden and Schwann both changed their opinions about the details of the origin of cells (41,49,53) (Note 3).

Many investigators prior to Schleiden and Schwann had seen cells with a nucleus (2,41) but none had generalized their findings into the formulation that these two proposed. Rather writes ". . . in a class by themselves were the much more important . . . discoveries of Schleiden and Schwann, those of Schleiden on the origin of young plant cells from nuclei in mother cells and those of Schwann on the like mode of cell formation in animals, on the origin of all animal tissues from cells, and on the subsequent transformation of cells into tissues" (33,40,41). The generalization of Schleiden

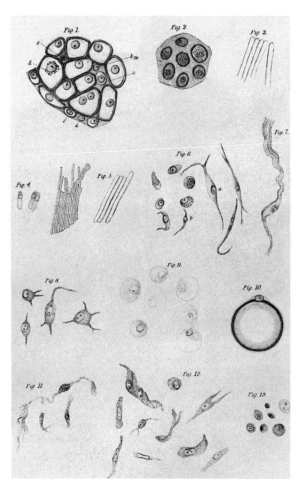

and Schwann indicated the "oneness" of biological life—the cells of animals and plants were similar in their fundamental structure (Note 4).

Cancer and the Cell Theory

With the rapid acceptance of the Cell Theory, obvious questions for those interested in cancer to ask were: from which cell comes the cancer cell? Can the cancer cell arise from a normal cell? Does the cancer cell arise de novo, or is there a transformation from a precursor? Can one recognize by microscopic examination cancer cells as distinct from normal cells?

Johannes Müller (1801–1858) focused attention on the cancer cell in 1838 with the publication of a monograph translated as, *On the Finer Structure and Forms of Morbid Tumors* (34) (Note 5). This was an attempt to form a practical classification of tumors. Müller was aware of the Cell Theory through his pupils. Using the corrected achromatic lens of the compound microscope and chemical tests, he attempted to establish histologic and cytologic criteria for distinguishing benign from malignant tumors. Such a distinction, he believed, would aid the practicing physician in the recognition and treatment of tumors.

Müller found that both benign and malignant tumors were composed of cells with nuclei. He was able to distinguish many tumors by their appearance to the naked eye, or with the aid of a magnifying glass (41), but whether they were benign or malignant could not be determined.

Müller examined many tumors by making slices of the tissue and studying histologically stained sections under the microscope. He concluded that

Figure 10-8
ANIMAL CELLS AND NUCLEI
Schwann's plate showing cells with nuclei in many cell types in amphibian larvae. (Plate III from Schwann T; Smith H, trans. Microscopic researches into the accordance in the structure and growth of animals and plants. London: Sydenham Society, 1847:226.)

Note 3: Schleiden, in a later book, continued to believe that new cells arose intracellularly from nuclei that were formed as needed from the mucous corpuscles that were part of the cell content. The new nuclei then give rise to new cells. The new cell was born in the fluid which arose from a blastoma, called a cytoblastoma, by a crystallization process in the liquid of the mother cell (49).

Schwann changed his original belief that cells arose from an intracellular nucleus to the belief that most cells arose extracellularly, from the "cytoblastoma" (blastoma) (41,53). The cytoblastoma hypothesis grew out of the "blastoma" concept that tissues were generated and nourished by diffusion through the blood vessel wall by a proteinaceous substance of the fluid part of the circulating blood (see chapter 9).

Note 4: In a meticulous scholarly review of the birth of the Cell Theory, Henry Harris, former head of the William Dunn School of Pathology at Oxford University, has questioned the historical acceptance of Schleiden and Schwann as the founders of the Cell Theory. Harris emphasizes the overlooked role of the Czech histologists Jan Evangelista Purkinje and Gabriel Gustov Valentin; the discovery of binary fission in multicellular plants by the Belgian botanist Barthelemy Dumortier; and the prior pre-Virchovian use of the phrase, "Omnis cellular e cellular" by the French histochemist Francois-Vincent Raspail and the Polish biologist who lived in Berlin, Robert Remak. Harris delivers justifiably harsh criticism against Schwann for the belief that cells arise extracellularly from a blastoma. Schleiden also receives criticism for believing that an intracellular blastoma gives rise to the new intracellular cell. Harris' exposition should be read by serious students of biology and historians of science (24a).

microscopic and chemical analyses were not definitive enough for the diagnosis of cancer: "microscopic and chemical analyses cannot, therefore, ever be expected to become diagnoses; it would be ridiculous to desire this or suppose it possible" (41). "The principle for classifying tumors into groups can be derived neither from fine structure alone nor from chemical composition.". He decided that one had to depend on the clinical behavior of the tumor in the patient in order to determine whether it was benign or malignant (Note 6).

It is ironic that Müller, the first person to apply the Cell Theory to the study of tumors through microscopy, was convinced that the microscope alone had no place in the diagnosis of tumors (40).

RUDOLPH VIRCHOW

Rudolph Virchow (1821–1902) was one of the most imposing figures in medicine in the latter half of the 19th century (fig. 10-9). Born in Pomerania, Prussia, the only son of a farmer, he was awarded a scholarship to study medicine in the Friedrich-Wilhelm Institute in Berlin in 1839. After graduation, Virchow developed an interest in two fields—microscopic anatomy and analytical chemistry—while also performing autopsies at the Charité Hospital in Berlin (1,40,62) (Note 7).

At the age of 25 years Virchow, with Johannes Müller, critically analyzed the concept of the origin of diseases proposed by Karl Rokitansky, a famous pathologist at the Allgemeines Krankenhaus in Vienna. To explain the mechanisms of action of the disease processes, Rokitansky had invoked a modification of the Humoral Doctrine, the blastoma

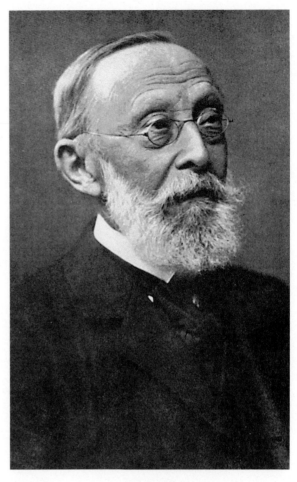

Figure 10-9
RUDOLPH VIRCHOW
Rudolph Virchow, the famous German pathologist, archeologist, and statesman, was a dominant figure in pathology and medicine in the last half of the 19th and the beginning of the 20th centuries. (Courtesy of the Director, Wellcome Historical Medical Museums, London.)

Note 5: Müller differed from Schleiden and Schwann about the origin of cells. He believed that benign and malignant tumor cells often arose from granules. The granules arose either de novo in the extracellular space or were discharged into the extracellular space when the mother cells ruptured. The granules were formed from a blastoma. He thus proposed a new version of the older blastoma hypothesis—granules arose from the blastoma and from the granules emerged nuclei and from the nuclei new cells were formed (41) (see chapter 9).

Note 6: Müller reached many sound general conclusions in his overall study of tumors (34). He visited many clinics and museums to examine pathologic specimens. The absence of clinical follow-up of patients after a diagnosis was made and Müller's own lack of cytologic experience prevented him from correlating the microscopic diagnosis and the subsequent clinical behavior of the tumor.

Note 7: Virchow established himself as a fearless investigator when, as a young pathologist, he was sent by the government to investigate a typhus epidemic in Silesia. He submitted a scathing report on the social conditions found in Upper Silesia in which he blamed the government for social and political conditions that led to the catastrophe. Later he was involved, in a minor manner, in the revolution for democracy which broke out in Berlin against the Prussian government in 1848. These activities did not endear him to the government and he was suspended from his post at the Charité. The students at the university rallied to his support and Virchow was reinstated on probation (1).

He is regarded as the greatest figure in the history of pathology. His death was symbolic of his active life; he broke a leg when, at the age of 80 years, he jumped off a street car. The fracture healed but he developed complications and died a few months later (1).

concept (see chapter 9). He speculated that as the tumors arose out of a blastoma they contained protein compounds in various states of oxidation. He postulated a complex theoretical system of chemical dyscrasias, each of which was the source of a specific disease (46). The criticism of Virchow and Müller was so vigorous and decisive, however, that Rokitansky soon gave up his hypothesis (Note 8).

Virchow accepted the chair of pathology at Würtzberg where he began to familiarize himself with many disease processes. He became aware of the phenomenon of mitosis, the division of a cell into two equal daughter cells, previously described. In addition, he recognized the different types of response of the connective tissues in diseases such as tuberculosis, syphilis, pyemic (pus) inflammation, degenerative diseases, and injuries. From this experience he developed great respect for the ability of the connective tissue to react and thought that the tissue had immense formative or generative potential (1).

Because of his increasing reputation, Virchow was called back to the University of Berlin where a new institute of pathology was built for him. Although he had originally believed in the blastema origin of cells, after his wide experience with many diseases, Virchow came to the belief that cells did not originate from an amorphous blastema coming from the blood (61).

Omnis Cellula E Cellula

Most importantly, Virchow concluded that there was no life except that propagated through direct succession of cell to cell, extending back to the fertilized ovum. His apt aphorism, "Omnis cellula e cellula" (All cells arise from other cells) indelibly imprinted this belief (1,58,61). "Where a cell arises, there a cell must have previously existed (omnis cellula e cellula), just as an animal can spring only from an animal, a plant only from a plant" (61). The concept did not originate with Virchow for others, including Remak, had suggested such a possibility (1,24), but Virchow was a vigorous prominent proponent of the idea and it came to be associated with his name (see Note 4).

Cellular Pathology

Of greatest importance to pathology and medicine was Virchow's concept that disease had its locus of action in the individual cell, his doctrine of Cellular Pathology. This was probably his most important contribution and is fundamental to the current concepts of medicine: that all diseases begin in the individual cell (1,61,62,65).

Virchow as a pathologist described a number of distinct types of cancer: leukemia (cancer of the blood), sarcomas (cancers of connective tissue), cancers of soft tissues, head and neck cancer, malignant melanoma of skin, chondrosarcoma (a cancer of cartilage), osteogenic sarcoma (a cancer of bone), and many others (1,59), including one of the earliest attempts at a systematic classification of brain and spinal cord tumors (66).

The Origin of Cancer from Connective Tissue

The Cell Theory and Cellular Pathology furthered progress in oncology since they implied that one could trace a cancer back to its origin in a precursor cell or cell type.

One of Virchow's mistakes was his belief that practically all cancers arose from the connective tissue, even those cancers found in areas in which the connective tissue was sparse or absent (61) (Note 9). He believed that the connective tissue cell

---

Note 8: Rokitansky was the most able descriptive gross pathologist of his day. He contributed greatly to an understanding of the gross pathology of diseases of the heart, lung, liver, and blood vessels as well as cancer and other less common afflictions (46). In regard to the etiology of cancer, his speculations were specious.

Note 9: Three circumstances were probably important to Virchow in causing him to believe that all cancers arose in connective tissues: 1) the remarkable variety of types of response of the connective tissue to different inflammatory agents; 2) the ability of some cells to change their physical appearance so that they resembled other types of cells, a process that he called "metaplasia" (Greek: change in form) (60); and 3) the occurrence of a tumor—the adamantinoma—which contained both epithelial and connective tissue elements. Much debate has occurred as to the origin of this tumor (40).

In regard to the origin of tumors from different types of tissue of the three germ cell layers (10), tumors containing tissue from two germ cell layers are rare, except in germ cell tumors themselves. There are rare cases of carcinosarcoma in which epithelial and connective tissues (from two different germ cell layers) are present. Since all cells, presumably, have a complete complement of DNA that potentially could produce any type of cell or cell product it would seem possible that in a perturbed cancer cell genome more than one gene function might be activated or released from suppression to cause additional transformation of cells from two different germ cell layers to cancer. It is surprising that tumors with an additional different type of tissue from a second or third layer of the purported generative layers of the embryo do not occur more often.

from which all cancers arose was a ubiquitous spindle-shaped cell which originated when a stimulus acted upon the reservoir of undifferentiated cells which were present in all organs. This cell, Virchow believed, was multipotential and had the ability to generate many different types of cancer, even those of an epithelial nature (61) (Note 10).

Because of Virchow's reputation, this concept was accepted for a short period by most medical scientists. However, the studies of Thiersch (56) and Waldeyer (64) showed convincingly that cancers of epithelial tissues were derived from epithelium, not from connective tissues (Note 11).

Cancer Metastases

In 1829, Recamier described a metastatic growth of cancer in the brain of a woman with cancer of the breast (42) and called it metastatic cancer. Virchow believed that metastases were not emboli of cancer cells from a primary cancer because their distribution did not always correspond to the usual vascular pathway taken by emboli traveling from organ to organ; it appeared to be

more random than if they were blood-borne. Virchow believed that a juice, a poison, was produced by cancer cells. It entered the blood and lymphatic systems and caused the production of a similar cancer in other organs, resulting in a metastasis (61). Virchow had already described pyemia, pus traveling in the blood stream from its source to another organ, and embolism, a blood clot traveling from a source to an organ.

In 1991, I. J. Fidler, at the M.D. Anderson Cancer Center, discovered that only certain cells in a tumor have the ability to metastasize. He identified metastatic regulating genes in the tumors of patients with recurrent disease that he believed might have predictive value regarding metastasis in certain cancers. The response of organs to metastasizing cells may differ (20,21).

For most cancers, the spread to regional lymph nodes pursues a stereotyped pattern. However, blood-borne metastases sometimes appear to be more random in their final location, probably because metastasis is a complicated phenomenon involving many factors, including host and organ responses (1,20,21,36) (Note 12).

Note 10: Virchow's lectures on tumors were published in three volumes which started to appear in 1863 (59). The second half of the third volume was to contain the important subject of epithelial cancer but no such lecture was published. The opposition to Virchow's hypothesis of the connective tissue origin of most cancers may have prevented him from committing his beliefs to print. Nevertheless, he continued to believe throughout his life that most carcinomas arose from connective tissue (1), now known to be an incorrect interpretation.

Note 11: In 1865, Carl Thiersch (1822–1895), a surgeon of Erlangen, used serial sections of over 100 tissue specimens of cancers of the skin, lips, and mouth, to demonstrate that the cancer arose in cells of the epithelium and only later involved the underlying connective tissue (56). The cancers were carcinomas, i.e., they arose in epithelium, they were composed of epithelial cells, and they were not derived from connective tissue cells.

In 1867, Wilhelm Waldeyer (Waldeyer-Hartz) (1836–1921), a pathologic anatomist studied cancer of the breast (64). His conclusions were the same as those of Thiersch: that the sole source of carcinoma cells was the normal epithelium of the breast. Connective tissue proliferation often accompanied the epithelial proliferation but was not the source of the common breast cancer.

The findings of Thiersch and Waldeyer were quickly verified and Virchow's concept of the connective tissue origin of cancer was generally disregarded.

Note 12: In 1949, George Pack and Robert Booher, surgeons at Memorial Hospital, New York City, reported a case of a 34-year-old man with a tumor of the left nostril. Biopsy revealed a malignant tumor (36). High voltage X-ray therapy and radium were given and there was complete remission. There was no evidence of metastasis. Twenty months later the patient sustained an injury to his penis. During sexual foreplay while he was sitting nude in a chair his companion, equally nude, threw herself unexpectedly onto his lap. A "fracture" of the erect penis occurred. There was severe pain, ecchymoses (bleeding into the tissues of the organ), and swelling which subsided. Two weeks after the trauma a nodule appeared at the site of the injury on the shaft of the penis and it grew in size. Four weeks later, a tumor 5 cm in diameter was present on the penis. The lesion was thought to be an unresolved organized blood clot, secondary to the trauma.

At operation, a tumor 3 cm in diameter was present at the dorsum of the lower third of the penis. The pathology report of the tumor of the penis was infiltrating malignant lymphoma, similar to the nose lesion. The patient died 6 months after discovery of the penile lesion.

Pack and Booher believed that the penile tumor was caused by entrapment of malignant cells from the blood stream by traumatic hemorrhagic tissue of the penis. Metastases to the normal penis are thought to be rare. The sites of metastases can be predicted in a statistical sense, in a large number of cases, but the case illustrates an unpredictable site of localization of a blood-borne metastasis.

The Etiology Of Cancer

Local continued irritation of normal cells was stressed by Virchow as the cause for the development of neoplastic cells. Gross mechanical trauma was believed to be a factor in some cases. A predisposition to the formation of neoplasms, hereditary or acquired (scar or chronic inflammation), was present in some organs which, when combined with local irritation such as chronic inflammation, produced tumors in these organs (1,59).

The emphasis on cancer being a local phenomenon caused by local conditions meant that extirpative surgery might be a cure; if the Humoral Doctrine were correct, surgery would have been futile.

Virchow's manifold interests and accomplishments indicate the prodigious energy, intellect, ability, and enthusiasm of the man. He was so prominent and such an authoritative figure that he was called the "Pope of Pathology" (Notes 13,14).

IN THE SHADOW OF THE POPE

Robert Remak (1815–1865), a pupil of Müller and a pathologist colleague of Virchow at the Charité Hospital in Berlin, was a clear-thinking, brilliant, independent individual. He concluded from his studies on embryology that there were three original layers of tissue in the embryo from which all tissues and all future organs developed, as did cancers (45). Remak wrote in 1852, prior to Virchow, that all cells, normal and abnormal, arose only from preexisting cells (44). Remak clearly stated that neoplastic cells were ultimately derived from normal cells through nuclear and cellular division. He also believed that carcinomas arose from epithelium, not from connective tissue (43) (Note 15).

ANAPLASIA

David von Hansemann (1859–1920), a pathologist in Berlin and a pupil of Cohnheim and assistant to Virchow, described in 1890 the concept of anaplasia (Greek: ana, backward; plasia, form), a characteristic of cancer (13,18,63). The increased growth of the cancer cell showed a loss of normal differentiation and reversal toward a more primitive form. von Hansemann believed that anaplasia and asymmetric mitoses (fig. 10-10) together were characteristics of the cancer cell, but they did not cause transformation. He postulated that some irritant acting on the anaplastic cells was necessary

---

Note 13: Because of his reputation, Virchow was involved in the diagnosis of a lesion of the throat which killed the German Emperor, Frederich III, the only member of the Hohenzollern family who was considered to be a liberal. He was Virchow's friend. The tissue from a biopsy of the larynx of the Emperor was interpreted by Virchow as showing no signs of malignant tumor and, unfortunately, this was interpreted by consultants as evidence that there was no throat cancer present and that an operation was unnecessary. Frederich died some months later of cancer of the larynx (1).

One wonders whether Virchow's demand that cancers could not be diagnosed unless there was invasion of adjacent tissues and the presence of a connective tissue stroma in the tumor, prevented recognition of a cancer that would be recognized by today's standards of diagnosis as a carcinoma of the larynx. It is possible, however, that the biopsy material sent to Virchow may not have contained any carcinoma in it. Trying to get a good representative biopsy specimen of the tumor of the larynx from such a patient must have been a formidable task for the surgeon.

Note 14: Virchow was active in medical societies, attended many international conferences, and gained worldwide prominence in the medical field. He was a co-founder of a pathology journal, still one of the prominent journals in pathology, and in 1903, in his honor, it was named *Virchow's Archives of Pathologic Anatomy, Physiology and Clinical Medicine*. He became an amateur archeologist, accompanying Schliemann on archaeological "digs," a member of the Prussian Diet, and a vigorous liberal exponent of democracy (1).

Bismarck, who was arming and unifying Prussia by "blood and iron," was constantly annoyed by the "little professor" and challenged him to a duel. Bismarck was an experienced duelist and Virchow, wisely, "declined the honor" (1). Virchow refused the honorary title of nobility—the privilege of using the "von" before his surname (1). He was not as receptive towards the increasing development of the field of bacteriology, particularly that of tuberculosis and diphtheria, as one would have expected, because he had experience with these diseases and had his own opinions about their pathogenesis (1).

Note 15: Ackerknecht states that Remak was a brilliant person, similar in many ways to Virchow, and became a Privatdocent the same year as did Virchow, although Remak was 6 years older. The reason for the delay was that Remak was Jewish and he refused to be baptized into the Christian religion. Under such circumstances, only the king, by a special decree, could grant him the position of Privatdocent. Remak eventually became the first Jewish Privatdocent in Prussia. Continued academic prejudice forced him to give up scientific research and he became a practicing neurologist, dying suddenly at the age of 50 years (1).

Because Rudolf Virchow was such a towering figure in pathology, anthropology, and medicine, his tremendous energy propelled his name and reputation throughout the world of biology and medicine. His apt phraseology, "Omnis cellula e cellula" resulted in his name becoming associated with that concept rather than that of Remak who had published the same concept (1) a few years before Virchow wrote his memorable maxim.

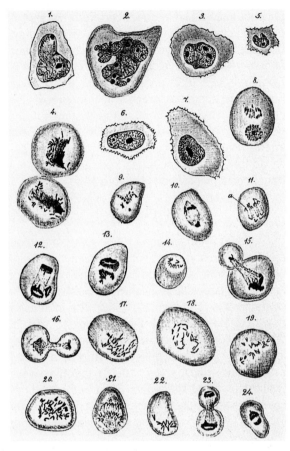

Figure 10-10
ASYMMETRIC MITOSES IN CANCER
D.F. von Hansemann believed asymmetric mitoses (figs. 4 and 8–24) were characteristic of, but did not cause, cancer. (Plate IX from von Hansemann DP. Ueber asymmetrische Zelltheilung in Epithelkrebsen und deren biologische Bedeutung. Arch pathol Anat Phys klin Med 1890:19:299–326.)

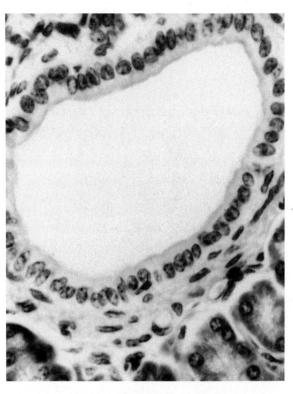

Figure 10-11
HISTOLOGIC TISSUE SECTION OF A
NORMAL DUCT OF THE HUMAN PANCREAS
The epithelial cells lining the duct are normal with basal oval nuclei and pale cytoplasm. These cells give rise to a ductal adenocarcinoma. Normal acinar cells are at the bottom. (Fig. 28.15 from Fawcett D.W. Bloom & Fawcett. A textbook of histology, 7th ed. Philadelphia: W.B. Saunders, 1986:728.)

to produce cancer (18,63). Anaplasia is seen in various degrees in carcinomas (figs. 10-11–10-14) (13), sarcomas (17), and other cancers.

ANGIOGENESIS AND TUMOR GROWTH

Cancer exerts its most devastating effects when it moves from its site of origin to invade local tissues and metastasizes to other organs. As the volume of metastatic cancer tissue increases it progressively robs normal organs of nourishment, oxygen, and vital elements.

Judah Folkman and associates of the Children's Hospital, Harvard Medical School, for many years emphasized the necessary concomitant growth of blood vessels (angiogenesis) with the growth of cancer. In a decrease or absence of vascular tissue there would be a corresponding lack of growth of the cancerous tissue (22). Folkman et al. studied the growth of blood vessels in the cornea of the eye of immunodeficient mice in which human cancers were growing. There was an inhibition of vascularity by a factor(s) in the bloodstream in the animals who had cancer of the prostate, colon, or urinary bladder (11). Angiostatin and endostatin, two substances which inhibited angiogenesis, were identified. The administration of these inhibitors caused regression of primary tumors to dormant microscopic lesions (35). Endostatin was administered to mice with lung cancer, a fibrosarcoma and a melanoma. After multiple treatment cycles, the tumors regressed and did not grow further after treatment was discontinued (4).

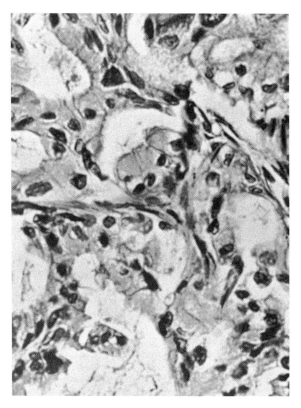

Figure 10-12
DUCTAL ADENOCARCINOMA OF PANCREAS

Fair attempt at gland formation. The nuclei of the cells vary in size, shape, position, and staining. Normal pancreas tissue is replaced by cancer cells. (Fig. 98 from Tumors of the exocrine pancreas. Atlas of Tumor Pathology, 2nd Series, Fascicle 19, Washington, D.C.: Armed Forces Institute of Pathology, 1984:117.)

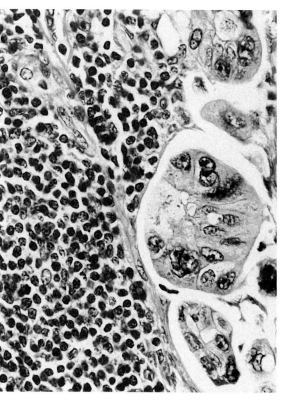

Figure 10-13
LYMPH NODE SHOWING METASTATIC
ADENOCARCINOMA IN SINUSOIDS

Poor attempt of cancer cells to form glands. (Fig. 124 from Tumors of the exocrine pancreas. Atlas of Tumor Pathology, 2nd Series, Fascicle 19, Washington, D.C.: Armed Forces Institute of Pathology, 1984:135.)

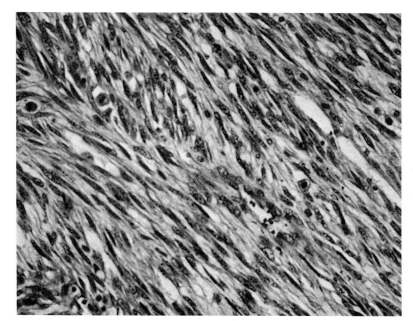

Figure 10-14
TYPICAL SPINDLE CELL SARCOMA
(FIBROSARCOMA)

Hypercellularity, irregular cellular pattern, and numerous mitotic figures. (Fig. 5-10 from Enziger FM, Weiss SW. Soft tissue tumors. St. Louis: C.V. Mosby, 1983:108.)

THE CELL AS THE SITE OF ORIGIN OF CANCER

The Cell Theory, the concept of "Omnis cellula e cellula," and Virchow's doctrine of Cellular Pathology focused attention on the cell as the site where transformation to cancer took place. No more could demons, evil spirits, blastomas, cancerous seeds, and black bile be seriously considered as causes of cancer.

REFERENCES

1. Ackerknecht EH. Rudolph Virchow. Doctor, statesman, anthropologist. Madison, WI: Univ. Wisconsin Press, 1953:13, 26, 29, 32, 34, 70–86, 98–185.
2. Baker JR. The cell theory. A restatement history and critique collection of articles 1948–1955. New York and London: Garland Publishing, 1988.
3. Blum F. Der formaldehid als Härtungsmittel. Vorläufige Mittheilung. Zeit Woch Med 1893;10:314–5.
4. Boehm T, Folkman J, Browder T, O'Reilly MS. Antiangiogenic therapy of experimental cancer does not induce acquired drug resistance. Nature 1997;390:404–7.
5. Bohmer F. Zur pathologischen Anatomie der Meningitis cerebro-medularis epidemica. Aerztl Intelligenzb Munchen 1865;12:539–50.
6. Bracegirdle B. A history of microtechnique. Ithaca, NY: Cornell Univ. Press, 1978:57–110, 128–30.
7. Bradbury S. Microscope. The evolution of the microscope. Oxford: Pergamon Press, 1967:3, 21, 22, 42–5, 68–103, 174–9, 201–3.
8. Brown R. On the organs and mode of fecundation in orchids and Asclepiadae. Trans Linn Soc 1833;16:685–738.
9. Cajal SR. Nuevo concepto de la histologia de los centros nerviosos. Rev Cienc Med 1892;18:457–76.
10. Carlson BM. Human embryology and developmental biology. St. Louis: Mosby, 1994:51–86.
11. Chen C, Parangi S, Tolentino MJ, Folkman J. A strategy to discover circulating angiogenesis inhibitors generated by human tumors. Cancer Res. 1995;55:4230–3.
12. Churchill TO. The life of Lord Viscount Nelson Duke of Bronte. London: T Benley, L Harrison, & JC Leigh, 1808:92–3.
13. Cubilla AL, Fitzgerald PJ. Tumors of the exocrine pancreas. Atlas of Tumor Pathology. 2nd Series, Fascicle 19. Washington, D.C.: Armed Forces Institute of Pathology, 1984.
14. Culling CF. Handbook of histopathological and histochemical techniques, 3rd ed. London: Butterworths, 1974.
15. Dobell C. Antony van Leeuwenhoek and his "little animals"; being some account of the father of protozoology and bacteriology and his multifarious discoveries in these disciplines. New York: Russell & Russell, 1958:17–105, 313–38.
16. Ehrlich P. Methodolische beitrge zur physiologie und pathologie der verschieaenen formen der leukocyten. Z Klin Med 1879;1:555–60.
17. Enziger FM, Weiss SW. Soft tissue tumors. St. Louis: Mosby, 1983.
18. Fawcet D.W. Bloom and Fawcett. A textbook of histology. New York: Chapman & Hall, 1993.
19. Feulgen R, Rossenbeck H. Mikroskopisch-chemischar Nachweiss einer Nucleinsaure vom Typhus der Thymonucleinsaure und die darauf beruhende elektive farbung von Zellkernen in mikrokopischen Praparaten. Hoppe-Seylers Z Physiol Chem 1924;165:203–48.
20. Fidler IJ. Cover and cover legend. Cancer Res 1999:59.
21. Fidler IJ. The biology of human cancer metastasis. Acta Oncologica 1991;30:668–75.
22. Folkman J. Seminars in Medicine of the Beth Israel Hospital of Boston. Clinical applications of research on angiogenesis. N Engl J Med 1995;333:1757–63.
23. Gerlach J. Mikroskopische Studien aus dem Gebiete der menschllchen Morphologie. Erlangen: Enke, 1858.
24. Goodsir J, Goodsir HD. Anatomical and pathological observations 2. Edinburgh: Macphail, 1845.
24a. Harris H. The birth of the cell. New Haven: Yale Univ. Press, 1999.
25. Hill J. The construction of timber from its early growth; explained by the microscope and proved from experiments in a great variety of kinds. London: published by the author, 1770.
26. Hodgkin TH, Lister JJ. Notice of some microscopic observations of the blood and animal tissues. Phil Mag NS 1827;2:130–8.
27. Hooke R. Micrographia: or some physiological description of minute bodies made by magnifying glasses with observations and inquiries thereupon. Lincolnwood, IL: Science Heritage, 1987:112–3.
28. Klebs E. Die Einschmelzunge-methode ein bertrage zur microscopischen Technik. Arch Mikr Anat 1869;5:164–6.
29. Lillie RD, ed. H.J. Conn's biological stains. Baltimore: Williams & Wilkins, 1977.
30. Lister JJ. On some properties in achromatic object glasses applicable to the improvement of the microscope. Phil Tans Roy Soc London 1830;130:187–200.
31. Majno G. The healing hand. Man and wound in the ancient world. Cambridge, MA: Harvard Univ. Press, 1975:138.
32. Milne-Edwards MH. Recherches microscopiques sur la structure intime des tissus organiques des animaux. Ann Sci Nat 1826;9:362–94.
33. Müller J. Jahresbericht ueber die Fortschritte der anatomisch physiologischen Wissenchaften in Jahre 1838. Med Arch Anat Physiol Wiss 1838:XCVI.
34. Müller J. Ueber den feineren bau und die formen der krankhaften geschwulste Berlin: G. Reimer, 1838.
35. O'Reilly MS, Boehm T, Shing Y, et al. Endostatin: an endogenous inhibitor of angiogenesis and tumor growth. Cell (United States) 1997;88:277–85.
36. Pack GT, Booher RJ. Localization of metastatic cancer by trauma. NY State J Med 1949;49:1839–41.
37. Pearse AG. Histochemistry theoretical and applied introduction, 4th ed. London: Churchill Livingstone, 1980:1–12.
38. Pickstone JV. Globules and coagula: concepts of tissue formation in the early nineteenth century. J Hist Med Allied Sci 1973;28:336–56.
39. Raspail FV. Dévelopment de la féculae dans les organes de la fructification des céréales et analyse microscopique de la féculae suivie d'experiences propres à en expliquier la conversion en gomme. Ann Sci Nat 1825;6:224–39, 384–427.

40. Rather LJ. The genesis of cancer: a study in the history of ideas. Baltimore: Johns Hopkins Univ. Press, 1978:84–8, 90–2, 100–4, 154–62.

41. Rather LJ, Rather P, Freirichs JB. Johannes Müller and the nineteenth century origins of tumor cell theory. Canton, MA: Science History 1986:14–7, 58, 68–9.

42. Récamier JC. Recherches sur le traiment du cancer. Par la compression methodique simple ou combinée. Sur l'histoire générale de la même maladie, vol 2. Paris: Gabon, 1829:107–10.

43. Remak R. In beitrag zur Entwickelungsgeschicte der krebshaften Geschwuelste. Deutsche Klinik 1854;6:170–4.

44. Remak R. Ueber extracellulare Entstehung tierischer Zellen und ueber vermehrung derselben durch Teilung. Arch Pathol Anat Phys Wiss Med 1852:49, 57.

45. Remak R. Untersuchungern uber die Entwickelung der Wirbeltiere. Berlin: G. Reimer, 1851–55.

46. Rokitansky K; Swaine WE, trans. Manual of pathological anatomy. London: The Sydenham Society, 1849–54.

47. Sandritter W, ed.; Kasten FH, trans. 100 years of histochemistry in Germany. Stuttgart: Schattauer, 1964.

48. Schleiden M. Beiträge zur Phytogenesis. Arch Anat Physiol Wiss Med 1838:137–76.

49. Schleiden M. Grundzüge der wissen schaftlichen Botanik Nebst einer methodologischen Anleitung als Anleitung zum Stadium der Pflanze, 1st ed. Leipzig: W Engelmann, 1842–1843:20–1, 267–8.

50. Schwann T. Fortsetzung der Untersuchung ueber die Uebereinstimmung in der Structur der Thiere un Pflanzen. Neue notizen aus dem gebiete der natur und heilkunde 1838;103:225–9.

51. Schwann T. Nachtrag zu den Untersuchung ueber die Uebereinstimmung in der Structur der Thiere un Pflanzen. Neue notizen uas dem gebiete der natur und heilkunde 1838;107:21–3.

52. Schwann T. Ueber die Analogie in der Structur und dem Wachstum der Thiere und Pflanzen. Neue Notizen aus dem Gebiete der Natur and Heilkunde 1838; no. 93:33–36.

53. Schwann T; Smith H, trans. Microscopical researches in to the accordance in the structure and growth of animals and plants. London: Sydenham Society, 1847:43–4.

54. Spicer SS. Histochemistry in pathologic diagnosis. New York: Marcel Dekker, 1987.

55. Stilling B. Neue Untersuchungen über den Bau des Ruckenmarks. Cassel: Hotop, 1859.

56. Thiersch C. Der Epithelialkrebs namentlich der Haut. Leipzig: Engelmann, 1865.

57. Thornton RJ. Account of a new machine invented by the late Mr. Custance for making vegetable cuttings for the microscope. Philosophical Magazine 1799;3:302–9.

58. Virchow R. Cellular-pathologie. Archiv Pathol Anat Physiol Klin Med 1855;8:1–39.

59. Virchow R. Die krankhaften Geschwülste. 3 vols. Berlin: A Hirschwald, 1863–1865.

60. Virchow R. Ueber Metaplasia. Arch Pathol Anat Phys Klin Med 1984;97:410–38.

61. Virchow. R; Chance F, trans. Cellular pathology as based upon physiological and pathological histology. Birmingham, AL: Classics of Medicine Library, 1978:27–8, 41–8, 218–9, 397–8, 462–72.

62. Virchow RL; Rather LJ, trans. Disease life and man: selected essays. Stanford, CA: Stanford Press, 1958.

63. von Hansemann DP. Ueber asymmetrische zelltheilung in epithelkrebsen und deren biologische Bedeutung. Arch pathol Anat Phys Klin Med 1890:119:299–326.

64. Waldeyer W. Die Entwickelung der Carcinome. Arch Path Anat Phys Klin Med 1867;41:470–523.

65. Wilson JW. Virchow's contribution to the cell theory. J Hist Med 1947;2:163–78.

66. Zulch KJ. Brain tumors: their biology and pathology. 3rd ed. Berlin: Springer-Verlag, 1986.

Additional Pertinent References

Gage SH; Richards OW, ed. Microscopy in America (1830–1945). Trans Am Microscopical Soc. 1964;4(Suppl.).

Hansen JL, Schrader WA, Cowan WR, Henderson JE, Richards OW, Purtle HR. The Billings microscope collection of the Medical Museum, 2nd ed. Washington, D.C.: Armed Forces Institute of Pathology, 1974.

Rooseboom M. Microscopium. Leiden, 1956.

Schlumberger HG. Origins of the cell concept in pathology. Arch Pathol 1944;37:389–407.

Turner GL. Micrographia historica. The study of the history of the microscope. Quickett Lecture. Proc Royal Microscopical Society 1972;7:2, 120–49.

✳ ✳ ✳

11
THE EMBRYONAL CELL REST HYPOTHESIS

In an unusual case report of bilateral kidney tumors in a child slightly over 1 year of age, Julius Cohnheim (1839–1889), of Breslau and Leipzig, a contributor of many discoveries in pathology, found a different type of cell than expected (fig. 11-1). Instead of a tumor made up of only malignant renal epithelial cells there were some cells which had "cross-striated muscle fibers." Such cells do not normally occur in the kidney but make up the voluntary muscle tissue of the body. Thus, not only were the tumors composed of malignant renal carcinoma cells but, in addition, contained malignant striated voluntary muscle cells (1). We now know that such striated muscle cells are part of the composition of cells in the malignant cancer of the kidney of childhood (Wilms' tumor).

Cohnheim's explanation was that as a result of an error in development during embryonic life the muscle germ cells were displaced from their usual position to an area in which the primitive cells that gave rise to the kidney were located. During development of the embryo the primitive muscle cells became incorporated in the kidney tissue and later gave rise to the two types of cancer cells. This became known as the "embryonal cell rest" hypothesis. Cohnheim expanded his findings into the suggestion that all tumors arose from displaced embryonal cells (2,6,9). He believed that heredity was a predisposing factor.

F. Durante, an Italian researcher, had published a similar hypothesis (3,4) a year before Cohnheim. Durante had observed that after the excision of birthmarks or moles in three patients, a "sarcoma" developed in the operative scar region. Microscopic examination of the lesion showed an angiomatous tissue and a stroma composed of round, oval, or fusiform cells. Durante believed that the latter cells represented incompletely differentiated embryonal cells which were irritated by the operation and this led to the formation of the sarcoma (Note 1).

Hugo Ribbert (1855–1920), a pathologist of Bonn, published a variation of the Cohnheim hypothesis. He believed that the focal isolation of embryonal cells was caused by the irregular growth of some tissues and a separation of these cells from their normal relationships. He believed that

there was tension between normal differentiated cells which prevented them from becoming neoplastic; the embryonal rest cells which were not under such tension were freed from such restraints, and thereby would be more prone to give rise to cancer (7–9).

As seen at autopsy, there are occasionally some embryonal rests present in the human body. Germinal cell tumors occur in organs outside the sex glands and may arise from displaced embryonal

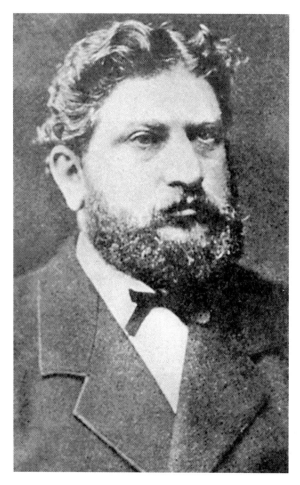

Figure 11-1
JULIUS COHNHEIM
A Berlin pathologist who made many contributions to pathology and proposed the "embryonic rest" hypothesis for the origin of cancer. (From Shimkin MB, Contrary to nature. Washington, D.C: U.S..Department of Health, Education, and Welfare, 1977:134.)

cells. Groups of cells known to have been displaced in embryogenesis, such as adrenal cells in the abdomen and thyroid tissue along the thyroglossal duct, do not usually become malignant. A small number of cancers might develop from embryonal rests but most do not (9). Probably the most cogent argument against the Cohnheim hypothesis is that in the earliest stage of most cancers seen today, carcinoma in situ, embryonal cell rests are not found.

REFERENCES

1. Cohnheim J. Congenitales querqestreiftes Muskelsarcom der Nieren. Arch Pathol Anat Phys Klin Med 1875;65:64–9.
2. Cohnheim J; McKee AB, trans. Lectures on general pathology, section II. London: New Sydenham Society, 1889;760–83.
3. Durante F. Nesso fisio-patologico tra struttura dei nei materni e la genesi di alcuni tumori maligni. Archivo di Memorie ed Osservazioni di Chirurgia Practica 1874;11:217–26.
4. Durante F; Columbo D, trans. Physical-pathological connection between congenital moles and the genesis of some malignant tumors. Archivo di Memorie ed Osservazioni di Chirurgia Practica, 1874;11:217–26.
5. Ewing J. Neoplastic diseases: a treatise on tumors, 2nd ed. Philadelphia: WB Saunders, 1922:94–7.
6. Rather L. The genesis of cancer: a study in the history of ideas. Baltimore: Johns Hopkins Univ. Press, 1978:169–74.
7. Ribbert H. Das Karzinom des Menschen sein Bau sein Wachstum seine Entstehung. Bonn: F Cohen, 1911.
8. Ribbert H. Die Entstehung des Carcinoms 55. Bonn: F. Cohen, 1905.
9. Wolff J; Ayoub B, trans. The science of cancerous disease from earliest times to the present. Canton MA: Watson, 1989:280–307.

Note 1: Durante concluded from his three cases that elements which conserved their embryonic anatomic characteristics (embryonal rests) in the adult organism, or regained them, represented the generating elements of every true neoplasm, especially malignant ones. He declared, ". . . it is impossible for me, at least for now, to demonstrate through anatomical and clinical observations the connection between the structure of epidermoidal congenital moles and the genesis of a sarcoma" (3,4). A very small percentage of some types of moles do give rise to a melanoma but other types of cancers do not arise from moles.

Wolff believes that Cohnheim did not know of Durante's report for if Cohnheim had been aware of it, he would have used it to bolster his hypothesis (9).

PART III
RECOGNITION OF THE VARIETIES
OF CANCER AND CARCINOGENS
(20TH CENTURY TO WORLD WAR II)

12

CHRONIC INFLAMMATION AS A CARCINOGEN

By the beginning of the 20th century, the Cell Theory and the Cellular Pathology doctrines had been generally accepted in biology and medicine, respectively. Medicine was involved mostly in the clinical problems of infectious diseases, at that time the most prominent diseases afflicting mankind. Although cancer was recognized clinically it did not constitute the major threat to life that it was to become in the latter half of the 20th century and it was not the principal focus of clinical, pathological, or medical interest and research. Cancer was looked upon as an uncommon disease, mostly of the elderly.

The pioneer surgical techniques for the extirpation of cancer had already been developed for gastrointestinal cancer by Theodor Billroth in Germany (19); tumors of the brain and spinal cord were being excised by Victor Halsey's neurosurgical approach in England (41); and William Halsted in the United States had devised his radical mastectomy for cancer of the breast (16). The techniques of these pioneer surgeons were beginning to be applied in cancer therapy throughout the world. Cancers were being treated by X ray and radium in institutions in France and throughout Europe (6,10,15), the United States (25), and in a few other countries. Pathologists were describing the characteristics of the cancer cell and defining the different types of cancers by their gross and microscopic appearance (3,11).

Bacteriology and immunology had revolutionized concepts concerning the cause of infectious diseases and many of them were being brought under control (5,33). Probably instigated by this success, researchers in the cancer field turned to the search for bacteria as possible causes of cancer.

BACTERIAL AND PARASITIC INFECTIONS AS CARCINOGENS

In the latter part of the 19th century, there began a flood of investigations as to whether a particular bacterium or parasite was associated with cancer. Earlier, cancer had been considered a contagious disease. "Epidemics" of cancer in towns or in "cancer houses" were described and related to various sources, such as infectious contamination of water or soil. A hospital for cancer patients was moved in 1779 from the town of Rheims, France, to a site outside the town to avoid the possibility of contagion (30).

Nicholas Tulp (1593–1674), the Dutch surgeon who commissioned Rembrandt to paint *The Anatomy Lesson*, wrote of the occurrence of breast cancer in a woman who had once been a nurse to a patient with breast cancer. The nurse's subsequent breast cancer was viewed as evidence for the contagiousness of cancer (31,37).

Zacutus Lusitanus (1575–1642), a physician of Portugal who settled in the Netherlands, reported that a woman who suffered from an ulcerated cancer of the breast for many years slept at night on the same couch with her three sons. All three were thought to have become affected with cancer. Five years after the death of the mother, two of the sons were said to have died of cancer of the breast but the third son survived after excision of the "cancer" by a surgeon. The cases were interpreted as proof of the contagiousness of cancer (22,31).

Until the end of the 19th century, and even into the 20th century, investigations into possible infectious causes of cancer continued. Suggestions were made that a particular bacterium, yeast, protozoa, insect, plant pathogen, or other organism caused cancer in man, animal, or plant. Wolff (42), Ewing (11), Henschen (18), and Triolo (36) have extensive reviews of the subject (Note 1).

There were a few specific parasites or bacteria that appeared to be the cause of cancer of a particular organ. The ova of the liver fluke, *Schistosoma hematobium*, appeared to be related to widespread cases of human bladder cancer in Egypt (12). A bacterium, *Bacillus tumefaciens*, caused the growth of a tumor of crown gall in plants (4,34). A parasite, *Clonorchis seninsis*, a liver fluke, seemed to be a causative factor in cancer of the bile ducts in the Orient (7). Viruses were not well known at the turn of the century, although Borrel had suggested that they might be the cause of cancer (see chapter 15) (2).

Folke Henschen, a pathologist at the Karolinska Institutet, Stockholm, Sweden, has summarized some of the research on the relationship of bacteria, fungi, and parasites to cancer. He also mentions the experimental attempts to validate Virchow's contention that chronic inflammation would produce cancer. None of the experiments could demonstrate more than epithelial proliferation; no cancers resulted (18).

In 1913 a Danish pathologist, Johannes Fibiger, reported that he had produced cancer in the stomach of rats by feeding them cockroaches that were infested with a parasitic worm (13,32). He later received a Nobel prize for his work. His findings were not verified subsequently by other scientists (Note 2).

CHRONIC INFLAMMATION AS A CARCINOGEN IN ANIMALS

Chronic inflammation, with its irritative stimuli, was thought by Rudolf Virchow to be a cause of cancer (38–40). Tumors were local events caused by "catalytic irritation that is the basis of neoplastic formations" (38). Predisposition of certain organs to become cancerous was also thought to be a factor (see chapter 10).

The Tar Cancer

A Japanese professor at the Imperial University of Tokyo, Katsusaburo Yamagiwa (1863–1930) (fig 12-1), had been a student of Virchow in Berlin and believed in the hypothesis espoused by Virchow that chronic irritation of an organ might produce cancer. Many attempts at inducing cancer by irritating substances had failed (18). Yamagiwa, with Koichi Ichikawa, began in 1914 to paint daily the inner surface of the ear of the rabbit with a solution of coal tar. Spontaneous tumor of the rabbit ear had not been reported. This was continued for a period of 2 years (43).

The earliest changes in the rabbit ear were ulcers, followed by scarring and thickening of the skin. The progressive microscopic changes seen in histologic sections of the skin of the ear were hyperplasia (increase in the number of cells); atypia of the cells (abnormal size, shape, or staining pattern); and finally, changes in the cells that warranted the diagnosis of cancer.

After 100 days of applying tar to the ear, skin tumors appeared in nearly all of the animals and in one animal 20 tumors developed. Eventually, 8 rabbits developed very early cancer, 16 showed early cancer, and 7 had fully developed cancer. Two animals of the last group had metastases to adjacent lymph nodes. The authors believed that the results confirmed Virchow's hypothesis that chronic irritation would cause a precancerous alteration in the epithelial cells and, if continued, might lead to cancer (21,43).

The results of the Yamagiwa and Ichikawa experiments were corroborated (1) but did not, at first, gain much attention in the oncologic world. After the Japanese investigators' results became known they were proposed for the Nobel Prize in 1926 (18) but the prize that year was given to Fibiger, the Danish investigator (8,13,29,30,32). Yamagiwa and Ichikawa never received a Nobel Prize for their outstandingly worthy contribution (Note 2).

CHRONIC INFLAMMATION AS A CARCINOGEN IN MAN

James Ewing (fig. 12-2), a pathologist at Memorial Hospital, a cancer hospital in New York City, was a leader in organizing the attack on cancer in the United

---

Note 1: Tuberculosis was often associated with Hodgkin's disease in the early 20th century and Ewing commented on the two diseases ". . . tuberculosis follows Hodgkin's disease like a shadow" but he appeared to be unconvinced that tuberculosis was the causal agent (11). Other bacteria have also been found in this disease from time to time (11,42), but no bacterium has been consistently isolated from the tissues of Hodgkin's disease. With the advent of a decrease in the incidence of tuberculosis in the United States, without a corresponding decrease of Hodgkin's disease, a causal relationship could not be sustained.

The Epstein-Barr virus has been shown to be present in a significant number of patients with Hodgkin's disease and other cancers but its high frequency in most populations makes it difficult to determine whether its presence is causal or incidental to the carcinogenesis process (see chapter 15).

Note 2: Clemmesen states that Fibiger was a meticulous investigator with integrity (8). The latter's photomicrographs show a papillomatous tumor occupying much of the stomach of the rat (13) which he believed to be a carcinoma with lymph node metastasis. The diagnosis of cancer has been questioned but there is no doubt that a benign papillary neoplasm was present. It has been suggested that the tumors of the rat stomach are caused by a vitamin A deficiency (30) or by contamination of the food by a fungus, *Fusarium,* which produces mycotoxins that are carcinogenic. Mycotoxins are now known to produce in the rat both benign and malignant tumors of the stomach (29). It is still uncertain as to the cause of the tumors produced by Fibiger.

The episode illustrates the difficulties besetting the cancer investigations of that period (1913) when pure rat strains were not available and little was known about vitamins and other necessary dietary components of foods for experimental animals or of the possible role of fungi as food contaminants and carcinogens.

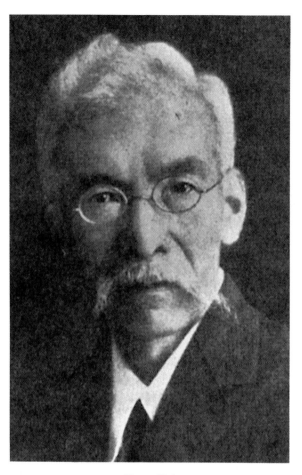

Figure 12-1
KATSUSABURO YAMAGIWA

Katsusaburo Yamagiwa, professor at the Imperial University of Tokyo, produced, with K. Ichikawa, cancer of the rabbit ear by painting the ear daily for 2 years with a solution of coal tar (21). (From Katsusaburo Yamagiwa (1863–1930). CA Cancer J Clin 1977;27:172–81.)

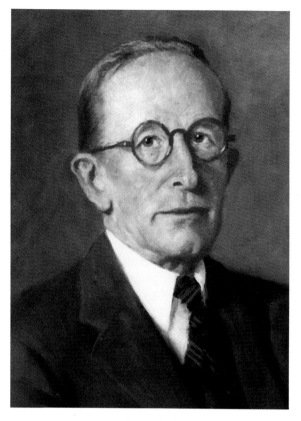

Figure 12-2
JAMES EWING

James Ewing, pathologist at Memorial Hospital, New York City, and author in 1919 of *Neoplastic Diseases,* a classic American textbook of oncology. He discovered a bone cancer, Ewing's sarcoma, which was named after him. (Author's photograph of portrait of Ewing.)

States (9,26,35) and the author in 1919 of a classic textbook on neoplastic diseases (11). He believed, with Virchow, that irritation from local chronic inflammation was the cause of most cancers (30).

The common source of cancer, Ewing believed, was a normal cell that had been transformed by chronic inflammation. "A process beginning as a simple inflammatory hyperplasia [increase in the number of cells] in the same individual gradually assumed neoplastic properties." Ewing believed that the changes of neoplasia were not merely a difference in degree from the hypertrophy of inflammation but that neoplasia was a distinct change, a loss of normal restraints to growth, whereas inflammation was an exaggerated response to external irritants

(11). "For the inception of many tumor processes chronic irritation acting upon normal cells seems to adequately explain the observed phenomena" (11). Ewing mentioned other agents that might be involved in maintaining the malignant state after its inception by chronic inflammation, a division into two major stages of carcinogenesis (11).

Ewing made an interesting general suggestion about the possible cause of cancer when he mentioned the "loss of normal restraint to growth" (11). Current emphasis on the loss of suppressor genes in some cases of cancer (see chapter 21) describes such a factor in more specific scientific terms (Note 3). Ewing believed that a local predisposition to tumor growth in an organ must be assumed to exist in order to account for the "capricious development of many neoplasms" (11). He was not impressed by the claim that heredity was an important factor in all human cancer although it appeared to be significant in some cases, as in the well known cancer families. The lack of reliable clinical statistics was the reason for his skepticism. He believed that mechanical trauma could be a factor causing cancer because of the inflammatory and reparative processes it instigated.

Rarely, chronic inflammation of a longstanding infected draining sinus tract or burn area has resulted in a squamous cell cancer originating from the epithelium lining these areas (20). The possibility of continued proliferation of the cells in the inflamed area leading to the expression of neoplastic changes secondary to gene mutations may explain these rare examples (see chapter 20).

Despite a great amount of effort expended, attempts to find specific organisms that cause human cancers have failed. In only a few types of cancer has a parasite been consistently found to be associated. Bacteria have not been proven to be carcinogenic. Viruses have been shown in recent years to cause practically all types of cancer in animals and a few types of cancer in humans (see chapter 15).

DISTINGUISHING FEATURES OF CANCER IN MAN

There are morphologic features of the cancer cell, discernible by microscopy, that distinguish it from normal embryonic and adult cells and from inflammatory and degenerate cells. Embryonic cells have relatively few or no adult cellular structural features or specific adult functions and they have a high proliferative rate. With a passage of time, they differentiate; i.e., they begin to take on the configuration and function of adult mature cells and decrease their rate of proliferation. When the carcinogenic process transforms normal cells to cancer cells, the

specific functions of the cell often decrease or stop and the cell's characteristic size and shape and nuclear chromatin pattern are altered towards the less differentiated embryonic cell, but usually some characteristics of the mature cell remain. In cancer there are typical abnormal changes in the nucleus of the cell that differ from the embryonic nucleus.

There generally is an inverse relationship between differentiation and carcinogenesis (24,44). This has been interpreted as indicating that cancer is causally linked to the loss of differentiation rather than it being an unrelated independent occurrence. In the Morris study of animal cancer of the liver, the tumor was well differentiated, and even its metastases were well differentiated (23); the question is thereby raised as to whether differentiation and carcinogenesis are inversely linked causally.

Diversity of Cell Types of Cancer

By the early years of the 20th century, textbooks of pathology described the different types of cancers by gross and microscopic appearance. In 1902, Max Borst of Würzburg (3) published drawings of the microscopic appearance of some types of human cancer. James Ewing emphasized, in a classic textbook published in 1919, that neoplasms of man were of widely diversified types. Cancer of childhood often differed from those of the adult. Biologic behavior and response to therapy also differed greatly in various types of cancer (11). German pathologists began a series of exhaustive microscopic anatomy autopsy studies typified by those of Henke-Lubarsch (17). The German surgeons earlier had begun investigating tumors. Surgical pathology started in Germany, but advanced more rapidly in the United States (28).

The microscopic classification of neoplastic lesions has proven of value in understanding the

---

Note 3: Ewing's experience with human cancers in a hospital devoted to cancer patients made him aware of the wide diversity of the kinds of cancer. From his own experience and a survey of the literature he described cancers of almost every type of tissue, organ, or cell, noting their microscopic appearance, routes of spread, response to surgical or radiation therapy, and the prognosis for the survival of the patient. He recognized a distinct bone cancer that bears his name, Ewing's sarcoma.

His book taught oncologists that cancer was not a stereotyped disease of a few types involving many organs but was composed of many different morphologic forms varying from organ to organ and even within the same organ. He was impressed with the curative and beneficial effect of radiation in some types of cancer and thought that the immune response was a significant factor in modifying the response to a few types of cancer (11). Some lesions in humans he described as "precancerous" would today probably be diagnosed as "cancer in situ."

Ewing was an outstanding leader in educating pathologists, physicians, and lay persons about cancer. He selected as his successor at Memorial Hospital, New York City, Fred W. Stewart. Stewart focused almost completely on the accurate microscopic diagnosis of cancer, becoming one of the finest cancer diagnosticians of his time and developing a school of surgical pathologists. He emphasized the importance of the diagnosis of cancer in its carcinoma in situ stage (14,28).

carcinogenic process and as a guide for the treatment of tumors. A recent textbook lists about 1,600 recognizable types of neoplastic lesions (27).

Classification of Neoplasms

By the early 20th century a histologic classification of cancers and a beginning definition of terminology had been achieved. The wide diversity of types of cancer was becoming apparent.

Neoplasm: An abnormal growth of new cells, benign or malignant, arising in an organ or tissue, e.g., in cells of the breast, lung, kidney, or connective tissue.

Benign: A neoplasm whose increase of cells is abnormal but is limited in that it does not invade adjacent structures or metastasize. It is usually not harmful to the general health of the patient, but may be removed or destroyed for cosmetic reasons, or if there is reason to believe that it may change into a malignant neoplasm.

Examples of benign tumors are: the relatively common leiomyoma (Greek: smooth muscle tumor) of the uterus ("fibroids") and the adenofibroma of the female breast, a benign neoplasm of epithelial and connective tissues.

Malignant (Cancer): A neoplasm whose growth is progressive, leading to invasion of tissues, spreading locally and/or to other organs (metastasis). In most cases, it would be fatal to the patient if not treated. An example is the cancer of the female breast. An exception is the common basal cell carcinoma of the skin which slowly invades tissue but very rarely metastasizes. It is removed or treated for cosmetic purposes.

Simplified Subdivisions of Cancer

Carcinoma: A cancer of epithelial cells, i.e., cells lining surfaces, ducts, tubules, and other organs (breast, pancreas, lung, colon, stomach, and kidney). The majority of cancers are carcinomas.

Adenocarcinoma: A carcinoma arising in the epithelial cells that form glands, e.g., pancreas (figs. 12-3–12-5).

Squamous Cell Cancer: A carcinoma arising from squamous cells, e.g., squamous cell cancer of the skin, pharynx, or larynx.

Basal Cell Cancer: A relatively innocuous cancer of the skin, arising in the basal cells.

Sarcoma: A cancer of connective tissue.

Fibrosarcoma: A cancer of fibroblasts, e.g., fibrosarcoma of the uterus (fig. 12-6).

Melanoma: A tumor of the skin, usually containing melanin, a black pigment. It may occur in areas other than the skin.

Osteogenic Sarcoma: A sarcoma arising in bone.

Malignant Lymphoma: A cancer of the lymphatic system.

Lymphocytoma: A cancer composed of malignant lymphocytes; also called non-Hodgkin's lymphoma.

Hodgkin's Disease: A cancer whose cell of origin is believed to be one of the cells of the lymphoid tissue.

Multiple Myeloma: A cancer arising in the plasma cells of the bone marrow.

Leukemia: A cancerous disease of the white cells of the bone marrow and blood, further defined as acute or chronic.

Myelogenous (Granulocytic) Leukemia: A cancer of the granulocytic cell line.

Lymphocytic Leukemia: A cancer of the lymphocyte line.

Neoplasms of Central and Peripheral Nervous System: *Astrocytoma:* A cancer of the astrocytes, the supporting tissue cells of the brain.

Neurofibrosarcoma: A cancer of the peripheral nerves.

Neoplasms Named After Individuals: Some neoplasms are named after the prominent individuals who first described or popularized them, e.g., Hodgkin's disease, a malignant lymphoma, after Thomas Hodgkin, a physician of Guy's Hospital; Ewing's sarcoma of bone, after James Ewing, a pathologist at Memorial Hospital, New York City; and Wilms' tumor, a cancer of the kidney in children named after Max Wilms, a surgeon at the University of Heidelberg.

There are many well known syndromes carrying the names of other investigators, particularly recently with the increased number of studies involving genetic syndromes.

Benign Tumors Changing to Malignant Tumors: Some benign tumors may change to malignant tumors over a period of time. Polyps of the colon, usually benign lesions, are examples that may become malignant.

The above classification has been greatly expanded since World War II, e.g., malignant lymphoma is divided into many subtypes depending on the cell of origin, such as the T-cell or B-cell lymphocyte. Further subdivisions by histologic and cytologic characteristics were greatly expanded and were correlated with clinical features such as prognosis.

REFERENCES

1. Bloch BT, Dreifuss SW. Ueber die experimentelle Er Zeugung von carcinomen mit lymphdrusen–und Lungen-metastasen durch Teerbestandteile. Schweiz. Med Wochenschr 1921;51:1035–7.

2. Borrel A. Le probleme du cancer. Bull Inst Pasteur 1907; 5:497, 545, 593, 641.

3. Borst M. Die Lehre von den Geschwülsten mit einem mikro-skopischen Atlas, 2 vols. Wiesbaden: Bergman, 1902.

4. Braun AC, Wood HN. Suppression of the neoplastic state with the acquisition of specialized functions in cells, tissues and organs of crown gall teratomas. Proc Natl Acad Sci USA 1976;73:496–500.

5. Bulloch W. History of bacteriology. London; Oxford Univ. Press, 1938.

6. Cade S. Malignant disease and its treatment by radium, vol 1. Baltimore MD: Williams & Wilkins, 1948.

7. Chatterjee KD. Parasitology (protozoology and helminthol-ogy) in relation to clinical medicine, 4th ed. Calcutta: Published by author, 1962:128–31.

8. Clemmesen J. Gongylonema and vitamin A in carcinogen-esis. Acta Pathol Microbiol Scand 1978;86:1–13.

9. Del Regato JA. James Ewing. Int J Rad Oncol Biol Phys 1977;2:185–98.

10. Dewing SB. Modern radiology in historical perspective. Springfield, IL: Charles C. Thomas, 1962.

11. Ewing J. Neoplastic diseases: a treatise on tumors, 2nd ed. Philadelphia: WB Saunders, 1922: 40–3, 103–25, 375.

12. Ferguson AR. Associated bilharziasis and primary malig-nant disease of the urinary bladder. J Pathol Bacteriol 1911;16:76–94.

13. Fibiger JA. Untersuchung über eine Nematode (Spiroptera sp. n.) und deren Fahigkeit papillomatose und cardinoma-tose. Geschwustbildungen im Magen der Ratte hervor-zurufen. Z Krebsforsch 1913;13:217–80.

14. Fitzgerald PJ. Fred W. Stewart. Memoir. Cancer 1991; 10:2419–21.

15. Glasser O. Dr. W.C. Roentgen. 2nd ed. Springfield, IL: Charles C. Thomas, 1958.

16. Halsted WS. Results of operations for the cure of cancer of the breast. Johns Hopkins Hosp Rep 1894;4:1–54.

17. Henke F, Lubarsch O. Handbuch der speziellen patho-logischen Anatomie und Histologie. Berlin Springer, 1924.

18. Henschen F. Yamagiwa's tar cancer and its historical significance. Gann 1968;59:447–51.

19. Hurwitz A, Degenshein GA. Theodor Billroth (1829–1894) and the rise of abdominal surgery. In: Milestones in modern surgery. New York: Hoeber-Harper, 1958:488–98.

20. Johnson L, Kempson RL. Epidermoid cancer in chronic osteomyelitis: diagnostic problem and management. J Bone Joint Surg 1965;47A:133–45.

21. Katsusaburo Yamagiwa (1863–1930). CA Cancer J Clin 1977;27:172–81.

22. Lusitanus Z. Praxis Medical Admiranda p. 31 ops. 124 (Appendix to Opera tome ii). Lugduni: Sumptibus Ioannis-Antonii Huguetan and Guillielmi Barbier, 1649.

23. Morris H, Wagner BP. Induction and transplantation of rat hepatomas with different growth rates (including "minimal deviation" hepatomas). In: Busch D, ed. Methods in cancer research. New York: Academic Press, 1968.

24. Pierce GB, Wallace C. Differentiation of malignant to be-nign cells. Cancer Res 1971;31:127–34.

25. Quimby EH. The first fifty years of the American Radium Society Inc. 1916–1966. Philadelphia: American Radium Society, 1967.

26. Robbins GF. James Ewing–the man. Mem Hosp Clin Bull 1978:11–14.

27. Rosai J. Ackerman's surgical pathology, 6th ed. St. Louis: CV Mosby, 1981.

28. Rosai J. Guiding the surgeon's hand. The history of Amer-ican surgical pathology. Washington D.C. Armed Forces Institute of Pathology, 1998.

29. Schoental R. Front. Gastrointestinal Res 1979;4:17–24.

30. Shimkin MB. Cancer hospitals. In: Contrary to nature. Wash-ington, D.C.: U.S. Department of Health, Education, & Welfare, 1977:245–6.

31. Shimkin MB. Contagiousness of cancer. In: Contrary to nature. Washington, D.C.: U.S. Department of Health, Education, & Welfare, 1977:69–70.

32. Shimkin M. Johannes Fibiger. Cover and cover legend. Cancer Res 1986:46.

33. Silverstein AM. A history of immunology. San Diego: Aca-demic Press, 1989.

34. Smith EF. Studies on the crown gall of plants in relations to human cancer. J Cancer Res 1916;1:231–309.

35. Stewart FW. Obituaries. James Ewing M.D. 1866–1943. Arch Path 1943;36:325–30.

36. Triolo VA. Nineteenth century foundation of cancer re-search advances in tumor pathology nomenclature and theories of oncogenesis. Cancer Res 1965;25:75–106.

37. Tulp N. Observatoines Medicae Lib. IV Amsteiredami L. Elzevirium, 1652:308–9.

38. Virchow R. Combinations–un ubergangsfahigkeit krank-hafter. Verhandlungen der physikalisch–medizinischen Gesellschaft zu Wuerzburg 1851;1:134–40.

39. Virchow R. Die Krankhaften Geschwuelste. Berlin: A Hirschwald, 1863;1:81.

40. Virchow R. Noch Einmal. Das Archiv fur Physiologische Heilkunde Archiv feur pathologischen Anatomie und Phys-iologie und fuer klinische Medizin 1860;17:126–38.

41. Walker AE, ed. A history of neurological surgery. Philadel-phia; Williams & Wilkins, 1951.

42. Wolff J; Ayoub B, trans. The science of cancerous disease. From earliest times to the present. Canton MA: Science History Publications, 1989:433–590.

43. Yamagiwa K, Ichikawa KJ. Experimental study of the pathogenesis of cancer. J Cancer Res 1918;3:1–29.

44. Yuspa SH, Kilkenny A, Roop DR. Aberrant differentiation in mouse skin carcinogenesis. In: Kakunaga T, ed. Cell differentiation genes and cancer. Lyon: International Agency for Research on Cancer, 1988: 3–19.

13
CHEMICAL CARCINOGENESIS

EXPOSURE TO CHEMICALS AND CANCER

Some investigators in the past suggested, with little or no evidence, that certain chemicals caused cancer, e.g., Paracelsus believed that both arsenic and calcothar gave rise to the malignancy (75) (see chapter 5). In the 17th century physicians became interested in the chemistry of the body and soon the language of the early chemists entered medicine. Words such as "ferments" (enzymes), "putrefaction," "acidity," and "acridity" were frequently used, as were "effervescents" and "volatile spirits" (87), but mention was still made of "spirits" and "cancer seeds."

In spite of the major contributions of Robert Boyle, an English investigator, to chemistry in the 17th century, Butterfield, a historian of science, believes that the great transformation of chemistry occurred in the closing decades of the 18th century (15). The composition of air and the role of oxygen in living substances occupied the interest of chemical investigators at this time. The chemical revolution occurred 100 to 150 years after the revolutions in mechanics and astronomy (15).

In the 19th century vitalism was the prominent concept in biology: that living organisms were characterized by a nonmaterial force or spirit that could not be defined by the laws of physics or chemistry. This vital force was believed to be the essential activating unit in animal and plant organisms and their products (71). When Frederick Wöhler (1800–1882), a German chemist at Göttigen, synthesized urea in the laboratory in 1828 from potassium cyanate and ammonium sulfate, the supposed distinction between living and nonliving matter disappeared because urea was thought to be synthesized only by living organisms. This laboratory experiment sped the demise of vitalism (58).

As early as 1825 chemical analysis was applied to histologic sections of tissue from organs by the French cytologist, F.V. Raspail. He stained the tissues with iodine to identify the presence of starch (85); other chemicals identified albumin, sugar, and protein (86). In 1829, Johann F. Lobstein, a German-born pathologist, reported that tumors contained albumin, fibrin, and gelatin (59).

In the 18th century it had been observed by physicians that persons with certain habits or occupations related to chemical substances seemed to have cancer more frequently than the rest of the population. The long use of snuff (powdered tobacco) was associated with an increased incidence of nasopharyngeal tumors (43,88). Other relationships noted were: that between cancer of the scrotum and a previous occupation as a chimney sweep (81); the seemingly increased prevalence of bladder cancer among the workers in an aniline dye factory (89); and the finding that persons who worked in an industry where they came into contact with coal tar and soot had a higher risk of scrotal skin cancer (102). In none of these cases was it known whether the cause of the cancer was a chemical compound itself or the effect of a chronic inflammation caused by the offending agent.

THE SEARCH FOR A SPECIFIC CHEMICAL CARCINOGEN IN TAR

In the 1920s, Ernest Kennaway (1881–1958) (fig. 13-1), a British biochemist, began the search for a specific substance that might be present in the coal tar that caused the cancer reported by Yamagiwa and Itchikawa (18) (see chapter 12). Joining the staff of the Research Institute of the Free Cancer Hospital in London, Kennaway began to collect samples of the complex hydrocarbon compounds known to be present in tar. These were applied to the skin of mice for over a 2-year period without the significant appearance of cancer.

Kennaway had read of Schroeter's work in which complex organic compounds might be formed at body temperatures and by this technique Kennaway isolated many of these compounds from coal tar and tested them on mouse skin. Of 496 animals, 110 developed cancers when natural and synthetic tars were applied. However, in none was a specific chemical compound identified as the carcinogen (50).

There was much frustration in the work of isolating possible carcinogens because the great number of hydrocarbons that might be present in tar precluded testing them all on animals for the production of tumors. W.V. Mayneord of the Kennaway

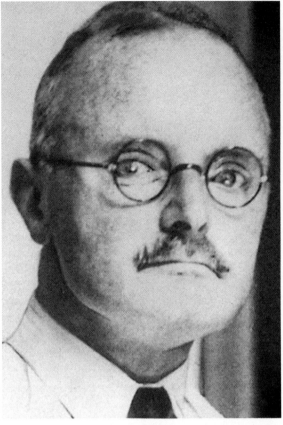

Figure 13-1
ERNEST KENNAWAY

Leader of the British group that isolated the carcinogen benzo[α]pyrene from coal tar. He was knighted. (From Shimkin MB. Contrary to nature. Washington, D.C.: U.S. Department of Health, Education, & Welfare, 1977:231.)

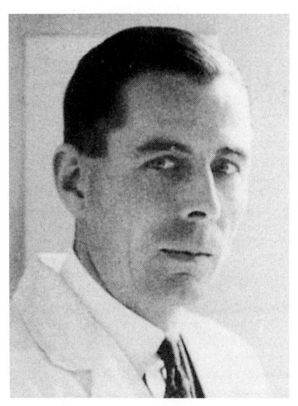

Figure 13-2
JAMES COOK

A British biochemist, James Cook sent a synthetic chemical, dibenz[α,η]-anthracene, to Kennaway for testing and it was found to be carcinogenic. It was the first synthetic chemical identified as a carcinogen. He was knighted. (From Shimkin MB. Contrary to nature. Washington, D.C.: U.S. Department of Health, Education, & Welfare, 1977:233.)

group noticed that the carcinogenic substances gave a blue-violet fluorescence when exposed to ultraviolet light or daylight. Spectroscopy showed that the carcinogens that fluoresced showed two distinct bands in the blue and violet regions of the spectrum, which the group called the "cancer bands." They realized that fluorescence might be used as a marker for screening out the compounds that were likely to be carcinogenic from the thousands of possible chemical compounds in tar (41). During the Kennaway group's studies at least two tons of pitch were fractionated by the Gas Light and Coke Company in Becton, England and the extract sent to Kennaway's laboratory for further fractional distillation.

The fluorescent spectrum findings directed attention to the benzanthracene type of molecular structure. J.W. Cook, a London biochemist (fig. 13-2), sent samples of polycyclic hydrocarbons for fluorescent spectroscopy to Kennaway's laboratory. A synthetic compound, 1:2:5:6-dibenzanthracene (now called dibenz[α,η] anthracene), tested by the Kennaway group, was found to be fluorescent and carcinogenic. This was the first synthetic chemical identified as a carcinogen (fig. 13-3) (19). Three other similar compounds were synthesized and proven carcinogenic, but the most potent was 1:2:5:6-dibenzanthracene.

A few years later Cook and others identified the carcinogen in coal tar as 1,2 anthracene (now known as benzo[α]pyrene [fig. 13-3]) (51). Benzo[α]pyrene was found to be the most highly carcinogenic compound tested; even when diluted in a concentration of 3 parts per 10,000 of solvent it produced skin cancer in mice.

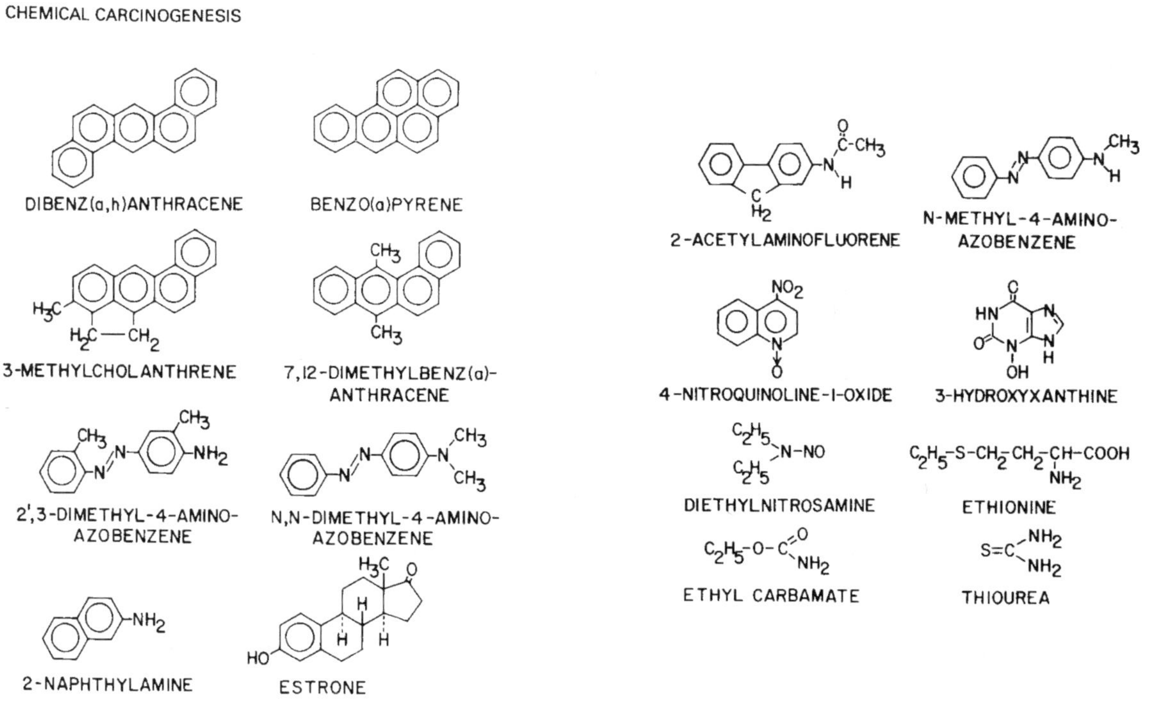

CHEMICAL CARCINOGENESIS

Figure 13-3
CHEMICAL STRUCTURE OF SOME OF THE BETTER KNOWN EXPERIMENTAL CARCINOGENS
(Modified from figs. 9–11 from reference 77.)

The identification of benzo[α]pyrene as the carcinogen in coal tar was a scientific achievement of the first magnitude and a most seminal event. It showed that cancer was not necessarily the result of a nonspecific irritative process but that it could be produced in an animal by a pure chemical compound. It initiated the examination of thousands of chemical compounds for their carcinogenic potential (Note 1).

STAGES OF CARCINOGENESIS

Initiation and Promotion

In the 1940s two groups, one at Rockefeller Institute, New York City, and the other at Oxford University, repeated the Yamagiwa method of producing a cancer using various tar products.

Peyton Rous (fig. 13-4) with his colleagues, J. Friedenwald, J. Kidd, and I. MacKensie of the Rockefeller Institute, were able to induce papillomas and carcinomas on the ears of rabbits using benzpyrene. With additional irritative effects on the tarred skin—punching holes in the irritated skin or applying turpentine or chloroform, to the area—they increased the number of papillomas and carcinomas, compared to control animals given benzpyrene applications alone (33,60,91).

The Rous group suggested that the original stimulus for the papillomas remained dormant in some cells and could be activated and heightened by the wounds, or turpentine or chloroform application, even months after the initial application of benzpyrene. They suggested that carcinogenesis could be considered as occurring in two steps, which they called "initiation" and "promotion" (34).

I. Berenblum and P. Shubik, of Oxford University, used the carcinogen DMBA (9:10-dimethyl-1:2-benzanthracene) painted on the mouse skin as the initiator and croton oil (73) as the promoter (6). With such a regimen, Berenblum and Shubik showed that there was a greater increase in the number of tumors produced in the mouse skin by

---

Note 1: The achievement of the Kennaway group was of a high order of scientific research. It is surprising that it did not receive a Nobel Prize.

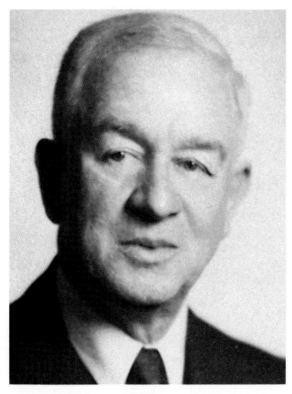

Figure 13-4
PEYTON ROUS

Peyton Rous of the Rockefeller Institute divided the process of carcinogenesis into two stages—initiation and progression. He earlier had discovered the Rous sarcoma and showed that it could be transmitted to other hens by means of a cell-free filtrate of the tumor. (Fig. 12 from Gross L. Oncogenic viruses, 3rd ed, Vol. 1. Oxford: Pergamon Press, 1983:127.)

DMBA and croton oil together than were caused by the carcinogen alone (6). Croton oil alone did not produce papillomas or cancers and when it was applied to the skin before the methylcholanthrene application there was no increase in papillomas or cancers over that produced by methylcholanthrene alone or by the combined action of the carcinogen and croton oil. Most promoting agents were shown to be tissue specific: they did not have to be activated and they were found to be nonmutagenic. Some carcinogens are complete carcinogens that do not require the additional action of a promoter. Some promoters when given for long periods of time give rise to a few neoplasms.

Since the work of the Rous and Berenblum groups it has been widely accepted that most cancers are the result of a multistage process, although there have been some objections or modifications to the original concept (31,45).

Promotion and Skin Carcinogenesis

One of the most productive approaches to the study of promotion has been the application of promoting agents to the skin of rodents. Squamous papillomas and squamous cell carcinomas are the most common skin tumors resulting from such applications.

Progress in the study of promotion occurred when a potent and frequently used promoter was isolated from croton oil; it was the phorbol ester TPA (12-0-tetradecanolphorbol-13-acetate). Extensive studies on mouse skin by Boutwell and associates of the University of Wisconsin showed that when the initiator urethan was given only once and was followed by the TPA promoter three times a week for some weeks thereafter, there was a marked increase in the number of tumors compared to when urethan was used alone (11,12). After 1 year, 40 to 60 percent of the animals given the initiator and promotor developed squamous cell carcinomas of the skin. If the promoting agent TPA was given alone, usually no malignant tumors occurred; if given before the initiating agent there was no increase of tumors over that produced by the initiator alone.

Boutwell et al. showed that the "memory" of initiation was essentially irreversible up to at least 1 year, i.e., there was an increase in the number of tumors produced if the promoter was added within a year after initiation. Younger animals retained the "memory" of the initiating compound longer than did older animals.

Promoting agents were thought by Boutwell and colleagues to exert their effects by altering the expression of genetic information by a derepression of certain genes, i.e., the removal of the influence of normally present inhibiting genes (11). They also suggested that promotion might be subdivided into two stages (11,12). Recent studies have strengthened this latter suggestion (96,97,113) with the finding that some TPA-like compounds may act only in the second stage of promotion.

Progression

Leslie Foulds, a British pathologist who studied breast cancer in mice, wrote two volumes of incisive criticism on the subject of neoplasia. He believed that initiation and promotion were part of a longer and more continuous process of carcinogenesis, which he called "progression" (31). Foulds spoke of the independent progression of different primary neoplasms in the same animal. Mentioned were independent progression of different characters of the same tumor; the clinical manifestation of the tumor occurring at any stage of progression and independently of size or clinical duration of the tumor; gradual or rapid progression in mouse breast cancer; all tumors not following the same path of development; and all tumors not always reaching an endpoint within the lifetime of the host (31).

It is now believed that progression occurs when the original initiated cell shows changes from normality to proliferation, with the appearance of atypical cells and chromosomal and nuclear changes, and, finally, when the cellular changes recognized as carcinoma in situ are present. A significant change comes about when the malignant cell acquires the property of invasiveness, extending into adjacent tissues and growing into lymphatic channels and blood vessels. Metastasis through blood and lymph vessels, as well as along some surfaces, may follow.

The growth of metastases is a complicated process which also involves the host reaction (9,28,109). In most cases, the growth of metastases in humans is progressive, unless altered by therapy. Rarely, metastases may lie dormant for some years and then suddenly begin to grow (1). Very rarely, spontaneous remissions of untreated metastases are reported, and even of the primary cancer, although many of these cases would not withstand critical evaluation (21).

LIVER CARCINOGENESIS

One of the most investigated fields in carcinogenesis has been that of liver cell cancer. In 1935, the Japanese investigators T. Sasaki and T. Yoshida reported the production of cancer in the rat liver with the azo dye o-amidoazotoluol (92). A year later R. Kinosita, also Japanese, produced liver cell cancer when he fed rats an isomer of o-amidoazotoluol, N N-dimethyl-4 amino-azobenzene (butter yellow) (fig. 13-3) (55). Since then the rodent liver cancer model has been a favorite for hundreds of experimental studies.

When metabolically activated, aromatic amines and alkylating agents can react with nucleic acids in the liver of rats. E. Farber and colleagues in Toronto discovered that 2-acetylaminofluorene (2AAF) and dimethylaminoazobenzene (DAB) were present in extracted ribonucleic acid (RNA) (24,63,64). 4-dimethyl-aminophenylazobenzene

was found to bind, preferentially, to liver ribosomal RNA (rRNA) (99). Later, binding to the deoxyribonucleic acid (DNA) of rat liver was demonstrated for 2AAF (fig. 13-3) (90).

A multitude of carcinogenic compounds of many types affecting many organs were discovered during the 1940s and 1950s, many of them known to possess toxic side reactions as well as being carcinogenic. In 1973, Peraino and associates introduced a new promoter, the sedative phenobarbital, which permitted lower dosages of the initiator to be used and avoided many of the toxic effects of liver carcinogens (76). When 2AAF (fig. 13-3) was fed to rats for 3 weeks a small number of the animals got cancer of the liver. Another group of rats was similarly treated with 2AAF but, in addition, was fed phenobarbital as the promoter for some months, and a much higher incidence of liver cell cancer occurred.

Other models of liver carcinogenesis were studied wherein a single dose of an initiator was given during liver regeneration following surgical resection of part of the liver, and phenobarbital was administered for some months. The partial resection of the liver set up a regenerative response that increased the tumor yield. Scherer and Emmelot in Holland (93), H. Pitot and the Wisconsin group (79), E. Farber and colleagues in Toronto (22), and others showed that many small heterogeneous foci of hyperplastic cells appeared in the liver, which upon application of histochemical techniques revealed a change in the activity of certain enzymes: a loss of activity of glucose-6-phosphatase (G-6-P) and adenosine triphosphatase (ATPase) and increased activity of gamma glutamyl-transpeptidase (GGTP). The areas with altered enzymes stained with basophilic dyes and were believed to contain cells in an early stage of the development of neoplasms.

Death of Cells in Liver Cancer—Apoptosis

Since Virchow, the process of cell death was looked at as a degenerative, passive necrosis imposed upon the cell by external forces and in which the cell itself played no active role (101). Textbooks of pathology have described the characteristics of necrosis following injury, vascular accidents, exposure to toxins and infectious agents, or to the insults of a nonphysiological environment, generally as a passive process. Trump and colleagues correlated morphologic and biochemical features of the necrotic process (100). Another type of cell death has been recognized by the embryologists who followed the growth of cells during embryogenesis and noted the focal disappearance of large numbers of cells as organs were formed and developed (35).

In 1970, Farber and colleagues suggested that death in some cell systems was an active process after they discovered that cycloheximide and other agents that inhibited protein synthesis could protect the intestinal epithelial crypt cells from the lethal effects of chemical agents and X rays. The protein inhibitors could not protect lymphoid cells from death. They concluded that the active metabolic response of the cell, protein synthesis, is necessary for the death of some cells (26).

In the 1970s and 1980s an active, self-programmed process of cell death was described by J. F. R. Kerr of the University of Queensland, Australia and colleagues. First designated as "shrinking necrosis" (52,53), the process was finally called "apoptosis" (Greek: "dropping off" or "falling off" of petals from a flower or leaves from a tree) (54,111). The process was said to be distinctive, recognized by light microscopic examination of the usual stained histologic sections of tissue, and further delineated by electron microscopy (54,110,111). Biochemical study of DNA extracted from the tissue, employing agar gel electrophoresis, was said to give a characteristic pattern, "laddering," of DNA fragmentation (98). There was an absence of the usual multicellular exudate characteristic of an inflammatory response.

Bursch and colleagues from the University of Vienna used a proliferation index and an apoptosis index to study rat liver tumors (37). Apoptotic activity gradually increased from normal liver cells, to preneoplastic foci, to adenoma, to hepatic carcinoma. At all stages the proliferative index was higher than the apoptotic index. Cancers obtained from the autopsies of 21 patients who died with liver cell cancer showed a marked increase of the proliferative index (24 times) and a smaller increase of the apoptotic index (7.5 times) over control values. The definitive extent and degree of apoptosis in many types of cancer has yet to be determined (see chapter 21).

Cell of Origin of Liver Parenchymal Cancer

Recently, attention has focused on the search for the cell of origin of liver cancer. Originally it was assumed that the mature differentiated liver parenchymal cell, the so-called hepatocyte, the parenchymal cell in the foci of hyperplastic nodules, was the cell of origin of liver cancer. It has been suggested that a precursor cell to the hepatocyte might give rise to liver cell cancer (95). A stem cell, possibly a cell called the oval cell, has been proposed as a cell that has the capacity to differentiate into the liver parenchymal cell, or into a cell of the bile duct system, and to give rise to liver parenchymal cell cancer. The cell of origin question has led to considerable debate as to its identity in liver carcinogenesis (23,27).

NITROSAMINES AND N-NITRO COMPOUNDS

In 1956, P. Magee and J.M. Barnes, British investigators, reported that a compound, dimethylnitrosamine (fig. 13-5), that they had studied for its liver toxicity, also caused liver tumors in rats (62). Later it was shown that in 40 animal species tested, tumors were produced by over 100 nitrosamines and other N-nitroso compounds. These compounds have an organ specificity that varies with their chemical structure, producing cancers of the liver, esophagus, stomach, pancreas, lung, bladder, and other organs (5,61).

The importance of the N-nitroso compounds lies in the fact that they may be produced in the normal human digestive system. The carcinogens can be formed by the nitrosation of a variety of secondary and tertiary amino compounds in the gastrointestinal tract. Nitrites in food or in human saliva can be converted by nitrosation into the carcinogens. Nitrates that occur in a significant percentage of the diet of man can be reduced to nitrites in the intestinal tract and these can then form with amines or amides in the bowel and result in carcinogenic nitrosamines or nitrosoamides, respectively (61).

It has been suggested that nitrosamines are involved in many human cancers, including the bilharzial bladder cancer in Egypt (40); nasopharyngeal, liver, and esophageal cancers in Hong Kong (30); esophageal cancer in Northern China (112); and gastric cancer in several parts of the world (16,107).

OTHER CARCINOGENS

There are animal models that can be used for the specific study of cancer of almost all organs. These studies usually require a specific chemical compound to be administered under certain conditions such

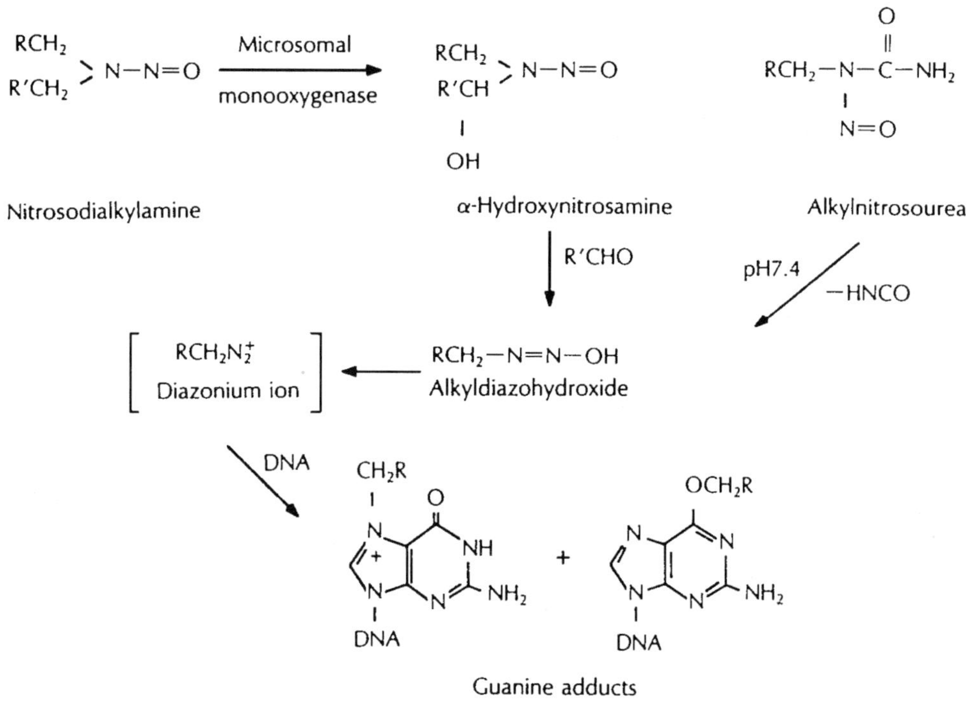

RCH_2
$R'CH_2$ $> N-N=O$ — Microsomal monooxygenase → RCH_2 $> N-N=O$ $R'CH$ | OH

$RCH_2-N-C-NH_2$ (with O double bond on C, and N=O on N)

Nitrosodialkylamine   α-Hydroxynitrosamine   Alkylnitrosourea

↓ R'CHO   pH7.4 / −HNCO

$RCH_2-N=N-OH$
Alkyldiazohydroxide

$\left[RCH_2N_2^+ \right]$
Diazonium ion ←

↘ DNA

Guanine adducts

Figure 13-5

CHEMICAL PATHWAY OF N-NITROSO COMPOUNDS

Diagram illustrating the metabolic chemical pathway of N-nitroso compounds and their formation of an adduct with guanine. (Fig. 7.14 from Tannock FF, Hill RP. The basic science of oncology, 2nd ed. New York: McGraw-Hill, 1992:110.)

as a particular strain of the animal, a distinctive route of administration, a definite dose schedule, and other factors. Usually one organ is most affected by the carcinogen but multiple organs may be affected when a single carcinogen is used. Organs in which cancers are commonly produced are skin, breast, lung, colon, bladder, prostate, and pancreas.

MECHANISMS OF ACTION OF CHEMICAL CARCINOGENS

Warburg Hypothesis

One of the important questions to answer when a compound has been shown to be carcinogenic is how does the carcinogen act to produce cancer— its mechanism of action. Otto Warburg of Berlin (fig. 13-6) was one of the important figures in biochemistry (56) who trained a generation of enzyme biochemists. He stimulated much progress in the biochemistry of tumors when in 1930 he proposed a hypothesis that appeared to explain carcinogenesis in chemical terms.

Warburg began studies in the 1920s on the respiration activity of cells from living tissue taken from animal and human cancers. He reported that in the absence of oxygen (anaerobiosis), and in an atmosphere of nitrogen, slices of tumor tissue utilized glucose and produced more lactic acid than did normal tissues. He believed that cancer cells differed from noncancer cells by their failure to suppress glycolysis in the presence of oxygen (56).

Warburg believed that the transformation of normal cells to cancer cells was caused by irreversible injury to the respiratory mechanism of the cells, which was compensated for by the cancer cell increasing its rate of glycolysis (103). Warburg's hypothesis stimulated hundreds of studies of the metabolism of all types of tumors. His work was an important step forward in the search for the Holy Grail of early cancer researchers, a single universal biochemical mechanism that was common to all neoplasms; a final biochemical common pathway in all cancers would make the search for the treatment of cancers simpler than if there were different metabolic pathways for each of many types of cancer.

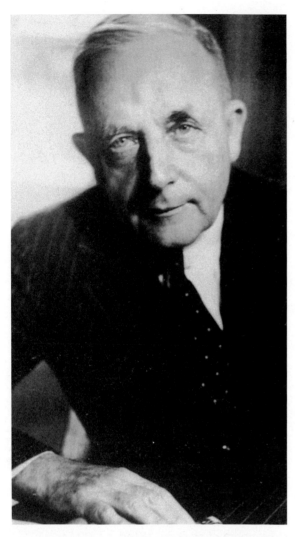

Figure 13-6
OTTO WARBURG

Otto Warburg was an outstanding enzyme chemist who trained many famous biochemists and performed early metabolic studies of cancerous tissues. (Frontispiece from Krebs H. Otto Warburg: cell physiologist, biochemist and eccentric. Oxford: Oxford Press, 1981.)

Sidney Weinhouse, a distinguished biochemist at Temple University and an editor of Cancer Research, reviewed Warburg's studies and stated, "there is no evidence either from Warburg's own observations or from those of his contemporaries that respiration in cancer is either quantitatively lower or fails to lower glycolysis" (105,106). The increased rates of glycolysis seen in many, but not all, neoplasms is viewed today as characteristic of the increased rate of growth in tumors and not the cause of the carcinogenic process (77).

Enzyme Convergence Hypothesis: Greenstein

In the 1940s and 1950s, Jesse Greenstein, a biochemist at the U.S. National Cancer Institute, compared the enzymes of many tumors and those of the normal tissues of the organ in which the cancer arose. Enzymes are proteins that facilitate chemical reactions but are not themselves consumed in the process. In 1954 he formulated the hypothesis that neoplasms in their progression to more malignant stages tended to converge to relatively simpler enzymatic patterns by the loss of many complex enzyme systems (38).

Later Henry Pitot and colleagues at Wisconsin University showed that in the hepatomas studied by Morris (see chapter 12) no lack of enzyme synthesis could be demonstrated. These authors found that the pattern of control of enzyme synthesis was unique to each tumor, essentially an antithesis of Greenstein's hypothesis (77).

Membron Concept

As a result of extensive study of the enzymes of nodules of breast cancer in mice and the serum of animals with regenerating liver nodules, Pitot and colleagues found that each nodule seemed to have its own unique pattern of biochemical heterogeneity and phenotypic variability that was characteristic of the cancer (80). This would imply that cancer might not be genetic in nature but the result of changes in some other nongenetic controlling structure. These investigators proposed that an epigenetic effect might be achieved by a structure composed of a functioning cytoplasmic polysome (a group of RNA ribosomes) with a cytoplasmic membrane (see chapter 18). Experiments showed that membrane-bound polysomes were more stable than the free ribosomes. The association of the membrane complex with a messenger RNA (mRNA), might add to the stability of the resultant "membron." This could be the site of action of carcinogens because of the importance of mRNA in the synthesis of protein. This concept implied an epigenetic mechanism for carcinogenesis.

The concept was in keeping with the then current biochemical thought, but advances in genetics and molecular biology placed more emphasis on genetic mechanisms (see chapters 18 and 19). Most recent research on methylation of nucleic acids has opened again the possibility that epigenetic factors may be very important in some cancers (see chapter 21).

Molecular Correlation Concept

George Weber, a biochemist at Indiana University, proposed that gene expansion and its variation in neoplasia can be deduced by determining the concentrations of specific key enzymes, the molecular correlation concept. He studied 40 enzymes that were found to correlate with the growth rate of tumors (104). Usually an increase in activity of anabolic enzymes and a decrease in that of catabolic enzymes occurred. There is a tendency for tumor tissue enzymes to respond less to normal controls but each tumor may exhibit a unique pattern of enzyme activation, with a great diversity of the patterns overall (78).

Deletion Hypotheses

In the 1940s the husband-wife team of Elizabeth and James Miller and their colleagues at the University of Wisconsin started a long, productive attempt to explain the metabolism of various carcinogens (fig. 13-7). They fed p-dimethylamino-azo-benzene to rats to produce liver cancer and found that the azo group became bound to proteins of the normal liver cells but not to the proteins of the liver tumors (68). A follow-up study of mouse skin painted with benz[a]pyrene also showed that the carcinogen, or some of its metabolites, was bound to protein (67). The Miller experiments led to their hypothesis that the binding of carcinogens to proteins might lead to the loss or deletion of critical proteins necessary for the regulation or control of growth, the "protein-deletion hypothesis" (68). Later work showed that many carcinogens also became bound to the DNA of cancer cells (66).

In 1973, V. Potter of the Wisconsin group suggested that there was a depletion of many catabolic degradative enzymes, a "catabolic depletion" in neoplasms (82). But with the use of the Morris "minimal deviation" tumor of liver cancer in rats (72) (a neoplasm that morphologically resembles normal liver) it became evident that the highly differentiated liver tumors deviated only slightly from the normal enzymatic patterns, even though the cells were malignant and gave rise to metastases (83).

Activation of Carcinogen— Proximate and Ultimate Carcinogens

In 1960, the Millers and Cramer reported that in the metabolism of the liver carcinogen AAF (2-acetylaminofluorene) there was hydroxylation of the

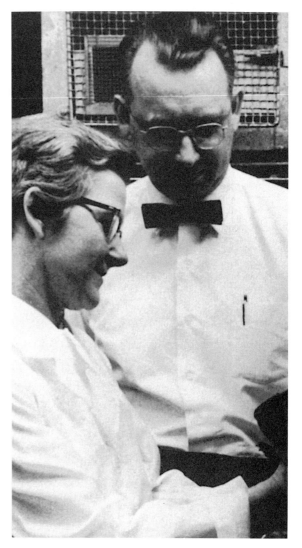

Figure 13-7
JAMES AND ELIZABETH MILLER
James and Elizabeth Miller, husband-wife biochemists of Wisconsin University, pioneered studies in chemical carcinogenesis. (From Shimkin MB. Contrary to nature. Washington, D.C.: U.S. Department of Health, Education, & Welfare, 1977:367.)

nitrogen of the acetylamino group (N-hydroxy-AAF) (70); this metabolite of AAF was later proven to be more carcinogenic than the parent AAF compound. The Miller group later showed that the N-hydroxy group of the N-hydroxy-AAF could be esterified to yield a highly reactive compound which would react with proteins, nucleic acids, amino acids, and nucleosides. They proposed that the carcinogenic metabolites were converted into electrophile reactants (chemicals with electrondeficient sites) that

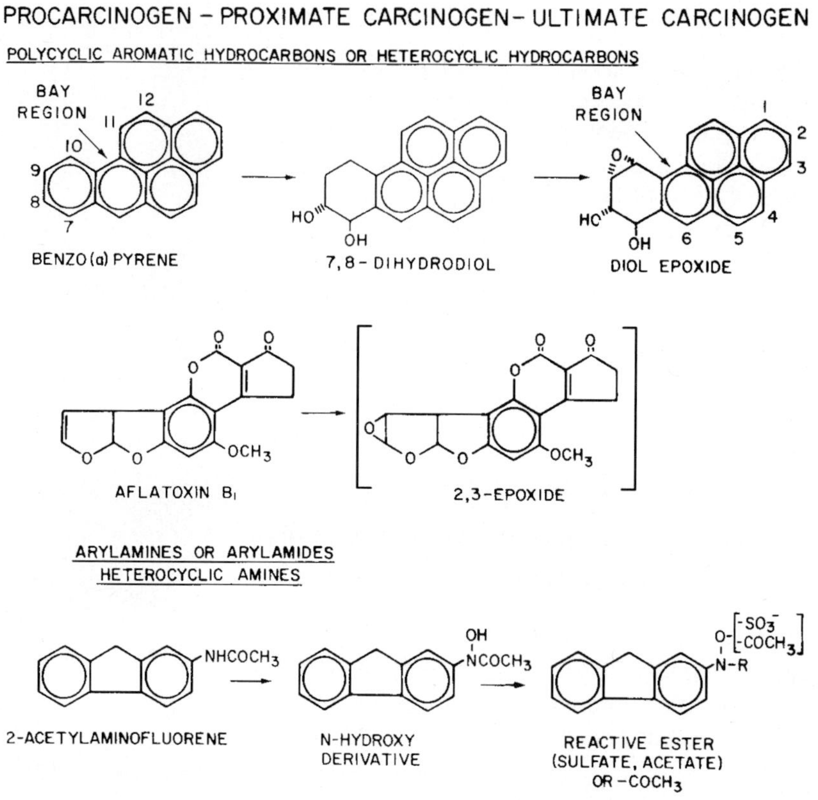

PROCARCINOGEN – PROXIMATE CARCINOGEN– ULTIMATE CARCINOGEN

<u>POLYCYCLIC AROMATIC HYDROCARBONS OR HETEROCYCLIC HYDROCARBONS</u>

BENZO (a) PYRENE   7,8– DIHYDRODIOL   DIOL EPOXIDE

Figure 13-8
JAMES AND ELIZABETH
MILLER'S CONCEPT
OF CARCINOGENESIS

The metabolism of a proximate procarcinogen to a proximate carcinogen to an ultimate carcinogen. (Modified from Miller EC, Miller JA. Searches for ultimate chemical carcinogens and their reactions with cellular macromolecules. Cancer 1981;47:2327–45.)

AFLATOXIN B₁   2,3–EPOXIDE

<u>ARYLAMINES OR ARYLAMIDES</u>
<u>HETEROCYCLIC AMINES</u>

2-ACETYLAMINOFLUORENE   N-HYDROXY DERIVATIVE   REACTIVE ESTER (SULFATE, ACETATE) OR –COCH₃

could interact with macromolecules such as DNA (66). It was later demonstrated that N-hydroxy-AAF was converted in rat liver to a sulfate, N-sulfonoxy-AAF, by a sulfotransferase in the cytosol of the liver cells. This sulfur compound reacted with nucleic acids and proteins (fig. 13-8) (69).

Many carcinogens are metabolized by organs of the body to compounds that are more carcinogenic than the parent compound; other carcinogens are direct carcinogens and do not require any further metabolic activity. The Millers suggested that in the former the metabolic process might be broken down into stages, the parent compound, the "proximate carcinogen," was metabolized to the "ultimate carcinogen." The latter acted with the target cell to transform it to a cancer cell (fig. 13-8) (69, 108). There may be more than one metabolite that can be considered an "ultimate" carcinogen (108). Some organs can metabolize proximate carcinogens to ultimate carcinogens while other organs cannot break down the proximate carcinogen; this may be one reason why some organs are susceptible to a carcinogen and others are not.

Cellular Adaptation Hypothesis of Farber and Rubin

The sequence of changes in the experimental liver cell cancer of the rat has been summarized by Emmanuel Farber of Toronto who has been a productive pioneer and leader in this field for many years (23,25). The carcinogen must provoke at least one episode of cell death and reparative cell proliferation in order to initiate the process of carcinogenesis. Carcinogens, in general, inhibit cellular proliferation and Farber suggested that one type of initiated liver cell might be a hepatocyte that had acquired resistance to the inhibition of proliferation caused by carcinogens.

Farber gave his rats an aromatic amine (2AAF) carcinogen for 2 weeks and then added the promoter (partial hepatectomy or carbon tetrachloride [CCl₄]). Within 10 days small nodules appeared throughout the liver. In time most of the nodules (90 percent) disappeared and were remodeled to normal-appearing liver cells. A small number of nodules remained that did not regress, and grew into larger nodules which were shown to be resistant to carcinogens in that they continued to proliferate. The nodules grew and proliferated into cancer of the liver. Because the liver cells in the nodule were resistant to the inhibitory action of the carcinogen, the model has been called the resistant hepatocyte (RH) model.

A special biochemical pattern was present in the resistant liver nodules: there were large decreases in total microsomal cytochromes P-450 and 65, and in several mixed-function oxygenase activities. The carcinogen was efficiently excreted. There were large increases in glutathione (reduced, oxidized, and bound) and many other compounds involved in the detoxification of metabolic derivatives. A special polypeptide was noted in the cytosol.

Farber and Harry Rubin, an outstanding virologist at the University of California, Berkeley, hypothesized that carcinogenesis involves the resistant hepatocyte and the physiologic cellular process of adaptation. They downplay the current emphasis on somatic mutation (25). Their hypothesis states that the first recognizable step in carcinogenesis is the resistance of the rare hepatocyte to the carcinogen's inhibition of proliferation; it is the precursor of the resistant cells of the liver nodule that did not regress after the initiating carcinogen was administered. The resistant cells had an increased ability to proliferate. Clonal expansion of the resistant nodules progressed further, and continued growth and proliferation led eventually to liver cancer. This is viewed by Farber and Rubin as an epigenetic process, at least in the early stages, and not dependent on multiple somatic mutations. It represents a normal physiologic adaptation of cells to exposure to hazardous environmental agents. An exception is granted for the oncogene retroviruses (see chapter 20).

The authors list many objections to genomic involvement in the early stages of carcinogenesis, many of which concern cell cultures, particularly of the initiated NIH3T3 cell line and the mouse embryo cell line 10T1/2. They believe that there is evidence in cell cultures against a mutational origin of both initiation and promotion (25).

Carcinogenesis of Polycyclic Aromatic Hydrocarbons

Since many of the carcinogens were polycyclic aromatic hydrocarbons, their metabolism has aroused considerable interest. Boyland, a biochemist of the Chester Beattie Institute, London,

suggested in 1950 that the active metabolite of benzo[α]pyrene was a diol epoxide which is bound preferentially to compounds more active in the transcription of genes (13,84).

In 1970, Jerina and colleagues at the National Institute of Health, Bethesda, Maryland, reported that an intermediate compound formed during the metabolism of the polycyclic hydrocarbon benzo[α]pyrene was an epoxide (a cyclic oxide) (47). Subsequently, many laboratories (17,48) reported studies that demonstrated that one of the epoxides, diasteromeric BP-7, 8-diol-9, 10 (fig. 13-9), was an ultimate carcinogenic metabolite of benzo[α]pyrene. This metabolite was 50 to 100 times more effective as a carcinogen in producing pulmonary tumors in mice than benzo[α]pyrene itself (17,48).

The benzpyrene model is believed to be representative of many other polycyclic aromatic hydrocarbons that are generally mutagenic and carcinogenic.

Complete Carcinogens

Not all carcinogens have to be activated to become effective. A complete carcinogen such as the very reactive alkylating agent N-methyl-N-nitrosurea is active in aqueous solution. Among other complete carcinogens are direct alkylating agents such as B-propio-lactone, nitrogen mustard, ethylenimine, and bis (chloromethyl ether). Ultraviolet radiation also acts as a complete carcinogen (113).

MUTAGENS AND CARCINOGENS

The use of animals in carcinogenesis research requires a long study period and great expense for the detailed administration of the carcinogen and care of the animals. Bruce Ames of the University of California at Berkeley devised a relatively simple and quick test to determine the ability of the suspected carcinogen to produce a mutation in a bacterium, *Salmonella typhimurium* (2). It was known that some carcinogens were mutagenic and many mutagens were carcinogenic.

Ames showed that mutagenesis generally paralleled carcinogenesis and recommended the use of the bacterial mutagenic test as presumptive evidence of carcinogenicity. This test is simple, quick, and inexpensive compared to the difficult, long, and expensive periods involved in testing compounds by animal experimentation (65). However, it has limitations because not all carcinogens are mutagens and not all mutagens are carcinogens.

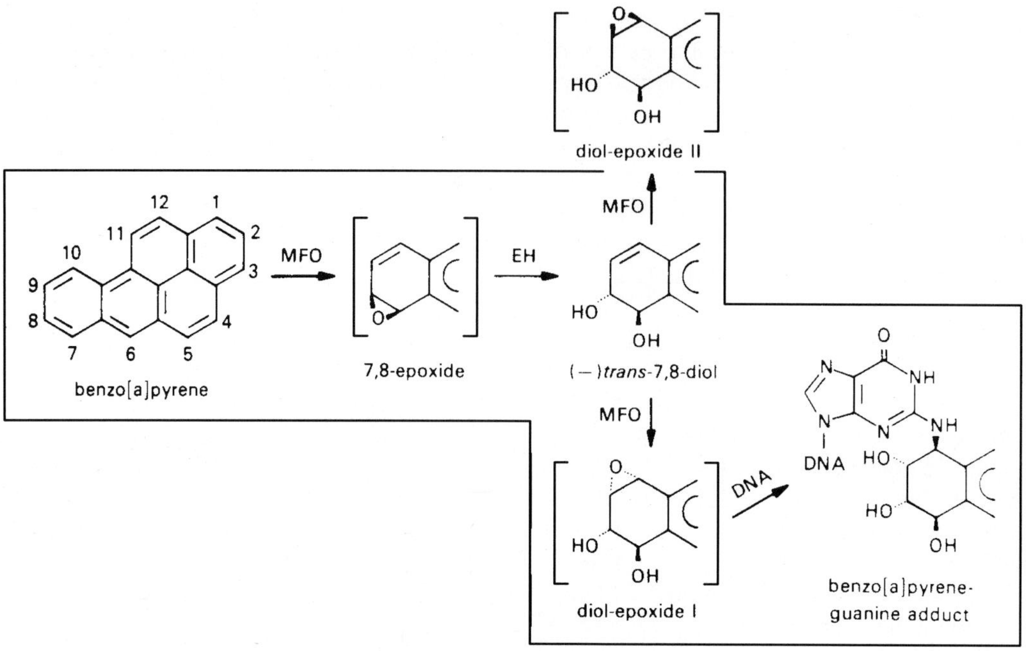

Figure 13-9

METABOLIC ACTIVATION OF BENZO[α]PYRENE AND FORMATION OF AN ADDUCT WITH GUANINE OF DNA

Metabolic activation of benzo[α]pyrene diol epoxides. Solid triangles and dashed lines indicate that substituents are toward and away from the viewer, respectively. MFO, mixed-function oxidase; EH, epoxide hydrase. (Fig. 2 from Yuspa SH, Poirrier M. Chemical carcinogenesis from animal models to molecular models in one decade. Adv Can Res 1988;50:25–70.)

CELL CULTURE CARCINOGENESIS

One of the most productive advances in carcinogenesis has been the application of carcinogens to cells growing in culture media, as reported by Y. Berwald and L. Sachs of Israel in 1965 (7). From the same laboratory, C. Borek developed specialized techniques for the growing of epithelial cells in a culture medium (10).

One may add potential carcinogens to the cells growing in the medium and then test the cells to determine whether they have been transformed from the normal state. The cells can be injected into animals of the same strain or "nude mice" (mice that have no thymus and are more receptive to transplants of tumors) to determine if they produce tumors. Chemical studies of carcinogenic metabolism can be carried out in the cells growing in a medium.

Daniel et al. have shown that metabolic profiles in cells of specific animal organs growing in culture media to which carcinogens are added are qualitatively similar to human cells grown in similar culture media (20). Harris et al. discovered that among

humans there might be a 100-fold variation in the quantitative capacity of tissues to metabolize a specific carcinogen (39). Conney et al. noted that in the liver biopsies of 10 patients with noncancerous diseases there was a difference of 6- to 9-fold between individuals in their ability to metabolize benzo[α]pyrene (17). The variation in the response of individuals to carcinogens is a factor that may determine why one strain of animals, or a human, may be susceptible to a carcinogen and another strain or human may not be.

NUCLEIC ACID ADDUCTS

The compound formed by the ultimate carcinogen or complete carcinogen and a macromolecule is called an adduct (fig. 13-9). Nucleic acids are assumed to be the major compounds upon which a carcinogen would form an adduct.

The covalent binding of the carcinogen to the DNA of mouse skin was shown by the British investigators P. Brookes and P. O. Lawley (14) to correlate with the carcinogenesis of several polycyclic hydrocarbons.

Guanine and adenine, the purines of DNA, are common sites of adduct formation. One of the most conspicuous examples of an adduct is that of the benzo[α]pyrene metabolite (Bp-7,8-diol-9,10-epoxide) which reacts almost exclusively with the 2-amino position of deoxyguanosine of DNA (fig. 13-9) and becomes the ultimate carcinogen (46).

The yield of tumors of the thymus (thymomas) in mice induced by single doses of the alkyl carcinogens nitrosoureas showed a positive linear correlation with the extent of alkylation of guanine at the O-6 atom (32). Guanine is the nucleotide base of DNA often found to react most avidly with the "ultimate" forms of chemical carcinogens. The persistence of an O-6 ethylguanine adduct in the DNA of the rat brain appears to correlate with carcinogenesis of the central nervous system (36).

DNA adducts may have many effects on the genes including decreasing the stability of the DNA, distortion of the DNA helix, mispairing of bases during replication of the DNA, causing a base transition (a purine-pyrimidine change) or a conformation change, or other effects.

Methylation of Nucleic Acids

Many studies indicate that methylation (addition of a CH_3 group to a nucleotide base) plays a role in the function of the genome, the sum of the genes (49).

Injection of the carcinogen dimethylnitrosamine methylates the RNA of the rat liver at the N-7 and O-6 positions of guanine in the liver ribosomal RNA (rRNA) (74). Methylation of transfer RNA (tRNA) occurs when the carcinogen N-acetoxy-2-acetylaminofluorene reacts with tRNA in vitro (29). Because of the vital role of the various RNAs in protein synthesis such a change as methylation may have serious consequences for the proteins produced. P.O. Lawley, a British biochemist and a pioneer in carcinogenesis, has an excellent review of the subject (57).

RECEPTOR EFFECT

Cells have on their surface many receptors which bind specific substances such as hormones, antibodies, and compounds. Binding is necessary for these substances to react with the cell.

It has been shown that in mouse skin carcinogenesis, the promoter, TPA, joins with a cell receptor for protein kinase and activates its kinase function, adding phosphate to compounds. Protein kinase C is an enzyme involved in relaying extracellular signals across the cell membrane in order to regulate many calcium-dependent processes inside the cell. Signal transmission from the outside of cells to the internal cellular mechanisms may control the growth and/or division of the cell (8) (see chapters 20 and 21).

Signals from hormones, neurotransmitters, and some growth factors may be transduced across the cell membrane into the cell by means of the protein kinases. These transducers may open switches for growth and division. Since cell proliferation is an essential part of the carcinogenic process, an increase of signal transduction could be a trigger which sets off the proliferation process in some types of carcinogenesis.

PREVALENCE OF CHEMICAL AGENTS AND HUMAN CARCINOGENESIS

Since World War II many thousands of chemical compounds have been shown to produce cancers in animals and some have been demonstrated by epidemiological methods to be associated with a greater risk of cancer in humans. Shubik and Hartwell have published a list of over 10,000 compounds which have been shown to be carcinogenic (94). Not only organic compounds but also derivatives of chromium, nickel, beryllium, lead, and arsenic, as well as metallic films and plastics when imbedded into tissues are carcinogenic in animals (44). Some, such as vinyl chloride, have been found to cause cancer in humans (42).

As mentioned by Ames and colleagues, many ingredients that are carcinogenic, mutagenic, or both are present in natural substances such as plants and foodstuffs (3).

Individual Susceptibility to Carcinogens

In addition to exposure to carcinogens, individual susceptibility is an important factor in cancer risk. In a group of individuals exposed to essentially the same concentration of a carcinogen over the same time period, some will develop cancer and others will not. Excessive cigarette smoking does not cause cancer in all humans in a normal life span, even though the risk, overall, of getting lung cancer may be very high.

It is doubtful that all of the chemical substances listed as carcinogenic for animals are correspondingly carcinogenic for humans. Many that have been

Table 13-1

ANIMAL MODELS FOR CHEMICAL CARCINOGENESIS*

Target**	Species	Agents	Tumor Type
Skin	Mouse, rat	Nitrosamines, alkylating agents, aromatic amines, PAH	Squamous cell and basal cell carcinoma
Skin	Hamster, guinea pig	DMBA	Melanoma
Liver	Mouse, rat	Nitrosamines, aromatic amines, vinyl chloride, PAH	Hepatocellular carcinoma, angiosarcoma
Lung	Mouse, rat, hamster, dog	Nitrosamines, asbestos, PAH	Adeno and squamous cell carcinoma, mesothelioma
Breast	Mouse, rat, dog	NMU, aromatic amines, DMBA	Adenocarcinoma
Colon	Mouse, rat	Nitrosamines, DMH	Adenocarcinoma
Pancreas	Rat, hamster, guinea pig	Azaserine, nitrosamines	Adenocarcinoma, ductal carcinoma
Bladder	Mouse, rat, hamster	Aromatic amines, nitrosamines	Urothelial carcinoma

*Table 1 from Yuspa SH, Poirier M. Chemical carcinogenesis from animal models to molecular models in one decade. Adv Can Res 1988;50:25–70.
**Other target sites for chemical carcinogenesis include cervix, endometrium, esophagus, kidney, and brain.

proven to be carcinogens in animals have been given in very high concentrations over a relatively long period. Often only a particular strain of animal is susceptible to the carcinogen (Table 13-1). Humans may concentrate or metabolize substances in organs differently than animals do. Organs may differ in the types and amounts of enzymes available for metabolic activities. Repair and suppressor mechanisms may also differ greatly in different organisms and in different organs of the body.

Chemical carcinogenic experimentation has been invaluable in identifying the carcinogenic potential of many classes of chemical compounds. It has provided an understanding of many of the details of the mechanisms of action of many carcinogenic compounds and has suggested possible means of counteracting or preventing their action. Much of the information of chemical carcinogenesis has been obtained from animal experimentation. Reactions in animals can not always be directly extrapolated to humans, although many studies have shown similar results in both humans

and animals. The problem is in determining which animal results are germane to humans and which are not—a constant dilemma.

Cancer cells growing in a culture medium are much less expensive, give quicker results, and can be more extensively manipulated than the corresponding animal carcinogenesis models. Their use is limited because there is no host response in the culture medium model.

Most chemical carcinogens operate by undergoing direct covalent reactions with DNA. These are classified as genotoxic. Some require metabolic conversion into reactive forms (electrophiles) in order to react with DNA. The products of these reactions are DNA adducts and it is by such agents that cells are ultimately transformed.

Recent studies have deemphasized the concept that a single carcinogen, by itself, causes transformation in all cases. In most carcinogenic processes a combination of metabolic factors may be necessary to carry through a network of reactions that causes the transformation (4).

REFERENCES

1. Allen JC, Jaeschke WH. Recurrence of malignant melanoma in an orbit after 28 years. Arch Ophthal 1966;76:79–81.
2. Ames BN, Durston WE, Yamasaki E, Lee FD. Carcinogens are mutagens: a simple test system combining liver homogenates for activation and bacteria for detection. Proc Natl Acad Sci USA 1973;70:2281–5.
3. Ames BN, Gold LS. Too many rodent carcinogens: mitogenesis increases mutagenesis. Science 1990;249:970–1.
4. Arcos JC, Argus MF. Multifactor interaction network of carcinogenesis—a "tour guide." In: Arcos JC, Argus MF, Woo Y. eds. Chemical induction of cancer. Modulation and combination effects: an inventory of the many factors which influence carcinogenesis. Boston: Birkhäuser, 1995.
5. Bartsch H, O'Neill IK, Schulte-Hermann R, eds. International symposium on N-nitroso compounds. Relevance of N-nitroso compounds to human cancer. IARC Scientific Publ No. 8403005085. Lyon: International Agency for Research on Cancer, 1987.
6. Berenblum I, Shubik P. The role of croton oil applications, associated with a single painting of a carcinogen, in tumour induction of the mouse's skin. Br J Cancer 1947;1:379–82.
7. Berwald Y, Sachs L. In vitro transformation of normal cells to tumor cells by carcinogenic hydrocarbons. JNCI 1965;35:641–61.
8. Blumberg PM, Jaken S, Konig B, et al. Mechanism of action of the phorbol ester tumor promoters: specific receptors for lipophilic ligands. Biochem Pharmacol 1984;33:933–40.
9. Bock G, Whelan J, eds. Metastasis. Ciba Foundation symposium, 141. Chichester: Wiley, 1988.
10. Borek C. Epithelial in vitro cell systems in carcinogenesis. Ann NY Acad Sci 1983;407:284–90.
11. Boutwell RK. The function and mechanisms of promoters of carcinogenesis. CRC Crit Rev Toxicol 1974;2:419–43.
12. Boutwell RK. Some biological aspects of skin carcinogenesis. Progr Exp Tumor Res 1964;4:207–50.
13. Boyland E. The biological significance of metabolism of polycyclic compounds. Biochem Soc Symp 1950;5:40–54.
14. Brookes P, Lawley PD. Evidence for the binding of the polynuclear aromatic hydrocarbons to the nucleic acids of mouse skin: relation between carcinogenic power of hydrocarbons and their binding to deoxyribonucleic acid. Nature 1964;202:781–4.
15. Butterfield H. The origins of modern science, 1300–1800. London: G. Bell and Sons. 1951:111–23, 175.
16. Charnley G, Tannenbaum SR, Correa P. Gastric cancer: an etiological model. In: Magee PN, ed. Nitrosamines and human cancer. Banbury Report No. 12. Cold Spring Harbor: Cold Spring Harbor Laboratory, 1982:503–22.
17. Conney AH. Induction of microsomal enzymes by foreign chemicals and carcinogenesis by polycyclic aromatic hydrocarbons. G.H.A. Clowes Memorial Lecture. Cancer Res 1982;42:4875–917.
18. Cook JW. Ernest Lawrence Kennaway. In: Biographical memoirs of fellows of The Royal Society. Proc Royal Soc 1958;4:139–54.
19. Cook JW, Heiger I, Kennaway EL, Mayneord WV. The production of cancer by pure hydrocarbons. Proc Roy Soc Series B 1932;111:455–84.
20. Daniel FB, Schut HA, Sandwisch DW, et al. Interspecies comparisons of benzo(α)pyrene metabolism and DNA-adduct formation in cultured human and animal bladder and tracheobronchial tissues. Cancer Res 1983;43:4723–9.
21. Everson TC, Cole WH. Spontaneous regression of cancer: a study and abstract of reports in the world medical literature and of personal communications concerning spontaneous regression and malignant disease. Philadelphia: WB Saunders, 1966.
22. Farber E. Cellular biochemistry of the stepwise development of cancer with chemicals. G.H.A. Clowes Memorial Lecture. Cancer Res 1984;44:5463–74.
23. Farber E. On cells of origin of liver cell cancer. In: Sirica AE, ed. Cell types in hepatocarcinogenesis, 1992:1–28.
24. Farber E, Marroquin F, Stewart GA. On the binding of N-2-fluorenylacetamide and other carcinogens to cellular nucleic acids [Abstact]. 148th National Meeting of Am Chem Soc 1962:38C.
25. Farber E, Rubin H. Cellular adaptation in the origin and development of cancer. Cancer Res 1991;51:2751–61.
26. Farber E, Verbin RS, Lieberman M. Cell suicide and cell death. In: Aldridge A, ed. A symposium on mechanisms of cancer development. New York: MacMillan, 1972:163–73.
27. Fausto N, Lemire JM, Shiojiri N. Oval cells in liver carcinogenesis: cell lineages in hepatic development and the identification of facultative stem cells in normal liver. In: Sirica AE, ed. The role of cell types in hepatocarcinogenesis. Boca Raton: CRC Press, 1992:89–108.
28. Fidler IJ. Tumor heterogenicity and the biology of cancer invasion and metastasis. Cancer Res 1978;38:2651–60.
29. Fink LM, Nichimura S, Weinstein IB. Modifications of ribonucleic acid by chemical carcinogens. 1. in vitro modifications of transfer ribonucleic acid by N-acetoxy-2-acetylaminofluorene. Biochemistry 1970;9:496–502.
30. Fong LY. Possible relationship of nitrosamines in the diet to the causation of cancer in Hong Kong. In: Magee PN, ed. Nitrosamines and human cancer. Banbury Report No. 12. Cold Spring Harbor: Cold Spring Harbor Laboratory, 1982:473–85.
31. Foulds L. Neoplastic development, vol 1. London: Academic Press, 1969:69–89.
32. Frei JV, Swenson DH, Warren W, Lawley PD. Alkylation of deoxyribonucleic acid in vivo in various organs of C57BL mice by the carcinogens N-methyl-N-nitrosourea, N-ethyl-N-nitrosourea and ethyl methanesulphonate in relation to induction of thymic lymphoma. Some applications of high-pressure liquid chromatography. Biochem J 1978;174:1031–44.
33. Friedewald WF, Rous R. The determining influence of tar, benzpyrene, and methylcholanthrene on the character of the benign tumors induced therewith in rabbit skin. J Exp Med 1944;80:127–44.
34. Friedewald WF, Rous P. The initiating and promoting elements in tumor production. J Exp Med 1944;80:101–26.
35. Glucksmann A. Cell death in normal vertebrate ontogeny. Biol Rev 1951;26:59–86.
36. Goth R, Rajewsky MF. Persistence of 06-ethylguanine in rat-brain DNA: correlation with nervous system-specific carcinogenesis by ethylnitrosourea. Proc Natl Acad Sci USA 1974;71:639–43.
37. Grasl-Kraupp B, Ruttkay-Nedecky B, Mullauer L, et al. Inherent increase of apoptosis in liver tumors: implications for carcinogenesis and tumor regression. Hepatology 1997;25:906–12.
38. Greenstein JP. Biochemistry of cancer. New York: Academic Press, 1954.

39. Harris CC, Trump BF, Grafstrom R, Autrup H. Differences in metabolism of chemical carcinogens in cultured human epithelial tissues and cells. J Cell Biochem 1982;18:285–94.

40. Hicks RM. Nitrosamines as possible etiologic agents in bilharzial bladder cancer. In: Magee PN, ed. Nitrosamines and human cancer. Banbury Report No. 12. Cold Spring Harbor: Cold Spring Harbor Laboratory, 1982:455–85.

41. Hieger I. The spectra of cancer-producing tars and oils and of related substances. Biochem J 1930;24(2):505–11.

42. Higginson J, Muir CS, Munos N. Human cancer: epidemiology and environmental causes. Cambridge: Cambridge Univ. Press, 1992.

43. Hill J. Cautions against the immoderate use of snuff. London: Baldwin and Jackson, 1761.

44. Hueper WC, Conway WD. Chemical carcinogenesis. Springfield, IL: Charles C. Thomas, 1964.

45. Iversen OH, ed. Initiation, promotion: critical remarks on the two-stage theory. In: Theories of carcinogenesis. Washington: Hemisphere Publishing, 1988.

46. Jeffrey AM, Jennette KW, Blobstein SH, et al. Benzo[α]pyrene-nucleic acid derivative found in vivo: structure of a benzo[α]pyrene tetrahydrodiol epoxide-guanosine adduct [Letter]. J Am Chem Soc 1976;98:5714–5.

47. Jerina DM, Daly JW, Wilkop B, Zaltman-Nirenberg P, Udenfriend S. 1.2-naphthalene oxide as an intermediate in the microsomal hydroxylation of naphthalene. Biochemistry 1970;9:147–56.

48. Jerina DM, Sayer JM, Yagi H, et al. Highly tumorigenic bay-region diol epoxides from the weak carcinogen benzo[c]-phenanthrene. Adv Exp Med Biol 1982;136A:501–23.

49. Jones PA, Buckley JD. The role of DNA methylation in cancer. Adv Cancer Res 1990;54:1–23.

50. Kennaway EL. Experiments in cancer-producing substances. Br Med J 1925;2:1–4.

51. Kennaway E. Identification of carcinogenic compound in coal tar. Br Med J 1955;2:749–52.

52. Kerr JF. A histochemical study of hypertrophy and ischemic injury of rat liver with special reference to changes in lysosomes. J Pathol Bact 1965;90:419–35.

53. Kerr JF. Shrinkage necrosis: a distinct mode of cellular death. J Pathol 1971;105:13–20.

54. Kerr JF, Wyllie AH, Currie AR. Apoptosis: a basic biological phenomenon with wide ranging implications in tissue kinetics. Br J Cancer 1972;26:239–57.

55. Kinosita R. Researches on the carcinogenesis of the various chemical substances. Gann 1936;30:423–6.

56. Krebs H. Otto Warburg: cell physiologist, biochemist and eccentric. Oxford: Oxford Press, 1981.

57. Lawley PD. Historical origins of current concepts of carcinogenesis. Adv Cancer Res 1994;65:17–111.

58. Lipman TO. Wöhler's preparation of urea and the fate of vitalism. J Chem Education 1964;41:452–8.

59. Lobstein JG. Traité d'anatomie pathologique. Paris: Levrault, 1829:399, 403.

60. MacKenzie I, Rous P. The experimental disclosure of latent neoplastic changes in tarred skin. J Exp Med 1941;73:391–416.

61. Magee PN, ed. Nitrosamines and human cancer. Banbury report, no. 12. Cold Spring Harbor: Cold Spring Harbor Laboratory, 1982:577–8.

62. Magee PN, Barnes JM. The production of malignant primary hepatic tumours in the rat by feeding dimethylnitrosamine. Br J Cancer 1956;10:114–22.

63. Marroquin F, Farber E. The apparent binding of radioactive 2-acetylaminofluorene to rat-liver ribonucleic acid in vivo. Biochem Biophys Acta 1962;55:403–5.

64. Marroquin F, Farber E. The in vivo labeling of liver ribonucleic acid by p-dimethylaminoazobenzene-11-C14 (DAB). Proc Am Assoc Cancer Res 1963;4:41.

65. McCann J, Choi E, Yamasaki E, Ames BN. Detection of carcinogens as mutagens in the Salmonella typhimurium microsome test. Assay of 1300 chemicals. Proc Natl Acad Sci USA 1975;72:5135–9.

66. Miller EC. Some current perspectives on chemical carcinogenesis in humans and experimental animals. Cancer Res 1978;38:1479–96.

67. Miller EC. Studies on the formation of protein-bound derivatives of 3,4-benzpyrene in the epidermal fraction of mouse skin. Cancer Res 1951;11:100–8.

68. Miller EC, Miller JA. The presence and significance of bound aminoazo dyes in the livers of rats fed p-dimethylaminoazobenzene. Cancer Res 1947;7:468–80.

69. Miller EC, Miller JA. Searches for ultimate chemical carcinogens and their reactions with cellular macromolecules. Cancer 1981;47:2327–45.

70. Miller JA, Cramer JW, Miller EC. The N- and ring-hydroxylation of 2-acetylaminofluorene during carcinogenesis in the rat. Cancer Res 1960;20:950–62.

71. Moore FJ. A history of chemistry, New York: McGraw-Hill, 1918:120, 127.

72. Morris HP, Wagner BP. Induction and transplantation of rat hepatomas with different growth rate (including, "minimal deviation" hepatomas). Methods Cancer Res 1968;4:125–52.

73. Mottram JC. A developing factor in experimental blastogenesis. J Pathol Bacteriol 1944;6:181–7.

74. O'Connor PJ, Capps MJ, Craig AW, Lawley PD, Shah SA. Differences in the patterns of methylation in rat liver ribosomal ribonucleic acid after reaction in vivo with methyl methanesulfonate and N, N-dimethylnitrosamine. Biochem J 1972;129:519–28.

75. Pagel W. Paracelsus: an introduction to philosophical medicine. In: The era of the renaissance, 146. Basel: Karger, 1988.

76. Peraino C, Fry RJ, Staffeldt E, Kisieleski WE. Effect of varying the exposure to phenobarbital on its enhancement of 2-acetylaminofluorene-induced hepatic tumorigenesis in the rat. Cancer Res 1973;33:2701–5.

77. Pitot HC. Fundamentals of oncology, 2nd ed. New York: Marcel Dekker, 1981:159–93.

78. Pitot HC. Metabolic controls and neoplasia. In: Becker FF, ed. Cancer, a comprehensive treatise, 3 vols. New York: Plenum Press, 1975:3:1331–3.

79. Pitot H, Barsness L, Goldsworthy T, Kitagawa T. Biochemical characterisation of stages of hepato-carcinogenesis after a single dose of diethylnitrosamine. Nature 1978;271:456–8.

80. Pitot HC, Shires TK, Moyer G, Garrett CT. Phenotypic variability as a manifestation of translational control. In: Busch H, ed. The molecular biology of cancer. New York: Academic Press, 1974:523–34.

81. Pott P. Chirurgical observations relative to the cataract, polypus of the nose, the cancer of the scrotum, the different kinds of rupture and the mortification of the toes and feet. London: Hawes, Clarke and Collins, 1775.

82. Potter VR. Biochemistry of cancer. In: Holland JF; Frei E, eds. Cancer medicine. Philadelphia: Lea & Febiger, 1973.

83. Potter VR. Transplantable animal cancer, the primary standard [Editorial]. Cancer Res 1961;21:1331–3.

84. Pullman A, Pullman B. Electronic structure and carcinogenic activity of aromatic molecules. New developments. Adv Cancer Res 1955;3:117–69.
85. Raspail FV. Développement de la fécule dans les organes de la fructification des créles, et analyse microscopique de la fécule, suivie d'experiences propres a en expliquier la conversion en qomme. Ann Sci Nat 1825;6:224–39, 384–427.
86. Raspail FV. Neues Reagens zur Unterschiedung des Zuckers, Oeles, Eiweisstoffes und Harzes. Notizen aus dem Natur und Heilkunde 1829;24:129–36.
87. Rather L. The genesis of cancer. A history of ideas. Baltimore: Johns Hopkins Univ. Press, 1978:30.
88. Redmond DE Jr. Tobacco and cancer: the first clinical report, 1761. N Engl J Med 1970;282:18–23.
89. Rehn L. Ueber Blasentumorem bei Fuchsinarbeitern. Arch Klin Chir 1895;50:588–600.
90. Roberts JJ, Warwick GP. Azo-dye carcinogenesis. The reactions of 4-hydroxymethylaminozobenzene with cytosine derivatives. Int J Cancer 1966;1:107–17.
91. Rous P, Kidd JG. Conditional neoplasms and subthreshold neoplastic states. J Exp Med 1941;73:365–90.
92. Sasaki T, Yoshida T. Experimentelle Erzeugung des Lebercarcinoms durch Fütterung mit o-Amidoazotoluol. Virchows Arch [A] 1935;295:175–200.
93. Scherer E, Emmelot P. Foci of altered liver cells induced by a single does of diethylnitrosamine and partial hepatectomy: their contribution to hepatocarcinogenesis in the rat. Eur J Cancer 1975;11:145–54.
94. Shubik P, Hartwell JL. Survey of compounds which have been tested for carcinogenic activity. 3rd ed. (1957) and 4th ed. (1969), Supplements 1 and 2, respectively. Washington, D.C. GPO, Public Health Service Publication 149. Updates 1961–1967 and 1970–1971.
95. Sirica AE, ed. The role of cell types in hepatocarcinogenesis. Boca Raton: CRC Press, 1992.
96. Slaga TJ. Multiple skin tumor promotion and specificity of inhibition. In: Slaga TJ, Sivak A, Boutwell RK, eds. Mechanisms of tumor promotion and cocarcinogenesis, vol 2. 1984:189–96.
97. Slaga TJ, Fischer SM, Nelson K, Gleason GL. Studies on the mechanism of skin tumor promotion: evidence for several stages in promotion. Proc Natl Acad Sci USA 1980;77:3659–63.
98. Spencer SJ, Cataldo NA, Jaffe RB. Apoptosis in the human female reproductive tract. CME Review Article 14, Obst Gyn Survey 1996;51:314–23.
99. Sporn MB, Dingman CW. 2-acetamidofluorene and 3-methylcholanthrene: differences in binding to rat liver deoxyribonucleic acid in vivo. Nature 1966;210:531–2.
100. Trump BF, Valigorsky JM, Dees JH, et al. Cellular change in human disease. A new method of pathological analysis. Human Pathol 1973;4:89–109.
101. Virchow R; Chance F, trans. Cellular pathology, 1858. London, John Churchill. Birmingham, AL: The classics of medicine library, 1978:316–9.
102. Volkmann R. Ueber Theer und Russkrebs. Berliner klin Wochschr 1874:11:218– .
103. Warburg O. The metabolism of tumors: investigations from the Kaiser Wilhelm Institute for Biology. New York: Richard R. Smith, 1931.
104. Weber G. Enzymology of cancer cells. N Engl J Med 1977;296:486–93.
105. Weinhouse, S. Glycolysis, respiration and anomalous gene expression in experimental hepatomas: G.H.A. Clowes Memorial Lecture. Cancer Res 1972;32:2007–16.
106. Weinhouse S. The Warburg hypothesis fifty years later. Z Krebsforsch Klin Onkol Cancer Res Clin Oncol 1976; 87:115–26.
107. Weisburger JH, Horn CL. On the factors associated with esophageal and gastric cancer in man. In: Magee PN, ed. Nitrosamines and human cancer. Danbury Report No. 12. Cold Spring Harbor: Cold Spring Harbor Laboratory, 1982:523–8.
108. Weisburger JH, Williams GM. Metabolism of chemical carcinogens. In: Becker FF, ed. Cancer, a comprehensive treatise. New York: Plenum, 1975:185–431.
109. Welch DR, Bhuyan BK, Liotta L, eds. Cancer metastasis: experimental and clinical strategies. New York: Alan Liss, 1986.
110. Wyllie AH. Apoptosis. The 1992 Frank Rose Lecture. Br J Cancer 1993;67:205–8.
111. Wyllie AH, Kerr JF, Currie AR. Cell death: the significance of apoptosis. Int Rev Cytol 1980;68:251–306.
112. Yang CS. Nitrosamines and other etiological factors in the esophageal cancer in northern China. In: Magee PN, ed. Nitrosamines and human cancer. Banbury Report No. 12. Cold Spring Harbor: Cold Spring Harbor Laboratory, 1982:487–501.
113. Yuspa SH, Poirier M. Chemical carcinogenesis from animal models to molecular models in one decade. In: Klein G, Weinhouse S, eds. Advances in cancer research. New York: Academic Press, 1988:25–70.

Additional Pertinent Reference

Ord MG, Stocken L. Foundations of modern biochemistry. A multi-volume treatise. Vols. 1–4. Stamford, CT: Jai Press. 1995–1998.

✳ ✳ ✳

14

RADIATION AND CARCINOGENESIS

X RADIATION

In the last 5 years of the 19th century a remarkable series of discoveries in physics was made in Europe that was to have a profound effect on science, medicine, and world history. The first of these occurred in the quiet town of Würzburg, Germany, where a minor laboratory incident was to have a major effect on the diagnosis, treatment, and understanding of human cancer.

At the University of Würzburg, in 1895, Wilhelm Conrad Roentgen (1845–1923) (fig. 14-1), Professor of Physics, was working alone late in the afternoon in his darkened laboratory when he noted a weak shimmering green light on a bench about 3 feet away from a glass vacuum tube through which he had passed an electrical current (29). The glass tube was showing the effects of an electric current pulsing through it; thin sparks 4 to 6 inches in length were visible inside the glass tube.

Although such sparks in a glass tube had been known by physicists for some years, a green light at a distance from the tube was not part of the recognized phenomena. When Roentgen turned the current on and off, a corresponding appearance and disappearance of the distant green light occurred.

When the laboratory was lighted, Roentgen saw that the object on the bench giving off the green light was a screen containing fluorescent material. Roentgen and other physicists knew from experience that cathode rays could not produce effects more than a few millimeters from the end of the glass tube. There was only one conclusion that Roentgen could draw from these findings: there was something other than cathode rays coming from the discharging tube that was causing the fluorescence on his distant screen. He recognized that this was a new phenomenon that should be thoroughly investigated. He called the new radiation, "X (unknown) rays" (20,70) (Note 1).

Confirmation of Roentgen's findings was quick and decisive, and he soon became widely known throughout the world for his discovery of "invisible rays" (29) which would permit the observer to see inside the human body.

Clinical Effects of X Radiation

It soon became apparent that X rays had a pronounced effect on normal skin and on some diseases of the skin. Physicians used X rays to treat tuberculosis (lupus) and cancers of the skin with successful results. By 1903 there were over 50 articles in the scientific literature reporting the use of X rays in the treatment of cancer (62). Eventually, X irradiation was used as a primary method of treatment for cancers of the uterus,

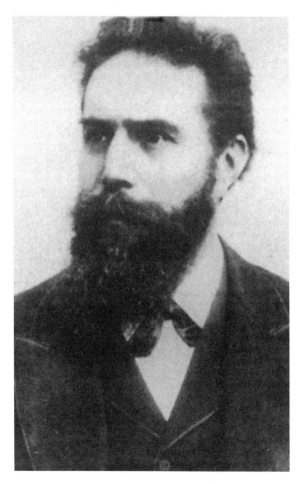

Figure 14-1
WILHELM CONRAD ROENTGEN
Wilhelm Conrad Roentgen, discoverer of X rays. (Frontispiece from Glasser O. Dr. W.C. Roentgen. 2nd ed. Springfield, IL: Charles C. Thomas, 1958.)

oropharynx, and some widespread cancers, e.g., leukemia and malignant lymphoma. In many institutions, prior to World War II, X ray treatment was the most commonly used form of therapy for some cancers. With technical developments, X rays were eventually used to treat cancers of internal organs.

Soon after the discovery of X rays, it was noticed that those who exposed their hands to the X ray beam to test the strength of the rays got dermatitis of the hands (88). In 1902, E. Frieben, a German scientist, reported the presence of a cancer in an ulcer caused by radiation. The patient was a technician who demonstrated X ray tubes for 4 years by holding his hand in the X ray beam. His carcinoma of the skin of the dorsum of the hand was associated with metastases in a regional lymph node (26). By 1909, a number of cases of skin cancer in X ray workers had been found in both the United States and England (39). Subsequently, bone marrow and blood cell changes were found in irradiated humans and by 1911, five radiologists had developed leukemia (Table 14-1) (94).

H.C. Marsh, a radiologist in the United States, discovered that 14 of 299 radiologists (about 5 percent) dying between 1928 and 1948 had leukemia; during the same period only 0.5 percent of nonradiologist physicians died of the disease (48). A later study (1981) showed that the mortality rate from cancer in British radiologists was 75 percent above that of medical practitioners, but there was little evidence of this excessive risk in those entering the specialty after 1921 (81). A study of radiologists in the United States showed that those entering radiology prior to 1940 had a 15-fold excess of leukemia above that of pathologists and bacteriologists who had little or no exposure to X rays. Radiologists entering the specialty from 1940 to 1969 had no increase in the incidence of leukemia above comparable control groups (52).

Table 14-1
EARLY REPORTS OF RADIATION INJURY FOLLOWING ROENTGEN'S DISCOVERY OF THE X RAY IN 1895*

Date	Type of Injury	Reported By
1896	Dermatitis of hands	Grubbe
1896	Smarting of eyes	Edison
1896	Epilation	Daniel
1897	Constitutional symptoms	Walsh
1899	Degeneration of blood vessels	Gassman
1902	Cancer in X-ray ulcer	Frieben
1903	Inhibition of bone growth	Perthes
1903	Sterilization	Albers-Schonberg
1904	Blood changes	Milchner and Moose
1906	Bone marrow changes	Warthin
1911	Leukemia in five radiation workers	Jagic
1912	Anemia in two X-ray workers	Belere

*Table 1 from Upton AC. Historical prospectives on radiation carcinogenesis. In: Upton AC, Albert RE, Burns FG, Shore RE, eds. Radiation carcinogenesis. New York: Elsevier 1986:2.

Transformation of Benign to Malignant Lesions

X rays were used for the treatment of benign lesions for many years throughout the world. In some cases benign lesions that had been irradiated later transformed into malignant lesions. In 1948, Cahan and colleagues from Memorial Hospital, New York City, reported that 11 patients whose benign lesions were treated with X irradiation were found at subsequent examination to have a malignant lesion (10).

Note 1: Before his discovery of X rays, Roentgen had a distinguished career in experimental physics (30). In his studies of X rays Roentgen found that a thick sheet of lead stopped virtually all rays. The rays were decreased in intensity by substances of increased density or thickness: heavy metals absorbed the rays much more than did a book, wood, or a thin sheet of tinfoil. The intensity of fluorescence from his detector was inversely proportional to the square of the distance between the discharge tube and the fluorescent screen (20).

Within 2 months of his initial observation Roentgen prepared a scientific report for publication which, translated from the German, was entitled: "On a new kind of rays, a preliminary communication" (70). Confirmation of Roentgen's findings was quick and widespread.

Honors rapidly came from all over the world to Roentgen, as well as international publicity. In 1901 he was awarded the first Nobel prize in physics. Roentgen refused to apply for a patent for his discovery believing that it should be free to all mankind. His Nobel prize money was donated to the University of Würzburg for scientific research (29). Roentgen's discovery is an example of Pasteur's well-known dictum that chance favors the prepared mind.

Irradiation of "Enlarged" Thymus and Thyroid Cancer

In 1950, Benedict Duffy and the author, at Memorial Hospital, New York City, reported that 10 of 28 children with cancer of the thyroid, a rare cancer in children, had been subjected previously to X irradiation for an "enlarged thymus" (Note 2). We suggested a possible causal relationship between the radiation and the appearance of the cancer (21, 22). The thyroid at the time was considered an organ with relatively greater resistance to the effects of X rays than most other organs.

C. L. Simpson, a British pathologist, with L. H. Hempelman, a radiobiologist at the University of Rochester, New York, later studied 2,800 cases of "thymic" irradiation in children, almost all less than 1 year of age. There were 30 cases of thyroid cancer and 59 benign thyroid neoplasms in the irradiated children, whereas in 500 nonirradiated siblings there was only one case of thyroid cancer and 8 cases of benign thyroid neoplasms (79,80).

A number of programs were then instituted in the United States to recall patients subjected earlier to radiation treatment in childhood for benign lesions of the head and neck area. In the Chicago area it was estimated that more than 70,000 patients had received such radiation in the 1940s and 1950s (18,19). At one hospital, 5,266 patients had been given X radiation to the head and neck region, usually to the tonsillar area. Of the 2,578 patients contacted or examined, 7 percent had thyroid cancer and 12 percent had benign neoplastic lesions (73); usually, thyroid cancer comprises only about 1 to 2 percent of all cancers in the United States (15). Thyroid cancer in young patients has a relatively high 5-year survival rate, over 90 percent (1).

L. Hempelman, a radiobiologist of the University of Rochester, New York, devoted many years to a follow-up of children who had been irradiated in infancy. With R. Shore of New York University Medical School and colleagues, he analyzed a group of 2,650 infants who were irradiated for an "enlarged thymus" and 4,800 of their nonirradiated siblings as controls. The cases were followed for an average of 29 years. The relative risk in the irradiated group was about 45 times greater for thyroid cancer and 15 times greater for benign thyroid adenoma than in the nonirradiated controls. An increased risk for both benign and malignant thyroid tumors remained for at least 40 years after irradiation (78).

Similar long-term results have been reported in survivors of the atomic bombings of Nagasaki and Hiroshima more than 30 years later (61,65,97) (Note 3). The risk for thyroid cancer in Nagasaki individuals was greater for those who received irradiation when they were under 30 years of age than in victims who were over 30 years (61,65). Wakabayashi et al., Japanese investigators, have recorded a highly significant increase of clinically evident thyroid cancer in the Nagasaki survivors of the atomic bomb 14 to 33 years later (97).

There have been many studies of the effects of the administration of radioactive iodine (^{131}I) for the diagnosis and therapy of noncancerous diseases of the thyroid (57). No significant increase in the risk of thyroid cancer has been found in investigations of large numbers of adult patients (40).

Recently, it has been reported from Memorial Hospital, New York City, that 55 percent of all patients with osteogenic sarcoma had been previously exposed to X rays (44).

"Ringworm" X Irradiation and Thyroid Cancer

E. Modan, E. Ron, and colleagues in Israel discovered that X ray treatment of the scalp for "ringworm" (Tinea capitis) in Jewish children emigrating to Israel

---

Note 2: The weights of the "normal" thymus (a gland of lymphatic tissue in the chest) had been determined by weighing the thymus from children who were autopsied in hospitals. These children usually died from infections or neoplastic diseases. What was not known at the time was that many diseases, particularly chronic ones, caused atrophy of the thymus. Thus, the atrophic gland was considered to be a normal thymus. An X ray of normal children or those with an acute disease showed a normal thymus that was interpreted as an enlarged thymus.

It was believed that an "enlarged thymus" might give rise to obstruction of the pulmonary tract and, thereby, pulmonary disease. X-ray therapy was delivered to the "enlarged" thymus to shrink it down to "normal" size. Thousands of children had irradiation of an "enlarged" thymus in order to reduce it to what was believed to be the normal size.

Note 3: A study conducted in New York City by Shore et al. matched irradiated patients with Tinea capitis to similar control patients treated with topical medication only (77). The results showed no difference in the incidence of thyroid cancer. However, in the irradiated group there were seven patients with a tumor of the thyroid, diagnosed as a thyroid adenoma. This study is at variance with others on the subject, perhaps because of the designation of the thyroid nodules as adenomas rather than carcinomas.

gave rise to an excess of thyroid cancer (54,71). The relative risk for the development of thyroid cancer was 5.4 times greater in irradiated children than in nonirradiated controls. Subgroups of Jewish children had different incidences of the tumor (77).

X Irradiation of the Fetus in Utero

In England, Alice Stewart and colleagues reported an excess of leukemia and other cancers in children who had been irradiated in utero: their mothers had received diagnostic X ray examinations of the pelvis during pregnancy (85–87). The risk of cancer was about doubled in children whose mothers were irradiated compared to the expected incidence for children of unirradiated mothers.

Examination of children who died of leukemia or other childhood cancers before the age of 10 years in England showed that those who had received radiation in utero had a greater risk of leukemia than the unirradiated control group. Other studies have also suggested a higher relative risk for leukemia in children who received radiation in utero (56) but a higher risk for other cancers was not found.

Recent studies of Japanese children who survived irradiation in utero in the Hiroshima and Nagasaki atomic bombings did not show an increase of leukemia or childhood malignancies (57). For conservative risk evaluation it had been assumed that fetal or prenatal radiation increases the risk of childhood cancer until the child is 10 years of age, but not thereafter (32). Children have shown, however, a significant increase in microcephaly (Greek: small head) and mental retardation if they were irradiated during the 8th to the 25th week of gestation (32).

Arthritis and Radiation

In the 1930s and 1940s in Britain, about 14,000 patients with a form of arthritis of the spine, ankylosing spondylitis, were given radiation therapy to the spine to relieve their pain. An increased incidence of leukemia has been reported in these patients (7,17). This study has been criticized for lack of a proper control group—patients with similar arthritis who received no radiotherapy (32).

RADIOACTIVITY

The discovery of radioactive decay of some elements has been of great use in the diagnosis and treatment of diseases and has played an im-

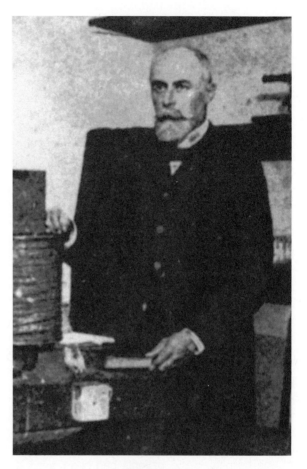

Figure 14-2
ANTOINE HENRI BECQUEREL

Antoine Henri Becquerel, the discoverer of radioactivity. (From Shimkin MB. Contrary to nature. Washington, D.C.: U.S. Department of Health, Education, & Welfare, 1977:184.)

portant role in radiobiology. Radioactivity was discovered, like X rays, through an unusual conjunction of events: the observance by a critical, trained mind of an unique laboratory event and a thorough investigation of its cause.

Antoine Henri Becquerel (1852–1908) (fig. 14-2) was born in Paris into a family in which both his father and grandfather were physicists, prominent in research and teaching. Becquerel's father, Edmund, had studied phosphorescence, a phenomenon whereby substances continued to emit light after the cessation of the activation energy input. Henri was testing uranium salts. He exposed the uranium to sunlight and measured the effect produced by the sun using an underlying photographic plate shielded from the rays of the sun by being wrapped in black paper. On a cloudy day when sunlight was lacking the experiments were postponed. The uranium salts rested on top of the shielded photographic plate and the preparation was put aside. Later the film was developed and showed a darkening of the photographic emulsion equal to that produced when the sun was shining on the uranium sample. Becquerel investigated further and proved that uranium itself, not the sunlight radiation, caused the darkening of the photographic plate. Uranium compounds constantly darkened the photographic plate whether the room was sunlit or in darkness.

Like Roentgen, Becquerel realized that he was witnessing something unique: the uranium salts were constantly emitting a new, different form of energy. He investigated the unexpected event and showed that a new type of radiation, not the X rays of Roentgen, was coming from uranium (3,6). The phenomenon was later given the name, "radioactivity," by Marie Curie. Becquerel's report in 1896 in the Compt. Rendu Academie des Science occupied about one page (3). His discovery did not receive the immediate worldwide attention that Roentgen's finding did but the discovery was recognized by the award of a Nobel prize in physics which he shared with Pierre and Marie Curie.

Eventually, radioactive isotopes of uranium were isolated and became important in the development of the atomic bomb and nuclear energy. Radioactive isotopes became available for medical and scientific investigations and resulted in many discoveries in the metabolism of normal and diseased tissues of animals and humans. The effects of Becquerel's discovery on science, medicine, and world history were originally not as apparent as those of Roentgen, but with the development of radioactive isotopes, the atomic bomb, and nuclear energy, they may have had an even greater effect on science and world affairs.

The Curies and Radium

Another discovery in physics at the turn of the century, that of radium, was to have an important direct effect in the cancer field, mostly in the therapy of cancer. Pierre and Marie Curie, husband and wife and French scientists, are well known throughout the world because of this and other important scientific discoveries and because of their heroic struggle with disease and poverty (16,20). Their story has been told in magazines, books, and in a motion picture.

Becquerel had invited Marie Curie to study the emanations from uranium and in April, 1898, she announced the probability that there was a new element in pitchblende (a native oxide of uranium found in black, pitch-like masses) which contained powerful radioactivity. By July 1898, she and Pierre Curie suspected that there were at least two elements present in uranium that were radioactive. They named them "polonium" (after Madame Curie's native land) and "radium." In 1902, small amounts of a pure radium salt were isolated (20) (Note 4).

Therapeutic Effects of Radium

After the German scientists Walkhoff and Giesel announced in 1900 that radium had physiological effects, Pierre Curie exposed his arm to radiation. A burn-like lesion appeared and had not completely healed 52 days later. Bequerel and Marie Curie had also received skin lesions from sealed tubes of radium in close contact with skin. Pierre Curie studied the effect of radium on animals and, impressed with its destructive power, collaborated with the French physicians to determine its effect on diseased cells and tissues. It was found to cure some tumors, including cancer. The use of radium for the treatment of cancer began (16).

Note 4: Pierre Curie had achieved recognition in scientific circles at an early age with his equally talented brother at the Sorbonne for their studies on piezo-electricity (electricity generated by pressure, as in certain crystals). Madame Curie (Marya Sklodowska) (1867–1934), born in Warsaw, Poland, was a precocious child and had a brilliant career in the gymnasium but had to go to France for university studies because the universities in Poland were closed to women. In 1891, at the age of 24 years, Madame Curie started her education in Paris at the Sorbonne and by 1894 had received master degrees in physics and mathematics. In 1885 she and Pierre Curie were married (20).

After her husband's tragic death Marie Curie continued her research on radium, wrote a textbook on radioactivity, and was awarded a second Nobel prize in 1911. In 1914, the Radium Institute in Paris, long planned, was finished, with Madame Curie as director of the research branch. In 1922 she was elected to the French Academy of Science, to which she had been denied admission earlier, by acclamation and received many honors from around the world. She died in 1934 after having developed cataracts, a chronic dermatitis in her hands, and aplastic anemia, all probably caused by her exposure to radioactivity over many years (16).

Radium (^{226}Ra) is a radioactive element with a half-life of 1,622 years. It decays through a cascade of daughter isotopes to a stable form of lead. It gives off short range alpha and beta particles and high energy gamma rays that are used clinically for therapy. Radium gives off a gas, radon, which can be collected in thin gold tubes that can be sealed and cut into small pieces, "seeds," and these can be planted in the tumor tissue. Radon gives off the same rays as does radium but has a short half-life of 3.85 days. The implanted tubes remain in the tissue after irradiation. Other forms of delivery were also used (67). If given orally or intravenously radium concentrates in the bones of humans or animals and becomes potentially carcinogenic.

Radium therapy developed extensively in France, throughout England and Europe, and later in the United States (67). Thousands of patients were cured of some types of cancer and many thousands received temporary amelioration of advanced cancers (9). After World War II radium was supplanted by other forms of therapy.

Deleterious Effects of Radium

As with X rays, there were deleterious effects from the use of radioactive elements. Often, technicians handling radium in hospitals developed dermatitis of the hands and those who had worked 10 years or more handling radium often had cancerous changes superimposed on their chronic dermatitis (9), sometimes with loss of fingers, a hand, or rarely, an arm.

The Watch Dial Painters. The tragic story of young women in the 1920s who were employed in a New Jersey plant painting with a luminous substance the numbers on the dial of watches, indicated the potential danger of ingested radioactive heavy elements (82). The paint contained radium and its daughter radioactive substances which made the dial figures glow in the dark. The women pointed the tip of the brush which had been dipped in the luminescent solution of radium by withdrawing the brush through their clenched teeth. In the pro-

cess they swallowed and absorbed some of the radioactive radium and its daughter metabolites, such as mesothorium, which were eventually deposited in their bones.

In a series of autopsies of the young women, Dr. Harrison Martland, a medical examiner in New Jersey, pointed out the wide distribution of the absorbed radioactive substances in bones, teeth, and vertebrae. He found osteogenic sarcomas in 4 of 18 girls autopsied. Other women workers eventually died of radiation-induced bone cancer (49–51). A few died of cancer arising from bones of the paranasal sinuses, the skull, and the mastoid area (25,64,84).

In 1971, a registry of patients who had been exposed to radium was set up by Austin Brues and colleagues at the Argonne National Laboratory (8,25). The group had found a second watch dial painting factory in Illinois. They also discovered in a state mental hospital in Illinois, patients who had been given radium intravenously for schizophrenia. A third group comprised patients who had been given radium salts as a stimulatory tonic. Over 5,000 individuals were included in these groups (8,25). Malignant tumors of bone were the most prominent cancers discovered but blood dyscrasias including leukemia also developed (Note 5).

Thorium

Another radioactive heavy element, thorium (^{232}Th), was introduced into radiography in 1928 by K. Frick and colleagues, radiologists in Germany (11). Thorium outlined the reticuloendothelial system, most of whose cells are contained in the spleen, liver, bone marrow, and lymph nodes. Its high atomic number (Z) made thorium opaque to X rays. After the patient swallowed a solution of colloidal thorium dioxide (Thorotrast) it was taken up by the phagocytic cells of the reticuloendothelial system. An X ray of the abdomen revealed the Thorotrast in the liver and spleen. An increase or decrease in the size of these organs could be determined by examination of the X ray film.

Note 5: In the group of watch dial painters in Illinois there were approximately 185 workers who were studied by whole body gamma-ray spectroscopy and skeletal radiography (8). Forty-one of these developed 44 malignant tumors, mostly bone sarcomas or fatal blood dyscrasias (25). Eight developed rare cancers of the paranasal sinuses, skull, and mastoid bone; 4 of those with cancer of the skull were diagnosed 34 to 41 years after beginning work as dial painters (25).

Forty-one young adult patients in a mental hospital received weekly injections of radium for therapy. Of the 36 who were studied, 3 developed cancer of the sphenoid sinus or mastoid bone and 1 had an osteogenic sarcoma of the right tibia (25).

Of 37 patients who had radium administered by their personal physicians, prescribed as a tonic to improve general health, 16 developed malignant tumors or blood dyscrasias (13 had bone cancer and 2 had blood dyscrasias) (8,25). The majority of the bone tumors were osteogenic sarcomas.

Thorium, however, is radioactive, with a half life of 1.4^{10} (over 10 billion) years. In its decay thorium gives off alpha and beta particles as well as gamma rays which could damage not only the macrophage cells that engulfed the particles, but also adjacent cells and tissues.

In 1948, Harold MacMahon, professor of pathology at the Tufts University Medical School, Boston, and coworkers reported a case of angiosarcoma of the liver associated with the presence of Thorotrast granules. They suggested a causal relationship between the two (47). Angiosarcoma of the liver is, otherwise, a rare cancer.

Thorotrast was given intravenously to over 50,000 patients worldwide. de Sylva Hortega, a Portuguese pathologist, collected over 1,000 cases in which neoplasms were believed to have been caused by radiation from the injected thorium (41,42, 55). The incidence of liver cancer and leukemia was six times greater than expected in patients receiving the injected thorium than in control patients.

Van Kaick and colleagues, German investigators, studied about 6,000 patients in West Germany who had been given Thorotrast for cerebral angiography and 6,000 patients in hospitals who were used as controls (95). The ratios of cancers in organs in the Thorotrast group compared with the cancers in organs of the control group were: liver, 88:6; bone marrow, 16:1; skeleton, 2:0; lungs, 24:25; spleen, 0:0; the last two organs apparently were not affected by Thorotrast. Janet Vaughan of Oxford University has reviewed the neoplastic effects of radiation on the human skeleton (96).

The lessons of radium and thorium ingestion or injection in humans alerted the medical profession and government agencies to the toxicity and carcinogenicity of the radioactive heavy elements and such usage has been abandoned.

Atomic Bombing of Japan and Cancer

After the atomic bombs were exploded in World War II over Hiroshima and Nagasaki, Japan, in August 1945, a committee of American and Japanese scientists and physicians (The Atomic Bomb Casualty Committee) was set up to study the radiation effects in the survivors. Its successors and other agencies have made extensive studies of the effects of these bombs (57,65,82,93,97).

The most dramatic oncogenic effect of the bombing was the appearance within 2 to 4 years of

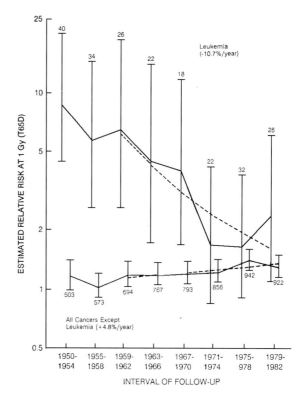

Figure 14-3
COMPARATIVE RELATIVE RISK OF MORTALITY FROM LEUKEMIA AND ALL CANCERS OTHER THAN LEUKEMIA IN JAPANESE A-BOMB SURVIVORS, 1950–1982, IN RELATION TO TIME AFTER IRRADIATION

The number of deaths in each interval of follow-up and 99 percent confidence intervals are indicated. A high incidence of leukemia occurred shortly after the bombing but decreased thereafter. There was a far greater interval (years) between the bombing and the peak appearance of other types of cancer (57). (Fig. 5.2 from National Research Council Committee on the biological effects of ionizing radiation: the health effects of exposure to low levels of ionizing radiation. Washington D.C.: National Academy of Sciences, 1990:244.)

an increased incidence of leukemia in the survivors; it reached a peak about 5 to 7 years after the bombing and had decreased considerably by 20 years (fig. 14-3) (53). Significant increases in incidence of other cancers followed thereafter, slowly over many years, particularly cancers of the thyroid, breast, lung, and stomach. Suggestive increases in the incidence of cancer of the colon, urinary tract, and multiple myeloma also were noted (97). Most of the cancers of the solid organs did not begin to appear until 10 years later; the latency period of most radiation-induced solid tumors was 25 to 30 years (32).

Cancer from Accidents in Nuclear Power Stations

Accidents in atomic energy plants that have released radioactivity have occurred in the United States, England, and Russia. The most catastrophic, a nuclear energy plant in 1986 in Chernobyl exploded, releasing far more radiation than occurred in Hiroshima and Nagasaki combined. Among the long-lived radioactive elements released were cesium, strontium, and plutonium. Radioactive isotopes of iodine were also released and became a public health menace because of their incorporation into the thyroid gland of exposed individuals, particularly children (79).

From the Nagasaki and Hiroshima experience it would be expected that radiation-induced cancers would exceed the normal incidence in the survivors of the Chernobyl accident who were exposed to heavy local fallout of radioactivity. Since thousands of people were exposed to varying amounts of radioactivity it is likely that there will be a significantly increased incidence of some cancers as the population ages (2). Recently, an increased incidence of cancer of the thyroid in children, assumed to be the result of absorbed radioactive isotopes of radioactive iodine, has been reported in the republic of Belarus, formerly the Byelorussian Soviet Socialist Republic, which is adjacent to Chernobyl (58).

RADIOBIOLOGY

Early in the 20th century the effects of X radiation were examined in bacteria, yeasts, plants, and animals. Soon it was apparent that relatively low doses of radiation had harmful effects on cell growth, mitosis, regeneration, and other functions. High doses could kill cells, tissues, and many organs very quickly. The effects, however, differed from species to species, from organ to organ, and from cell type to cell type. Different types and energies of the radiation have varied effects on tissues, organs, and cells.

Types of Radiation and Effect on Tissues

Biological tissues are exposed primarily to two forms of radiation: 1) X (gamma) rays are electromagnetic forms of energy delivered in a stream of photons or packets of energy; and 2) particles of energy: electrons, which are negatively charged particles; protons, positively charged, relatively

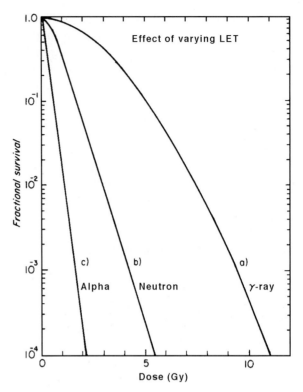

Figure 14-4

MAMMALIAN CELL SURVIVAL CURVES AFTER IRRADIATION WITH VARYING DOSES OF LET (LINEAR ENERGY TRANSFER)

a = ^{60}Cobalt X rays; b = neutrons; and c = alpha particles. A higher LET value gives a lower survival rate. Alpha particles result in a lower survival rate than neutrons or X rays. (Fig. 8.10 from Tannock IF, Hill RP. The basic science of oncology. Toronto: McGraw-Hill, 1992:125.)

massive particles; neutrons, with a mass similar to that of the proton but carrying no electrical charge; and alpha particles, which are the heavy nuclei of the helium atom (32,83).

The important reaction of radiation on biological tissues is that of ionization: the ejection of one or more orbital electrons from the atom or molecule of the target tissue. Ionization releases a large amount of energy locally, enough to break chemical bonds. An indirect effect of radiation is the interaction with water to produce free radicals (91).

Linear Energy Transfer (LET) and Relative Biological Effectiveness (RBE)

In order to understand the relative efficiency of various forms of radiation, a term, "linear energy transfer" (LET), which measures the deposition of energy per unit of path length of the ray or particle,

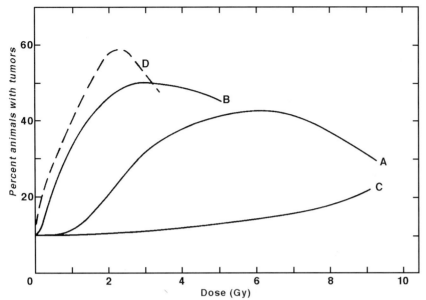

Figure 14-5
TUMORS PRODUCED IN
MICE BY DIFFERENT
DOSES OF RADIATION
Contrast curve A (single dose of low LET radiation) with curve B (single dose of high LET radiation). Curve C represents tumors produced by fractioned low LET radiation and curve D the tumors produced by fractioned high LET radiation. (Fig. 7-16 from Tannock IF, Hill RP. The basic science of oncology. Toronto: McGraw-Hill, 1992:119.)

is used, e.g., an alpha particle has a higher LET than an electron because of the greater mass of the alpha particle (fig. 14-4). Radiation of a higher LET produces more neoplasms than radiation of a lower LET (fig. 14-5) (91).

Because equal energies of different types of ionizing radiation do not produce equal biological effects, the term, "relative biological effectiveness" (RBE) has been introduced. X ray effects are used as the standard to which other forms of energy are referred (91).

Biological Response to Irradiation

The sensitivity of the tissue, organ, or cell to radiation is an important factor in evaluating the effects of radiation on biological tissues. Casaret has divided cells into four groups in which sensitivity is determined by cell death (72):

Group I cells are the most sensitive and represent the stem cell for the self-renewing systems, e.g., the hematopoietic cells, crypt cells of the intestine, and skin basal cells.

Group II cells divide regularly but also differentiate and mature, as occurs in hematopoietic cells in intermediate stages of differentiation. This group contains the spermatogonia and spermatocytes of the testes.

Group III cells are relatively resistant to radiation and are long-lived, undergoing significant division only under certain circumstances, e.g., liver cells after surgical partial resection.

Group IV comprises cells which are highly differentiated and normally don't divide; the neuron of the brain is an example of this group. They are considered to be the most resistant of cells.

Connective tissue cells are intermediate: some cells are very sensitive and other cells are greatly resistant to radiation. Some exceptions to these rules occur.

In 1906, Claudius Regaud, professor of histology of the Faculty of Medicine and J. Blanc at Lyon, observed that radiation of the rat testes affected the least differentiated cells, spermatogonia, more than the differentiated cells, the spermatozoids (68). Jean Begonié and Louis Tribondeau of France verified these findings and proposed a law that the effects of radiation on cells were greater the more their reproductive activity, the longer their mitotic phase, and the less their differentiation (4). There are many exceptions to this "law," e.g., the small lymphocyte which does not divide is killed by radiation, and the law does not predict the sensitivity to radiation of many tissues. However, proliferating tissues, in general, are more susceptible to radiation damage than are differentiated tissues.

Whole Body Irradiation

The biological effects of irradiating a whole organism, animal or human, differ greatly from those when radiation is applied to a single organ, tissue, or cell. Whole body irradiation may produce far greater

Table 14-2

EARLY EXPERIMENTAL RADIATION-INDUCED CANCERS*

Author (Date)	Radiation or Isotope	Species	Type of Tumor
Marie et al. (1910)	X ray	Rat	Sarcoma, spindle cell
Marie et al. (1912)	X ray	Rat	Sarcoma, spindle cell
Lazarus-Barlow (1918)	Ra**	Mouse, rat	Carcinoma of skin
Bloch (1923)	X ray	Rabbit	Carcinoma
Bloch (1924)	X ray	Rabbit	Carcinoma
Goebel and Gerard (1925)	X ray	Guinea pig	Sarcoma, polymorphous
Daels (1925)	Ra	Mouse, rat	Sarcoma, spindle cell
Jonkhoff (1927)	X ray	Mouse	Carcinoma-sarcoma
Lacassagne and Vinzent (1929)	X ray	Rabbit	Fibrosarcoma, osteosarcoma, rhabdomyosarcoma
Schurch (1930)	X ray	Rabbit	Carcinoma
Daels and Biltris (1931)	Ra	Rat	Sarcoma of cranium, kidney, spleen
Daels and Biltris (1931)	Ra	Guinea pig	Sarcoma of cranium, kidney, spleen
Daels and Biltris (1937)	Ra	Chicken	Carcinoma of biliary tract, osteosarcoma
Schurch and Uehlinger (1931)	Ra	Rabbit	Sarcoma of bone, liver, spleen
Uehlinger and Schurch (1935–47)	Ra, Ms-Th	Rabbit	Sarcoma of bone, liver, spleen
Sabin et al. (1932)	Ra, Ms-Th	Rabbit	Osteosarcoma
Lacassagne (1933)	X ray	Rabbit	Sarcoma, spindle cell, myxosarcoma
Petrov and Krotkina (1933)	Ra	Guinea pig	Carcinoma of biliary tract
Sedginidse (1933)	X ray	Mouse	Carcinoma, spindle cell
Ludin (1934)	X ray	Rabbit	Chondrosarcoma

*Table 3 from Upton AC. Historical prospectives on radiation carcinogenesis. In: Upton AC, Albert RE, Burns FG, Shore RE, eds. Radiation carcinogenesis. New York: Elsevier 1986:6.
**Ra = radium; Ms-Th = mesothorium and thorium.

damage per unit of radiation than the same amount of radiation applied to a single organ. From 300 to 400 rads, 3 to 4 Gy (Gray units), of X (gamma) radiation delivered to the entire body will cause the death of about half of the irradiated persons.

Whole body irradiation damages or kills reparative and regenerative cells, thereby inhibiting or preventing them from repairing damage (32). Injury to the bone marrow and immune system hinders an immune response. Injury to the gastrointestinal mucosa permits the ever-present bacteria in the lumen of the bowel to gain entrance to the tissues of the bowel wall and the blood stream and spread infection to other parts of the body. Recently, less energetic whole body irradiation has been used successfully for many types of neoplasia to destroy much of the bone marrow, after which normal bone marrow cells are injected to repopulate a normal marrow in the patient.

Therapeutic radiation to an individual organ (other than the bone marrow) usually does not seriously affect adjacent organs or the immune system. Occasionally, organs in the line of fire of therapeutic radiation were the site of malignant change years later. Modern techniques have decreased greatly such risks.

Radiation-Induced Cancer and Organ Sensitivity

It was shown early in the 1920s and 1930s that many types of cancer could be produced in animals by radiation (Table 14-2). Since then cancers of most organs of animals have been induced by radiation. In the human, the tissues most sensitive to radiation are the bone marrow, lung, thyroid in children, and female breast.

Individuals who have certain genetic defects, e.g., xeroderma pigmentosa, Bloom's syndrome,

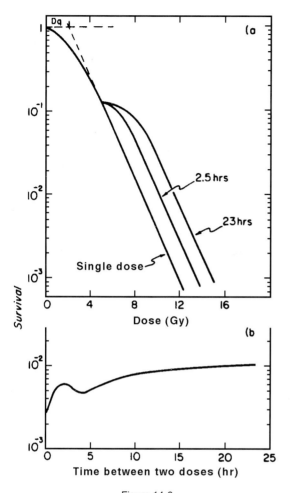

Figure 14-6
FRACTIONATION OF THE DOSAGE OF X IRRADIATION
    Pauses between fractions of irradiation permit repair of sublethal damage to tissues compared to when the entire dose is given at one time. (Fig. 15.14 from Tannock IF, Hill RP. The basic science of oncology. Toronto: McGraw-Hill. 1992:269.)

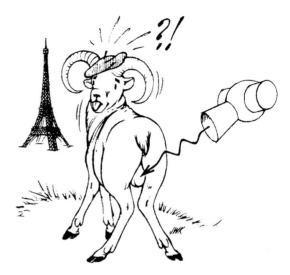

Figure 14-7
FRACTIONATED THERAPY
    Conventional multifraction radiotherapy was based on experiments with rams. They could not be sterilized with a single dose of X rays without extensive scrotal skin damage, whereas if the radiation were delivered in daily fractions sterilization was possible without skin damage. The testes were regarded as a model of a growing tumor and skin as the dose-limiting normal tissue. (Fig. 12.1 from Hall EJ. Radiobiology for the radiologist. 3rd ed. Philadelphia: JB Lippincott, 1988:240.)

Fanconi's anemia, Cockayne's syndrome, and ataxia telangiectasia, exhibit an increased sensitivity to radiation-induced injury (91). Some are also susceptible to an increased incidence of cancer.

Dosage Response

    High dosages of radiation are usually more efficient in producing tumors in animals than low dosages (fig. 14-5) (91). Even a relatively low single dose of radiation, 0.15-8.0 Gy, when given to the whole body may increase the frequency of both benign and malignant lesions in many animals, including dogs, monkeys, and rats (89) (Note 6).

    If a relatively low or moderate total dose of radiation is given in multiple fractions (fractionated dosage) rather than in one application, the effect is an increase of cell survival because during the intervals between doses, repair of damage to cells occurs (fig. 14-6). The well-known effect of one high dose versus repeated low doses of radiation to the ram testicle graphically illustrates this (fig. 14-7) (32). There is little effect on tumor production by fractionizing the dosage of high LET, implying that the lack of repair occurs because of irreparable damage or destruction of some integral part of the repair system when high LET radiation is used.

Note 6: Stoner irradiated 12,000 female mice with 1 to 4 Gy of X ray and followed them during their complete lifetimes (89). The following sensitivities to the production of cancer were noted: highest sensitivity, thymus and ovary; moderate sensitivity, pituitary, uterus, breast, myelopoietic tissue, lung, and Harderian gland; low sensitivity, bone, skin, stomach, liver, and gastrointestinal tract. The order of these sensitivities varied with the age and strain of the mouse, the level of repair enzymes, and other host factors.

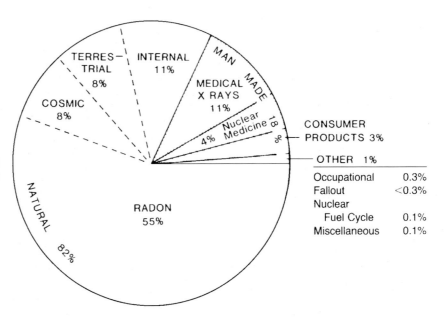

Figure 14-8

PERCENT CONTRIBUTION OF SOURCES OF NATURAL AND MAN-MADE RADIATION TO THE EFFECTIVE DOSE EQUIVALENT IN THE U.S. POPULATION

(Fig. 9.1 from Travis EL. Medical radiobiology, 2nd ed. Chicago: Year Book, 1989:187.)

Animal Experimentation

Soon after the introduction of X rays, tumors were produced in animals, mostly sarcomas of the connective tissue. In time, practically all types of tumors similar to those occurring in man were reproduced in animals using different animal strains and different dosages of radiation (94).

One of the early malignant lesions caused by X rays in animals was leukemia. In the 1930s, Jacob Furth, then a pathologist at Cornell University Medical College, New York City, irradiated mice and obtained a strain that was prone to develop leukemia (28). The strain, AKR, was later shown by Ludwig Gross, a virologist (see chapter 15) to harbor a leukemogenic virus (30). The activation of a latent virus by irradiation and the subsequent appearance of leukemia has been a major development regarding concepts in experimental animal carcinogenesis (100).

Natural Radioactivity

There are many natural sources of radiation which may affect biological organisms (fig. 14-8): cosmic rays from outer space; normal organ concentrations of radioactive elements in animals and humans, e.g., potassium (^{40}K), carbon (^{14}C), tritium (^{3}H); and radon (^{222}Ra), a gas released from the radium residing in rocks and soil. Ultraviolet radiation from the sun is commonly recognized as a cause of skin cancer (38).

Man-Made Radioactivity

The radiation exposure from diagnostic medical and dental X ray examinations has decreased in the last few decades because of more efficient X ray equipment and film emulsions. Exposure to radiation from fallout after the detonation of atomic bombs, radiation associated with the manufacture of nuclear bombs, and exposure resulting from nuclear power installation accidents are potentially carcinogenic events.

The massive explosion in Unit 4 of a nuclear power station in Chernobyl, Ukraine, in April 1986 (2) caused some deaths, many injuries, and the exposure of thousands of people in the immediate areas in the Ukraine and nearby republics to heavy fallout radioactivity. Significant fallout involved other parts of Russia (27,102), Scandinavia, and some other countries. The increased incidence of thyroid cancer in children in areas adjacent to Chernobyl has been mentioned earlier.

The relative contribution of various sources of radiation to the total exposure of man is shown in figure 14-8 (92).

MECHANISM OF ACTION OF RADIATION UPON BIOLOGICAL TISSUES

The effects of relatively high energy radiation on biological organisms have been more extensively studied than relatively low energy effects because the former are more quickly apparent, more dramatic, and easier to measure. High energy radiation kills cells or organisms by irreversibly damaging DNA (deoxyribonucleic acid) or the enzymes necessary for its repair, so that the life of the organism cannot be sustained. Low or moderate LET radiation acts mainly indirectly.

Free Radical Damage

Since about 90 percent of biological matter is composed of water (H_2O) much of the effect of radiation involves changes in water ionization:

$$H_2O \rightarrow H_2O^+ + e^-$$
$$H_2O^+ + H_2O \rightarrow H_3O^+ + OH\bullet$$

H_2O^+ decays to the hydroxyl $OH\bullet$ free radical whose hydrogen atom has one unpaired electron. It has been estimated that about two thirds of the damage caused by irradiation to mammalian cells is caused by the $OH\bullet$ radical (32,34,35).

The ground state of the oxygen molecule (O_2) is a radical with two unpaired electrons; upon removal of one electron (as by radiation) the superoxide radical O_2^- is produced. This can be formed in almost all aerobic cells.

Excess oxygen can damage cells, but there are mechanisms to repair the damage. Superoxide dismutase (SOD) is an enzyme that uses O_2^- as a substrate and then destroys the radical. Various molecules can scavenge free radicals, or, like vitamin E, act as antioxidants (fig. 14-9).

A system generating the superoxide radical O_2^- could produce hydrogen peroxide (H_2O_2) by nonenzymatic means or by the action of superoxide dismutase (SOD). H_2O_2 has no unpaired electron and therefore is not a radical but is very reactive. It damages some bacteria and animal cells; other bacteria and algae generate and release large amounts of H_2O_2.

The damage done by superoxide (O_2^-) and hydrogen peroxide (H_2O_2) is probably not caused directly by these two compounds but possibly by their conversion into the more highly reactive compounds, hydroxyl ($OH\bullet$) and hydroperoxyl ($OH\bullet_2$). The latter free radicals can attack compounds such as fatty acids directly. The hydroxyl radical ($OH\bullet$) could lead to modifications of purines or pyrimidines or to the breakage of DNA strands (35,36).

Oxidants have been implicated in the promotional phase of carcinogenesis and in cell transformation (101). Tumor promotion by croton oil promoters such as PMA (phorbolmyristic acetate) may

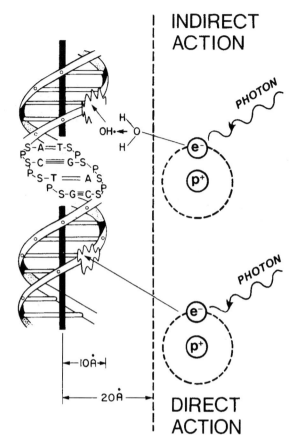

Figure 14-9
DIRECT AND INDIRECT DAMAGING
EFFECTS OF RADIATION ON DNA

In indirect action a secondary electron (e^-) reacts with H_2O to produce free radicals, e.g., $OH\bullet$ which causes damage to DNA. In direct action the secondary electron (e^-) acts directly with the DNA. (Fig. 1-7 from Hall EJ. Radiobiology for the radiologist. 3rd ed. Philadelphia: JB Lippincott, 1988:11.)

act, in part, by accelerating production of O_2 and H_2O_2 (34). Halliwell and Gutteridge suggest that oxidants could be involved in the initiation, promotion, or progression of carcinogenesis (34).

Intracellular Effects of Radiation

Many of the advances in the study of radiation carcinogenesis have occurred because of the ability to grow normal and irradiated cells in culture medium (5). The complex cell reactions that are possible after irradiation are illustrated in figure 14-9. Nuclear damage may give rise to damage to the nucleotide bases and loss or change in the sequence of the nucleotides. This could seriously affect cellular function.

Damage of the structure of strands of DNA can occur. Single strand breaks are not as important as double strand breaks in DNA; the latter are more difficult to repair. Cross-linking of DNA in the same strand, between two complementary strands, or to a completely different DNA molecule may occur. There could also be a covalent linkage with a protein (fig. 14-10) (90,92).

Chromosomal damage is also important in radiation effects. Breaks in the chromosomes, or a loss of part of a chromosome (deletion), may occur. After breakage, some chromosomes have "sticky" ends and fuse with other chromosomes with "sticky" ends, resulting in the formation of abnormal chromosomes. Translocations of bits of chromosomes to other chromosomes or to different parts of the same chromosome may cause changes in the sequence of DNA nucleotides (see chapter 20). Radiation produces characteristic changes in chromosomes such as acentric fragments, dicentric rings, and anaphase bridges (90,92).

Biochemical Changes

By the 1960s, many investigators had studied the changes in X-irradiated tissues. These are summarized by M.G. Ord and L.A. Stocken, Oxford biochemists, as follows (59): release of bound DNAase II from mitochondria; a need for added cytochrome C for mitochondrial oxidation and phosphorylation; decreased oxidative phosphorylation; inhibited nuclear formation of nucleotide triphosphates; and inhibited DNA synthesis.

Subsequently, Ord and Stocken showed that radiation uncouples nuclear and mitochondrial phosphorylation in some tissues, resulting in an alteration in ATP (adenine triphosphate) synthesis and carbohydrate metabolism, leading to radiation-induced interphase death (60). Decreases in NAD^+ and NADPH appeared to be the underlying mechanism.

The cyclic nucleotides, adenosine (cAMP) and guanine (cGMP), are important in mediating the activities of hormone release and other important functions. A high dose of whole body irradiation decreased both cAMP and cGMP concentrations in the brain of a rat from 30 to 65 percent within 10 minutes (43).

The cell cycle is also affected by irradiation: the latter induces a block in the G2 phase and a prolongation of the S period (90) (see chapter 18).

Apoptosis, a programmed process of cell death, may be induced by radiation (99). Since apoptosis

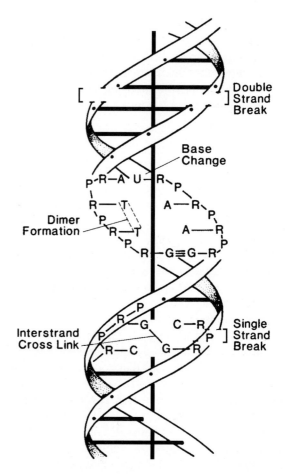

Figure 14-10
SOME TYPES OF INJURY TO DNA FROM RADIATION
(Fig. 2.2 from Travis EL. Medical radiobiology, 2nd ed. Chicago: Year Book, 1989:35.)

might be considered as a factor balancing the proliferation of cells, and proliferation is one of the features of cancer cells, radiation may cause an increase of cell death by this means, as well as by the direct damaging effects of radiation (see chapter 21).

DNA Repair

In 1911, C. Regaud and T. Nogier of the University of Lyon, while attempting to sterilize rams with X rays, found that a dose causing sterilization also led to destruction of the scrotum. However, if the same dose was divided into three doses with a 15-day interval between irradiations, sterilization was achieved without serious damage to the scrotum (fig. 14-7) (69). This suggested that damage was repaired during the intervals.

Repair after ultraviolet light (UV) irradiation was studied by R. Setlow and colleagues of Oak Ridge National Laboratories. They showed that UV radiation caused the formation of thymine dimers, i.e., the production of thymine-thymine pairs instead of the normal adenine-thymine pairs (37,74,75). Other dimers less often formed were cytosine-uracil, uracil-thymine, and cytosine-thymine (Note 7) (36).

Recovery of Organisms

Upon plotting the survival of hamster ovarian cells in culture medium against radiation dosage, T.T. Puck and P. Marcus of the University of Colorado found that the percentage of cells surviving radiation correlated to the logarithm of the dosage (66). This study indicated that a quantitative relationship existed between the absorbed dosage of radiation and the surviving fraction of tumor cells in an in vitro system.

M. M. Elkind of the National Cancer Institute, Bethesda, Maryland, suggested that the "shoulder" at the beginning of the curve formed when survival of cells was plotted against dosage of X rays indicated that repair of some of the damage had occurred (23). This was demonstrated by dividing the total dosage into fractions and allowing an interval of a few hours between administration of the fractions. The resultant survival curve showed that a higher percentage of cells survived when a fraction of the total dose was administered repeatedly than when the total dosage was applied at one time (fig. 14-6).

Elkind and Sutton found that cells in a culture medium that survived irradiation rapidly repaired their lesion and the repair did not appear to be attenuated by repeated cycles of radiation (24).

Enzymatic Repair

Repair of DNA damage has been found to be a normal process whereby intracellular enzymes remove abnormalities and replace defects in the DNA.

UV irradiation-caused linkage of two nucleotides to form an abnormal dimer, most often the thymine-thymine pair, can be excised by enzymes and the defect filled in with a patch of the proper nucleotide by other enzymes to restore the proper alignment of nucleotides. To replace the abnormal dimer, the intact, uninjured complementary strand of DNA is used as a template from which the original sequence is restored.

At least four different enzymes are required in the repair process: an endonuclease to cut the damaged DNA strand, an exonuclease to remove the damaged DNA, a polymerase to synthesize the new DNA, and a ligase to restore the continuity of the DNA strand. Such a process has been well characterized in bacteria but is not so clear in mammals (14).

Another type of repair is the excision of an abnormal base by a specific DNA enzyme, glycosylase (13). Excision is then followed by the actions of an endonuclease, an exonuclease, a synthesis of DNA by a polymerase, and a restoration of the continuity of the DNA strand by the ligase (Note 7).

In other types of repair, e.g., postreplication repair, bypass or toleration of the abnormal dimer after normal replication may occur. The abnormal dimers may be bypassed and repaired at a later time by synthesis of new DNA. These processes may give rise to error because of the presence of the abnormal dimer in the template used for the new DNA synthesis.

Radiation-produced abnormalities in the DNA of the affected somatic cells may persist during the life of the organism but are not transmitted to the cells of the progeny. Radiation-produced changes in the germ cells may be transmitted to the progeny's germ cells. Individuals lacking repair enzymes (12), or with chromosomal defects (12,98), have an associated predisposition for cancer.

Recent Studies of DNA Injury and Repair

Recent investigations of DNA injury and repair have focused mainly on single- and double-strand DNA breaks and their repair. Lankinen and Vilp of the University of Tampere, Finland, found that gamma irradiation of individual bone marrow cells from a ^{137}Cs (Cesium 137) source gave rise to single-strand DNA breaks, which were dose-dependent. When the cells were incubated at 37°C a fast initial repair phase was followed by a slower rejoining of the single-strand breaks. A higher dosage

---

Note 7: The lesion in ultraviolet radiation is repaired by a process called photoreactivation. A photoreactivating enzyme, photolyase, binds to the dimer, and upon exposure to visible light the enzyme uncouples the dimer and converts the nucleotides to their original state. Mammalian cells are less able to perform photoreactivation than lower forms of life because they have lower levels of photolyase (37,74).

required a significantly longer time for repair. Human blood granulocytes and lymphocytes showed similar breaks and repairs as did the human bone marrow cells (46).

C. G. Poirier and colleagues of the Cross Cancer Institutes, Edmonton, Canada, studied DNA-dependent protein kinase and poly (adenosine diphosphate [ADP]-ribose polymerase), two enzymes known to be involved in the response of mammalian cells to ionizing radiation. The enzymes are believed to be activated by binding to radiation-induced single-strand DNA breaks. The authors concluded that the chemical nature of the DNA at the 3' and 5' termini in the double-strand breaks did not influence the response of the DNA-dependent protein kinase. Single- and double-bond breaks activated poly (ADP-ribose polymerase) with about equal efficiency, but because of their greater number, single-stranded breaks dominated the response (63).

Gunz et al. of the University of Zurich, Switzerland, investigated the mechanism of nucleotide excision repair (NER) (31). They tested the ability of NER to recognize a bulky modification that either stabilized or destabilized the DNA double helix. They found a marked difference in the efficiency by which the helix-destabilizing and -stabilizing adducts sequestered NER factors. The authors concluded that the human NER is primarily targeted to sites at which the secondary structure of DNA is destabilized. They suggested that an early stage of recognition of DNA

damage involved a thermodynamic probing of the duplex. The convergence of biochemistry, genetics, and radiobiology has been reviewed by Jeggo of the University of Sussex, England (45) and Hall of Columbia University (33).

The scientific, medical, and sociologic fallout from the seminal discoveries of Roentgen, Becquerel, and the Curies has been profound. From Roentgen's discovery of X rays came not only diagnostic and therapeutic tools in oncology and medicine but the subsequent technique of X ray diffraction which has revealed the atomic structure of biological tissues.

Application of the radioactive isotopes that resulted from Becquerel's discovery delineated many pathways in animal and human metabolism, including cancer. The awesome development from Becquerel's discovery, the atomic bomb of World War II, caused thousands of deaths and devastation in Hiroshima and Nagasaki; it also ended World War II, thereby probably saving thousands of lives. Much of the atomic bomb arsenal built up during the "Cold War" has not yet been destroyed.

The long latent period from irradiation to the occurrence of cancer, often as long as decades in man, is an important intriguing phenomenon not yet understood. Radiobiology has contributed greatly to oncology through its fundamental studies of growth, replication, DNA injury and repair, and the process of carcinogenesis.

REFERENCES

1. Akslen LA, Haldorsen T, Thorensen SO, Glattre E. Survival and causes of death in thyroid cancer: a population-based study of 2479 cases from Norway. Cancer Res 1991;51:1234–41.

2. Anspaugh LR, Catlin RJ, Goldman M. The global impact of the Chernobyl reactor accident. Science 1988;242:1513–9.

3. Becquerel H. Sur les radiations émises par phosphorescence. Compt Rend Acad de Sci 1896;122:420–1.

4. Bergonié J, Tribondeau L. Interprétation de quelques résultats de la radiothéraple et essai de fixation d'une technique rationelle (note presented by Dr. d'Arsonval). Compt Rend Acad Sci Paris 1906;143:983–5.

5. Borek C. Malignant transformation in vitro: criteria, biological workers and application in environmental screening of carcinogens. Radiat Res 1979;79:209–32.

6. Broca A. The work of Henri Becquerel. Washington, D.C.: Smithsonian Annual Report, 1908.

7. Brown WM, Doll R. Mortality from cancer and other causes after radiotherapy for ankylosing spondylitis. Br Med J 1965;2(5474):1327–32.

8. Brues AM, Kirsh IE. The fate of individuals containing radium. Trans Amer Clin Climatol Assoc 1976;84:212–8.

9. Cade S. Malignant disease and its treatment by radium, vol 1. Baltimore: Williams & Wilkins, 1948.

10. Cahan WG, Woodward HQ, Higinbotham NL, Stewart FW, Coley BL. Sarcoma arising in irradiated bone. Report of eleven cases. Cancer 1948;1:3–29.

11. Casper J. The introduction in 1928–1929 of thorium dioxide in diagnostic radiology. Ann New York Acad Sci 1967;145:527–9.

12. Chaganti RS, Schonberg S, German J. A manifold increase in sister chromatid exchanges in Bloom's syndrome lymphocytes. Proc Natl Acad Sci USA 1974;71:4508–12.

13. Cleaver JE. Defective repair-replication of DNA in xeroderma pigmentosa. Nature 1968;218:652–6.

14. Cleaver JE. DNA damage and repair. In: Upton AC, Albert RE, Burns FJ, Shore RE, eds. Radiation carcinogenesis. New York: Elsevier, 1986:43–5.

15. Crousos GP. Thyroid tumors. In: Pizzo PA, Poplack DG, eds. Principles and practice of pediatric oncology. Philadelphia: JB Lippincott, 1989:741–3.

16. Curie E; Sheehan V, trans. Madame Curie, a biography. Garden City, NY: Doubleday, 1937:197–8.
17. Darby SC, Doll R, Gill SK, Smith PG. Long term mortality after a single treatment course with x-rays in patients treated for ankylosing spondylitis. Br J Cancer 1987;55:179–90.
18. DeGroot LJ, ed. Radiation-associated thyroid carcinoma. New York: Grune & Stratton, 1977.
19. DeGroot LJ, Paloyan E. Thyroid carcinoma and radiation. A Chicago endemic. JAMA 1973;225:487–91.
20. Dewing SB. Modern radiology in historical perspective. Springfield, IL: Charles C. Thomas, 1962:45–59, 225.
21. Duffy BJ, Fitzgerald PJ. Thyroid cancer in childhood and adolescence. Cancer 1950;3:1018–32.
22. Duffy BJ, Fitzgerald PJ. Thyroid cancer in childhood and adolescence: a report of 28 cases. J Clin Endocrinol Metab 1950;10:1296–308.
23. Elkind MM. Repair processes in radiation biology. Radiat Res 1984;100:425–49.
24. Elkind MM, Sutton H. Radiation response of mammalian cells grown in culture. I. Repair of X-ray damage in surviving Chinese hamster cells. Radiat Res 1960;13:556–93.
25. Finkel HJ, Miller CE, Hasterlick RJ. Radium-induced malignant tumors in man. In: Delayed effects of bone-seeking radionuclides. Salt Lake City: Univ. Utah Press, 1969:195–225.
26. Frieben A. Cancroids des rechten handruckens, das sich nach langdauernder einwirkung von Roentgenstrahlen entwickelt hatte. Fortsch Geb Roentgenstr 1902;6:106.
27. Furmanchuk AW, Averkin JL, Egloff B, et al. Pathomorphological findings in thyroid cancers of children from the republic of Belarus: a study of 86 cases occurring between 1986 ("post-Chernobyl") and 1991. Histopathology 1992;21:401–8.
28. Furth J, Furth OB. Neoplastic diseases produced in mice by general irradiation with x-rays. I. Incidences and types of neoplasms. Am J Cancer 1936;28:54–65.
29. Glasser O. Dr. W.C. Roentgen. 2nd ed. Springfield, IL: Charles C. Thomas, 1958:54.
30. Gross L. "Spontaneous" leukemia developing in C3H mice following inoculation in infancy with AK leukemic extracts, or AK-embryos. Proc Soc Exp Biol Med 1951;76:27–32.
31. Gunz D, Hess MT, Naegeli H. Recognition of DNA adducts by human nucleotide excision repair. Evidence for a thermodynamic probing mechanism. J Biol Chem 1996;271:25089–98.
32. Hall EJ. Radiobiology for the radiologist, 3rd ed. Philadelphia: JB Lippincott, 1988:12–3, 365–75, 389–9, 452–65, 493–4.
33. Hall EJ. What will molecular biology contribute to our understanding of radiation-induced cell killing and carcinogenesis? IRB Inter J Radiat Biol 1997;71:667–74.
34. Halliwell B, Gutteridge JM. Free radicals in biology and medicine. 2nd ed. Oxford: Clarendon Press, 1989:466–508.
35. Halliwell B, Gutteridge JM. Role of free radicals and catalytic metal ions in human diseases: an overview. In: Packer L, Glazer AN, eds. Oxygen radicals in biological systems. Part D. Methods in enzymology, vol. 186. New York: Academic Press, 1990:1–85.
36. Hanawalt PC. DNA repair comes of age. Mutat Res 1995;336:101–13.
37. Hanawalt PC, Setlow RB. Molecular mechanisms for repair of DNA. 2 vols. New York: Plenum Press, 1975.
38. Harley NH. Physics: environmental sources of radioactivity levels and interactions with matter. In: Upton AC, Albert RE, Burns FJ, Shore RE, eds. Radiation carcinogenesis. New York: Elsevier, 1986:23–42.
39. Henry SA. Cutaneous cancer in relation to occupation. Ann Royal Coll Surg Engl 1950;7:425–54.
40. Holm LE, Wiklund KE, Lundell GE, et al. Thyroid cancer after diagnostic doses of iodine 131: a retrospective cohort study. JNCI 1988;90:1132–8.
41. Horta JD. Late effects of thorotrast on the liver and spleen and their efferent lymph nodes. Ann NY Acad Sci 1967;145:676–99.
42. Horta JD, Da Motta LC, Tavares MH. Thorium dioxide effects in man–epidemiological, clinical and pathological studies (experience in Portugal). Environ Res 1974;8:131–59.
43. Hunt WA, Dalton TK. Reduction in cyclic nucleotide levels in the brain after a high dose of ionizing radiation. Radiat Res 1980;83:210–5.
44. Huvos AG, Woodard HQ, Cahan, WG, et al. Postradiation osteogenic sarcoma of bone and soft tissues. A clinicopathologic study of 66 patients. Cancer 1985;55:1244–55.
45. Jeggo PA. DNA-PK–at the crossroads of biochemistry and genetics. Mutat Res 1997;384:1–14.
46. Lankinen MH, Vilpo JA. Repair of gamma-irradiation-induced DNA single-strand breaks in human bone marrow cells: analysis of unfractionated and CD34+ cells using single-cell gel electrophoresis. Mutat Res 1997;377:177–85.
47. MacMahon HE, Murphy AS, Bates MJ. Endothelial cell sarcoma of liver following thorotrast injections. Am J Path 1947;23:585–611.
48. March HC. Leukemia in radiologists in a 20 year period. Am J Med Sci 1950;220:282–6.
49. Martland HS. Occupational poisoning in manufacture of luminous watch dials. JAMA 1929;92:466–73, 552–9.
50. Martland HS. Occurrence of malignancy in radioactive persons: a general review of data gathered in study of radium dial painters, with special reference to occurrence of osteogenic sarcoma and the interrelationship of certain blood diseases. Am J Cancer 1931;15:2435–516.
51. Martland HS, Humphries RE. Osteogenic sarcoma in dial painters using luminous paint. Arch Path 1929;7:406–17.
52. Matanoski GM, Seltser R, Sartwell PE, Diamond EL, Elliot EA. The current mortality rates of radiologists and other physician specialists: specific causes of death. Am J Epidermiol 1975;101:199–210.
53. Miller RW, Beebe GW. Leukemia, lymphoma and multiple myeloma. In: Upton AC, Albert RE, Burns FJ, Shore RE, eds. Radiation carcinogenesis. New York: Elsevier, 1986:245–60.
54. Modan B, Baidatz D, Mart H, Steinitz R, Levin SG. Radiation-induced head and neck tumors. Lancet 1974;1:277–9.
55. Monez E. L'Angiographie cérébral. Paris: Masson, 1934.
56. Monson RR, MacMahon B. Prenatal x-ray exposure and cancers in children. In: Boice JD Jr, Fraumeni JF Jr, eds. Radiation carcinogenesis, epidemiology and biological significance. New York: Raven Press, 1984:97–105.
57. National Academy of Science-National Research Council. Committee on the biological effects of ionizing radiation. Cancer in childhood following exposure in utero. In: Health effects of exposure to low levels of ionizing radiation (BEIR V). Washington, D.C.: National Academy of Sciences, 1990:281–98, 352–62.
58. Nikiforov Y, Gnepp DR. Pediatric thyroid cancer after the Chernobyl disaster. Pathomorphologic study of 84 cases (1991–1992) from the Republic of Belarus. Cancer 1994;74:748–66.
59. Ord MG, Stocken LA. The biochemical lesion in vivo and in vitro. In: Errera M, Forssberg A, eds. Mechanisms in radiobiology. New York: Academic Press, 1961:259–331.
60. Ord MG, Stocken LA. The radiosensitivity of rat thymocytes. Biochem J 1896;238:517–23.

61. Parker LN, Belsky JL, Yamamonto T, Kawanoto S, Keehn RJ. Thyroid carcinoma after exposure to atomic radiation. A continuing survey of a fixed population, Hiroshima and Nagasaki, 1958–1971. Ann Intern Med 1974;80:600–4.

62. Perthes G. Ueber den Einfluss der Roentgenstrahlen auf epitheliable Gewebe, in besondere auf das carcinom. Arch klin Chir 1903;71:955–1000.

63. Poirier GG, Povirk LF, Lees-Miller SP. Interaction of DNA-dependent protein kinase and poly (ADP-ribose) polymerase with radiation-induced DNA strand breaks. Radiat Res 1997;148:22–8.

64. Polednak AP. Bone cancer among female radium dial workers. Latency periods and incidence rates by time after exposure. JNCI 1978;60:77–82.

65. Prentice RL, Kato H, Yoshimoto K, Mason M. Radiation exposure and thyroid cancer incidence among Hiroshima and Nagasaki residents. Natl Cancer Instit Monogr 1982;62:207–12.

66. Puck TT, Marcus PI. Action of X-rays on mammalian cells. J Exper Med 1956;103:653–66.

67. Quimby EH. The background of radium therapy in the United States, 1906–1956. Am J Roent Rad Therapy Nuc Med 1956;75:443–50.

68. Regaud C, Blanc J. Actions des rayons X sur les diverses générations de la lignée spermatique: extrême sensibilité des spermatogies a les rayons. Compt Rend Soc de Biol 1906;61:163–5.

69. Regaud C, Nogier T. Stérilization röntgénienne total et définitive sans radiodermite, des testicules du Bélier adulte; conditions de sa réalization. Compt Rend Soc de Biol 1911;70:202–3.

70. Roentgen WC. Uebereine neve art vou strahlen. Sitzunasberichte der Würzburger physikal–medicin Gesellschaft. 1895:132–41.

71. Ron E, Modan B. Thyroid and other neoplasms following childhood scalp irradiation. In: Boice JD Jr, Fraumeni JF, eds. Radiation carcinogenesis: epidemiology and biological significance. New York: Raven Press, 1984:139–51.

72. Rubin R, Casaret GW. Clinical radiation pathology, vol 1. Philadelphia: WB Saunders, 1968:28–35.

73. Schneider AB, Favus MJ, Stachura ME, Arnold J, Arnold MJ, Frohman LA. Incidence, prevalence and characteristics of radiation-induced thyroid tumors. Am J Med 1978;64:243–52.

74. Setlow RB. Twenty five years of DNA repair. In: Castellani A, ed. DNA damage and repair. New York: Plenum Press, 1989:1–9.

75. Setlow RB, Carrier WL. The disappearance of thymine dimers from DNA. An error-correcting mechanism. Proc Natl Acad Sci USA 1964;51:226–31.

76. Setlow RB, Setlow JK. Evidence that ultraviolet-induced thymine dimers in DNA cause biological damage. Proc Natl Acad Sci USA 1962;48:1250–7.

77. Shore RE, Albert RE, Pasternak BS. Follow-up study of patients treated by x-ray epilation for Tinea capitis: resurvey of post-treatment illness and mortality experience. Arch Environ Health 1976;31:21–28.

78. Shore RE, Woodard E, Hildreth N, Dvoretsky P, Hemplemann L, Pasternack B. Thyroid tumors following thymus irradiation. JNCI 1985;74:1177–84.

79. Simpson CL, Hempelmann LH, Fuller LM. The association of tumors and roentgen-ray treatment of the thorax in infancy. Cancer 1957;10:42–56.

80. Simpson CL, Hempelmann LH, Fuller LM. Neoplasia in children treated with x-rays in infancy for thymic enlargement. Radiology 1955;64:840–5.

81. Smith PG, Doll R. Mortality from cancer and all causes among British radiologists. Br J Radiol 1981;54:187–94.

82. Stannard JN. Radioactivity and health: a history. Springfield, VA: National Technical Information Service. 1988:23–43.

83. Stanton R, Stinson D, Shahabi S. An introduction to radiation oncology. Physics. Madison, WI: Medical Physics, 1992:7–52.

84. Stehney AF, Lucas HF, Rowland RE. Survival times of women radium dial workers first exposed before 1930. In: Late biological effects of ionizing radiation. Proceedings of the symposium on the late biological effects of ionizing radiation. International Atomic Energy Agency. Vienna, 1978.

85. Stewart A, Kneale GW. Prenatal exposure and childhood cancer. Lancet 1971;1:42–3.

86. Stewart AM, Kneale GW. Radiation dose effects in relation to obstetric x-ray and childhood cancers. Lancet 1970;1:1185–8.

87. Stewart A, Webb J, Hewitt D. A survey of childhood malignancies. Br Med J 1958;1:1495–508.

88. Stone-Scott N. X-ray injuries. Am X-Ray J 1897;1:57–67.

89. Stoner JB. Radiation carcinogenesis. In: Becker FF, ed. Cancer: a comprehensive treatise, vol. 1. New York: Plenun Press, 1982:629–59.

90. Tannock IF. Cell proliferation. In: Tannock IF, Hill R, eds. The basic science of oncology. Toronto: McGraw-Hill. 1992:154–77.

91. Tannock IF, Hill RP. The basic science of oncology. Toronto: McGraw-Hill. 1992:52, 106–24, 130.

92. Travis EL. Medical radiobiology, 2nd ed. Chicago: Year Book, 1989:25–46.

93. United Nations Scientific Committee on the Effects of Atomic Radiation. Report to the General Assembly, with annexes. New York: United Nations, 1986.

94. Upton AC. Historical prospectives on radiation carcinogenesis. In: Upton AC, Albert RE, Burns FJ, Shore RE, eds. Radiation carcinogenesis. New York: Elsevier, 1986:1–10.

95. Van Kaick G, Lorenz D, Muth H, Kaul A. Malignancies in German thorotrast patients and estimated tissue dose. Health Phys 1978;35:127–36.

96. Vaughan J. Carcinogenic effects of radiation on the human skeleton and supporting tissues. In: Upton AC, Albert RE, Burns FJ, Shore RE, eds. Radiation carcinogenesis. New York: Elsevier, 1986:311–34.

97. Wakabayashi T, Kato H, Iketa T, Schull WJ. Studies of the mortality of A-bomb survivors. Report 7, part III. Incidence of cancer in the 1959–78, based on the tumor registry. Nagasaki Radiat Res 1983;93:112–46.

98. Wolff S, Carrano AV. Radiation-induced chromosome aberrations and cancer. In: Upton AC, Albert RE, Burns FJ, Shore RE, eds. Radiation carcinogenesis, New York: Elsevier, 1986:57–69.

99. Yamada T, Ohyama H. Radiation-induced interphase death of rat thymocytes is internally programmed (apoptosis). Int J Radiat Biol 1988;53:65–75.

100. Yokoro K. Experimental radiation leukemogenesis in mice. In: Upton AC, Albert RE, Burns FJ, Shore RE, eds. Radiation carcinogenesis. New York: Elsevier, 1986:137–50.

101. Zimmerman K, Cerutti P. Active oxygen acts as a promoter of transformation in mouse embryo C3H/1OT/C18 fibroblasts. Proc Natl Acad Sci USA 1984;81:2085–7.

102. Zurnadzhi IN, Bogdanova TI, Tron'ko ND, et al. Morphofunctional characteristics of malignant thyroid gland tumors in children from various regions of the Ukraine who had been victims of the Chernobyl nuclear power plant accident. Arkh Patol 1993;55:55–60.

15

VIRAL CARCINOGENESIS

VIRUSES

One of the most insidious enemies of mankind has been a group of agents that are so small, even smaller than bacteria, that they could not be seen, with rare exception, through the best microscopes available up to the 1950s. Only with the development of the electron microscope could one obtain photographs of most of these organisms—the viruses (fig. 15-1) (18).

One of the viral diseases, poliomyelitis, had been known for centuries for its lethality, mostly in children, or because of the muscular paralysis persisting in the survivors (45). President Franklin Roosevelt of the United States was one of the most conspicuous of the recent victims of the poliomyelitis virus. Smallpox was another virus that had been a scourge to mankind since Egyptian times and only recently has been eradicated from the human population (4,45).

A devastating virus, influenza, swept through the world in the second and third decades of the 20th century to cause the death of an estimated 20 million people; it still causes epidemic disease throughout the world although, fortunately, no epidemic as severe as that of 1918–1920 has recurred (45). The AIDS (acquired immunodeficiency syndrome) virus and its growing global infection of millions of persons is but the latest of the major afflictions caused by a virus (45).

A virus (Latin: poison) is an organism that has to live within cells and, with rare exception, cannot live outside them because it lacks the biochemical means to reproduce itself. The virus uses the replicative mechanisms of the host cell for this purpose. The virus may injure or kill the host cell or it may insert all or some of its genes into the host cell DNA and set up a live-in arrangement whereby it uses the host's cell genes for its own (viral) replication (18,45).

FILTERABLE AGENTS

A Russian botanist of St. Petersburg, Dimitri Ivanowski, was studying a disease of tobacco leaves, tobacco mosaic disease, in 1882 and found that the sap of the diseased leaves when filtered left a filtrate that remained infectious. The pores of the filter used were so small that they retained cells, parasites, and bacteria and prevented them from passing through with the juice (37). However, the infectious units of tobacco mosaic disease were so small that they easily passed through the pores of the filter and thus were called filterable agents.

In 1898, Martinus Beijerinek of the Netherlands confirmed Ivanowski's work and, in addition, showed that the infectious agent could multiply only in the leaves but not in the filtrate (5). The agent, a plant pathogen, was named the "tobacco mosaic virus" (fig. 15-1) (45).

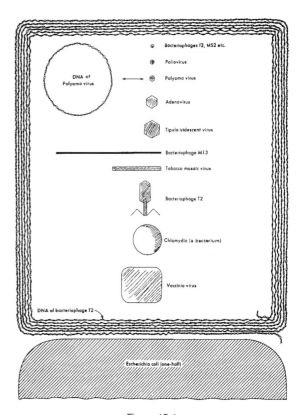

Figure 15-1
RELATIVE SIZES OF BACTERIA, VIRUSES, AND BACTERIOPHAGES

Schematic general design of some bacteriophages, viruses, and the bacterium *Escherichia coli*. The viruses and bacteriophages are drawn to scale. (Fig. 44.1 from Dulbecco R. The nature of viruses. In: Dulbecco R, Ginsberg HS, eds. Virology, 2nd ed. Philadelphia: JB Lippincott, 1988:3.)

The first human disease demonstrated to be caused by a filterable agent was yellow fever, a disease known for centuries. It was present in the United States Army troops in Cuba during the Spanish American War. The classic experiment of Walter Reed and the U.S. Army Commission used human volunteers in 1900 to prove that the virus was transmitted by the mosquito from human to human (3,45,54).

In 1908, two Danish pathologists, V. Elleman and O. Bang, showed that an agent extracted from leukemia cells of chickens, filtered free of cells and bacteria, could produce leukemia in other chickens (21). At that time the relationship of a virus to cancer was not recognized because leukemia was not considered to be a cancer.

Bacteriophage

Just as there were bacteria that infected animals and humans, there were agents that infected bacteria. A filterable agent that caused a disease in bacteria was found in the fluid extracts of bacteria by F.W. Twort of England in 1916 (45,65). The next year, F. d'Herelle of France described an agent in the dysenteric stools of cavalry troops in France that destroyed the bacillus causing the dysentery (17). Because the agent infected bacteria and destroyed them, they were called bacteriophages (Greek: bacteria eaters) (fig. 15-2). Bacteriophages (often shortened to phages) played a very important part in eventually attaining an understanding of the mechanisms of viral carcinogenesis (45) (Note 1).

Rous Sarcoma Virus (RSV)

Peyton Rous, of the Rockefeller Institute, in one of the most important discoveries in oncology, showed that a cell-free filtrate from an extract of a tumor in a Plymouth Rock hen could, when injected into a hen of the same species and litter, produce a cancer of connective tissue, a sarcoma (fig. 15-3) (26,56,57). The filtrate contained an agent, identified later as a virus of the ribonucleic acid (RNA) group, and it was named the Rous sarcoma virus (RSV) (fig. 15-4). The recognition of this virus was not only important in the field of virology, but provided the means whereby the transforming genes of the Rous sarcoma virus,

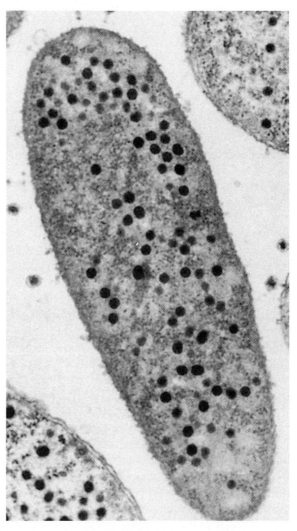

Figure 15-2
BACTERIOPHAGE: SMALL BLACK
SPHERES INFECTING BACTERIA
Electron micrograph of a bacterium (*E. coli*) infected with a bacteriophage (T4, black round dots). (From Levine AJ. Viruses. New York: Scientific American Library, 1992: 21.)

the genes that changed a normal cell into a cancer cell, were identified (68).

Neither the Danish report of Elleman and Bang nor that of Rous created much of a stir in the oncological world. James Ewing, a pathologist at Memorial Hospital, New York City, and a foremost authority on cancer in the United States, had objections to the

---

Note 1: Twort joined the British Army in World War I and upon his return after the war did not pursue his discovery (44,64). d'Herelle spent many years unsuccessfully attempting to use the bacteriophage as a therapeutic agent against bacterial infections (17,45).

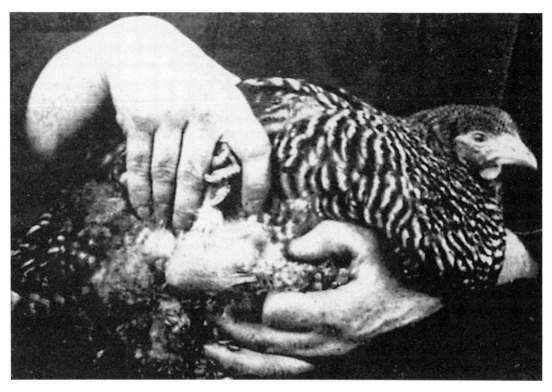

Figure 15-3
ROUS SARCOMA
Plymouth Rock hen displaying Rous sarcoma (white mass) the source of the Rous virus. (Plate LXVI from Rous P. Transmission of avian neoplasm (sarcoma of the common fowl). J Exp Med 1910;12:696–705.)

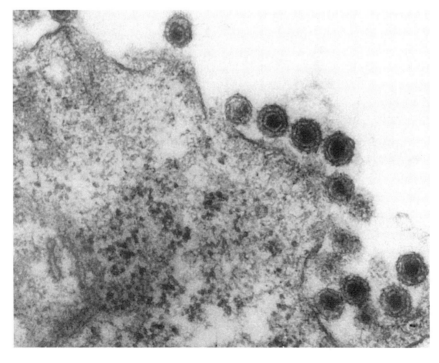

Figure 15-4
ROUS SARCOMA VIRUS
Rous sarcoma virus grown on chorioallantoic membrane of the rat. (Fig. 13A (X90,000) from Gross L. Oncogene viruses, 3rd ed. vol 1. Oxford: Pergamon Press, 1983:130.)

parasitic origin of cancer because of the numerous bacteria and parasites that had been suggested to be the causal agent of cancer in the late 19th and early 20th centuries, only to be shown subsequently not to be. He regarded the Rous tumor as a true animal cancer but he suggested that it was a chemical, not a living agent, that caused the sarcoma. He believed that living agents, with rare exceptions, had no relation to human cancer (24), but Rous maintained for years that a virus might cause some cancers in humans (24,58).

Shope Virus

In the early 1930s Richard Shope of the Rockefeller Institute reported that an infectious agent caused papillomas (benign warty lesions) of the skin of wild cottontail rabbits in Iowa. The agent was filterable, free of bacteria and cells, and could be isolated from the papillomas. When it was rubbed into the skin of other normal wild rabbits, it produced similar skin lesions (60).

Rous injected a sample of Shope's virus into rabbits of a different strain, a domestic species, but the virus seemed to have lost its infectivity and no papillomas appeared. Some months later, however, cancers of the skin developed. Rous attempted to isolate a virus from the skin cancers but failed (59). Much later it was shown that cells of the skin cancer produced in the experiment contained a part of the deoxyribonucleic acid (DNA) of the Shope papilloma virus which was integrated into the DNA of the host skin cells. Free virus was not present in the cell and thereby all attempts at that time to isolate virus from the cancer cells were unsuccessful.

Since all the cancer cells from the Shope papilloma virus had viral DNA incorporated in the same place on a specific chromosome, it was apparent that the origin of the cancer was a single cell and that the cell had replicated many times to give a clone of identical cancer cells. The experiment also showed that host cells of one animal strain might differ in their response in another animal strain of the same species.

The Shope papilloma virus was the first tumor virus shown to contain DNA (45).

FROG KIDNEY TUMORS

A kidney cancer commonly found in frogs of the New England lakes was demonstrated by Balduwin Lucké, a pathologist of the University of Pennsylva-nia, to be transmitted from frog to frog by a ground-up, lyophilized, cell-free extract of the tumor (48). The extract was thereby inferred to be a virus.

MILK FACTOR OF BITTNER

An important discovery by John Bittner of Yale University showed that cancer of the mouse breast was caused by a "factor" contained in the milk of nursing mothers. Suckling mice received the virus from the mother's milk and later developed breast tumors (8). The tumor was strain selective and hormone associated, i.e., only certain strains of mice were susceptible to the virus and hormones could affect susceptibility. Female mice developed breast cancer but castrated female and male mice did not (7). The experiment indicated the complex nature of cancer, that many factors, including hormones, are important in carcinogenesis.

The "milk factor of Bittner" is now known to be a virus, the murine mammary tumor virus (MMTV), an RNA virus (45).

"SPONTANEOUS" LEUKEMIAS

For many years it had been known that some strains of mice, e.g., the AKR and C58 strains, had a high incidence of "spontaneous" leukemia and so they were used as models for the study of human leukemia. Ludwig Gross, a virologist, was unable to transmit the AKR leukemia to adult mice of the C58 strain when he used filtered extracts from the leukemic organs of adult AKR mice. However, when he injected the filtered extracts into newborn mice of the C3H strain, 100 percent of the mice got leukemia when they reached adulthood. The mice could be successfully infected only during a short period after birth (31); soon after birth the mouse developed an immune system that prevented the transmission of the virus.

The virus causing mouse leukemia has been isolated and is called the murine leukemia virus (MLV). It is an RNA virus with a characteristic morphology as seen by electron microscopy (30).

Other Murine Viruses

In the 1950s and 1960s a large number of viruses were discovered that caused cancers in animals (30). These RNA viruses could replicate in fibroblasts in culture and did not kill the host cells in the process (Table 15-1).

Table 15-1

RETROVIRAL ONCOGENES*

Oncogene	Prototype Virus(es)	Species or Origin
abl	Abelson murine leukemia virus (Ab-MLV)	Mouse
erb A, *erb* B	Avian erythroblastosis virus (AEV)	Chicken
ets	E26	Chicken
fes, fps	Fuginami sarcoma virus (FuSV)	Chicken
	Snyder-Theilen feline sarcoma virus (St-FeSV)	Cat
	Feline sarcoma virus (GA-FeSV)	Cat
fgr, yes	Gardner-Rasheed feline sarcoma virus (GR-FeSV)	Cat
	Yamaguchi 73 sarcoma virus (Y73)	Chicken
	Esh sarcoma virus (ESV)	Chicken
fms	Susan McDonough feline sarcoma virus (SM-FeSV)	Cat
fos	FBJ-murine sarcoma virus	Mouse
	FBR-murine sarcoma virus	Mouse
mos	Moloney murine sarcoma virus (Mo-MSV)	Mouse
myb	Avian myeloblastosis virus (AMV)	Chicken
	E26	Chicken
myc	Myelocytomastosis-29 virus (MC29)	Chicken
	Mill-Hill-2 virus (MH2)	Chicken
	CMII/OK10 viruses	Chicken
raf	Mill-Hill-2 virus (MH2)	Chicken
	Murine sarcoma virus strain 3611 (MSV-3611)	Mouse
ras Ha	Harvey murine sarcoma virus (Ha-MSV)	Rat
	Rasheed rat sarcoma virus (RaSV)	Rat
(bas)	BALB murine sarcoma virus	Mouse
ras Ki	Kirsten murine sarcoma virus (Ki-MSV)	Mouse
rel	Reticuloendothelial virus strain T	Turkey
ros	UR2	Chicken
sis	Simian sarcoma virus (SSV)	Woolly monkey
	Parodi-Irgens feline sarcoma virus (PI-FeSv)	Cat
ski	SKV770	Chicken
src	Rous sarcoma virus (RSV)	Chicken

*Table 3.5 from Burck KB, Liu ET, Larrick JW. Oncogenes. An introduction to the concept of cancer genes. New York: Springer-Verlag, 1988:57.

The AKR strain of mice was interesting because in addition to a leukemia-producing virus, they harbored a second virus. It was called the polyomavirus (Greek: many tumor virus) because of the many types of tumor it produced (62). Surprisingly, the polyoma strain did not cause tumors in mice in the wild who already harbored the virus but only in laboratory animals who did not. In 1960, Peter Vogt and R. Dulbecco of California Technology showed that the murine polyomavirus was capable of transforming cells in culture (67).

Polyomavirus and another virus, the SV40 virus from the kidney of the rhesus monkey, were small viruses with considerable transforming ability and they proved to be very useful in the study of the transformation process. The SV40 virus was an unrecognized contaminant of the early Salk vaccine for poliomyelitis, which had been prepared from monkey kidney cells. Fortunately, it has not been carcinogenic for humans although it transforms rodent cells (45).

SARCOMA VIRUSES

In the 1970s, J. J. Harvey (33), J. B. Maloney (49), and W. H. Kirsten (39) discovered that mice that were infected with a weakly transforming RNA virus occasionally had a tumor from which a different virus could be isolated. These viruses not only transformed cells in culture but produced sarcomas in animals. The transforming ability of the sarcoma viruses was the direct result of the activity of specific viral genes, called oncogenes (Greek: tumor genes) (see chapter 20) (15).

REVERSE TRANSCRIPTASE

Bacterial genetic experiments by Joshua Lederberg and Norman Zinder had demonstrated that genetic information of DNA could be transmitted from one bacterium to another by a virus (16, 43,70). One of the problems arising from the hypothesis that RNA viruses caused cancer was the question as to how the RNA of the virus could be incorporated into the DNA of a host cell genome. The means was discovered, independently, by David Baltimore of the Whitehead Institute, Massachusetts Institute of Technology (MIT) (1) and Howard Temin of the University of Wisconsin (63). These investigators discovered an enzyme, called reverse transcriptase, which synthesized complementary DNA from the RNA virus. Portions of this complementary DNA were then incorporated into the host DNA as a provirus component. The proviral component replicated when the cell divided and

thereby continued its existence as part of the DNA of the cell. It could give rise to viral progeny, transform fibroblast cells into a sarcoma, or remain inactive (Note 2).

DNA VIRUSES AND HUMAN CANCERS

Retroviruses (RNA viruses) have been shown to be the cause of many cancers in animals and were suspected to be the cause of cancers in humans. Was any DNA virus responsible for human cancer?

Hepatitis B Virus and Liver Cancer

Clinical experience showed that liver cancer, primary hepatocellular cancer, often occurred in patients who lived in areas where infectious hepatitis (inflammation of the liver) was prevalent. Many patients with primary hepatocellular cancer gave a history of a previous attack of infectious hepatitis B, cirrhosis of the liver, or both. The association of hepatitis with liver cancer was thought to be a causal one. Results of epidemiologic investigations furthered the likelihood that the hepatitis B virus (a DNA virus) was the cause or at least involved in the process of liver carcinogenesis (45). Hepatitis B was one of the two viruses known to cause hepatitis. Recently a third virus, hepatitis C (originally called non-A, non-B) has been found and has become more prevalent (50). A delta hepatitis virus is also recognized (28).

The hepatitis B virus (HBV) (fig. 15-5) became accepted, from epidemiologic evidence, to be the agent probably involved in the production of human primary hepatocellular carcinoma (45). The cancer appeared most often in areas where infectious hepatitis type B was widespread, i.e., in coastal China, the sub-Sahara desert area of Africa, and other focal areas throughout the world.

Note 2: The term "reverse transcriptase" was used because the accepted route for protein synthesis was from the DNA of the gene to a messenger RNA (mRNA) to a ribosomal RNA (rRNA) to a protein:

DNA → mRNA → rRNA → PROTEIN.

In order for RNA to be incorporated into the DNA of the host cell a complementary DNA (cDNA) to the RNA was formed. The enzyme which made this conversion acted in a reverse direction than the enzymes involved in the normal pathway of DNA to mRNA to protein, i.e.:

$$\text{RNA} \xrightarrow[\text{transcriptase}]{\text{reverse}} \text{cDNA} \rightarrow \text{Proviral DNA Complex} \rightarrow \text{mRNA} \rightarrow \text{rRNA} \rightarrow \text{PROTEIN}$$

The independent discovery of the enzyme by Baltimore (1) and Temin (63) was not only important in molecular biology (see chapter 18) but also explained how RNA viruses might be incorporated into the DNA of the host cells. The Huebner and Todaro hypothesis of C-type RNA viruses as a cause of human cancers became more plausible when it was shown how RNA viruses might be incorporated into the DNA of the human genome.

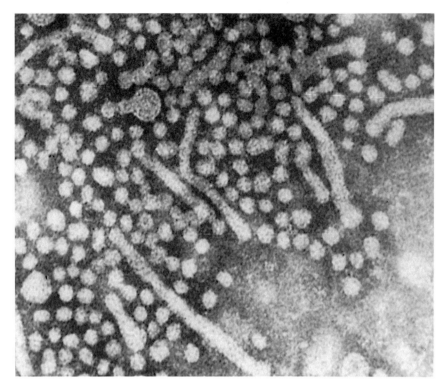

Figure 15-5
HEPATITIS B VIRUS
Hepatitis B virus is associated with human hepatitis and liver cell cancer. Virions, long filamentous and spherical particles, are shown. (From Levine AJ. Viruses. New York: Scientific American Library, 1992:187.)

The majority of the patients with primary hepatocellular cancer had antibodies in their serum to an antigen of the hepatitis B virus, an antigen residing on the surface of the virus, labeled HBsAG (hepatitis B surface antigen). The usual sequence of carcinogenic events is believed to be an acute infectious hepatitis caused by the hepatitis B virus, leading to chronic hepatitis, cirrhosis of the liver, and, finally, in a very small percentage of cases, liver cell cancer. The DNA sequences of the hepatitis B virus have been demonstrated to be integrated into the cellular DNA of some human liver cell carcinomas (45).

An effective vaccine has been prepared against the hepatitis B virus and is being used in many areas of the world where the incidence of the disease is high (19,45). It will be important to follow persons who have received the vaccine in these areas to determine whether they have a lower incidence of liver cancer than a comparable group that did not receive the vaccine.

More recently, hepatitis of the C type (formerly called non-A, non-B type) has become important (45). A study from Greece showed that in a high percentage of patients with primary hepatocellular cancer, both hepatitis B and hepatitis C antibodies are present (32).

A confounding factor in deciding with certainty about the causal relationship of the hepatitis B virus and hepatocellular cancer is the presence in some areas in which liver cell cancer is prevalent of a mycotoxin carcinogen, aflatoxin (AFB1) (see chapter 13). The fungus is a contaminant of spoiled animal feed. It has been suggested that the aflatoxin may be the agent causing the liver cancer.

Herpes Viruses

The herpes viruses, DNA viruses, were discovered early in the century; one type causes the common "cold sore" of the lip (herpes simplex virus 1 [HSV-1]). There are now seven known herpes viruses affecting humans, many of which affect animals as well (45).

One of the most interesting herpetic viruses related to cancer is the Epstein-Barr DNA herpes virus (EBV) (fig. 15-6) (27,45). This virus has been demonstrated to have a consistent relationship to Burkitt's lymphoma, a malignant lymphoma (cancer of the lymphatic system) among African children (fig. 15-7) (45). A British surgeon, Dennis Burkitt, studied the pattern of distribution of malignant lymphoma among African children and suggested a virus vector

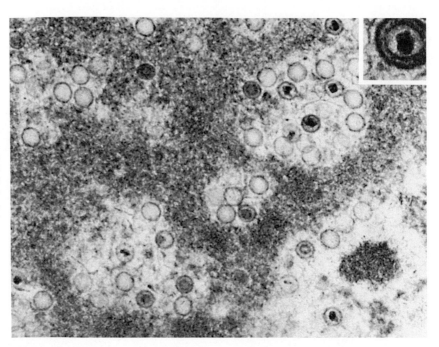

Figure 15-6
EPSTEIN-BARR VIRUS

Epstein-Barr virus (EBV) is associated with infectious mononucleosis, Burkitt's lymphoma, and squamous cell carcinoma (X70,000). Insert shows virus structure; mature virus particle with additional outer envelope (X164,000.) (Fig. 90 from Gross L. Oncogenic viruses. 3rd ed. vol 2. Oxford: Pergamon Press, 1983:931.)

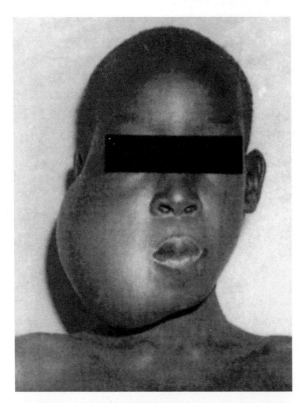

Figure 15-7
BURKITT'S LYMPHOMA

African boy with Burkitt's lymphoma showing swelling of the right side of lower face and jaw region. The cancer is an undifferentiated B-cell lymphoma. (Fig. 18.4 from Raven RW. The theory and practice of oncology. Park Ridge, NJ: Parthenon Press, 1990:280.)

(fig. 15-8) (14,16). Other British investigators, M. A. Epstein, B. O. Archong, and Y. M. Barr, isolated the Epstein-Barr virus from these tumors (23).

The Epstein-Barr virus is ubiquitous in humans. Werner and Dorothy Henle of Philadelphia showed that the virus caused infectious mononucleosis in young people (35). Lloyd Old and colleagues of the Sloan Kettering Institute found that the blood of patients with squamous cell cancer revealed a high incidence of reactivity to the Epstein-Barr virus antigen (52). George Klein of the Karolinska Institutet, Stockholm, Sweden, has given an interesting account of the symbiotic presence of the virus in normal individuals, in patients with infectious mononucleosis, in patients with B-cell lymphomas, and in patients with squamous cell cancer (40). The intriguing relationships of this virus present a complex puzzle, not yet completely understood (45).

Human Papilloma Virus

Another prominent virus of the herpes group is the human papilloma virus (HPV), of which 64 different types have been isolated from lesions of various parts of the body (45,71). Types 16, 18, 31, and 33 have been found in association with anogenital (uterine, cervix, anal, and rectal) cancers (71). The association is believed to be causal because the DNA of the virus is incorporated into the DNA of the cancer cells (Table 15-2). Harold zur

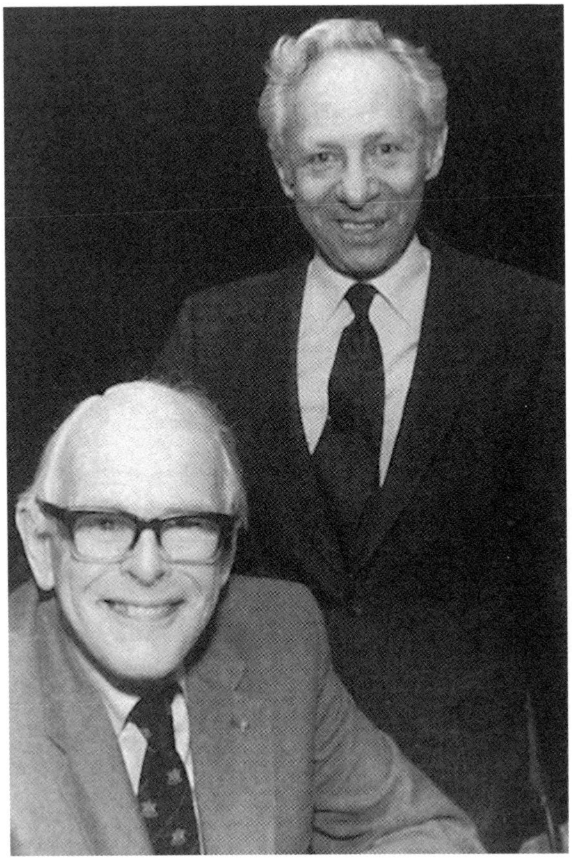

Figure 15-8
DENNIS BURKITT AND MICHAEL EPSTEIN
Dennis Burkitt, left, a British surgeon who described the clinical features of Burkitt's lymphoma in Africa and Michael Epstein (right), a British virologist who isolated the Epstein-Barr virus from cells of Burkitt's tumor. Both have been knighted. (From Levine AJ. Viruses. New York: Scientific American Library, 1992:77.)

Table 15-2
DNA TUMOR VIRUSES*

Papilloma Viruses
Multiple species including human, bovine, rabbit (Shope), equine, canine, elk, deer, sheep

Herpes Viruses
Alpha subfamily: herpes simplex 1 and 2; equine herpes virus type 1
Beta subfamily: cytomegalovirus (human)
Gamma subfamily: Epstein-Barr virus (human); Marek's virus (avian); *Herpesvirus saimiri* (squirrel monkey); *Herpesvirus ateles* (spider monkey)
Other: Lücké herpes virus (frog): *Herpesvirus sylvilagus* (rabbit)

Hepatitis B Family
Hepatitis B virus (human)
Woodchuck (*Marmota monax)* hepatitis virus
Ground squirrel (*Spermophilus beecheyi)* hepatitis virus
Duck hepatitis virus (domestic duck, Peking duck)

Polyoma Virus
Polyoma virus (murine)
Simian virus 40 (monkey)
BK virus (human)
JC virus (human)

Adenovirus
Human (at least 37 types), groups A, B, C, D, and E
Simian, bovine, murine, canine, avian, porcine, ovine, equine, tree shrew

*Table 3.1 from Burck KB, Liu ET, Larrick JW. Oncogenes. An introduction to the concept of cancer genes. New York: Springer-Verlag, 1988:40.

Hausen of the University of Heidelberg, Germany, who discovered the association of the virus and anogenital cancers, has estimated that about 20 percent of female and slightly less than 10 percent of male anogenital cancers are associated with human papilloma virus (71).

ACTIVATION OF LATENT VIRUSES

Radiation has many effects on cells, one of which is the activation of latent viruses hidden in the cell genome (see chapter 14). Henry Kaplan, a radiologist at Stamford University, and Ludwig Gross (29,46), a virologist of the U.S. Veteran's Service, New York City, were able to isolate a virus, called the radiation leukemia virus (RadLV), from a radiation-induced thymus lymphoma in mice.

Some tumors that were originally thought to be the result of radiation were later shown to contain viruses that were only activated by the radiation. The mouse mammary tumor virus (MuMTV) was found in breast tumors of mice following radiation (64). The osteosarcoma in mice produced following irradiation by the radioactive isotopes of strontium (^{90}Sr) and radium (^{224}Ra) was associated with the FBR virus (41).

The viruses activated by radiation are retroviruses. Their single-stranded RNA contains a reverse transcriptase enzyme which can synthesize a DNA provirus from the viral RNA. The incorporated provirus replicates with the host cell DNA and acts as a transforming agent (Note 2).

RNA VIRUSES

Only one group of the RNA viruses has the ability to transform normal cells of animals into cancer cells: the retroviruses (Table 15-1). They are characterized by the presence of a reverse transcriptase enzyme (see chapter 18). Neoplasms similar to those seen in man are produced by the retroviruses in species from fish to primates.

THE ONCOGENE CANCER (HUEBNER–TODARO) HYPOTHESIS

In 1969, after years of research with viruses, Robert Huebner and George Todaro, prominent virologists at the National Institutes of Health in Bethesda, Maryland, proposed a hypothesis concerning the origin of human cancer based on certain known facts (36):

1) C-type RNA virus particles have been found in almost all species of vertebrates examined (C-type refers to a classification of viruses by their size and configuration as seen by electron microscopy) (fig. 15-9).

2) C-type viruses have a role in the causation of "spontaneous" cancer of certain animal species. The DNA viruses (polyoma, SV40, and the adenoviruses) do not appear to be significant factors in the development of cancer in their natural hosts.

3) The types of cancer seen in the human where C-type viruses are not known to have a causative role are similar to those observed in mice and cats where C-type RNA viruses are known to be involved.

Huebner and Todaro suggested that cells of most or all vertebrate species have C-type RNA virus genomes that are vertically transmitted from parent to offspring. They postulated that:

". . . there exists a unique class of viruses present in most, and perhaps all, vertebrates that play[s] an important etiologic role in the development of tumors in these animals. The unique property transmitted from animal to progeny animal and from cell to progeny cell is a repressed viral genome. While full viral expression can occur, we postulate that more frequently there is only partial expression, with perhaps only the gene of the virus expressed being that responsible for transforming the cell into a tumor cell (the oncogene). The new hypothesis predicts that both spontaneous cancers and cancers induced by chemical and physical agents will be the result of expression of the oncogenes(s) of covert C-type RNA virus."

The Huebner-Todaro oncogene hypothesis postulated that cancer was an event determined by

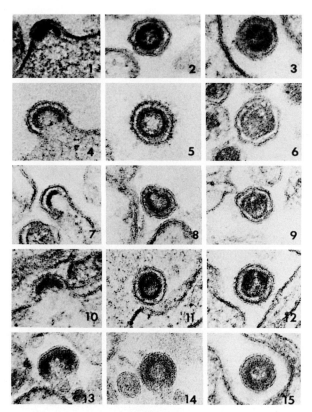

Figure 15-9
C-TYPE VIRUS
Electron microgram of C-type virus found in human placenta and in the placentae of rats and rhesus and baboon monkeys. The C-type virus was the basis for the Huebner-Todaro hypothesis that a virus caused human cancer (X165,000). (Fig. 100 from Gross L. Oncogenic viruses. 3rd ed, vol. 1 Oxford: Pergamon Press, 1983:1034).

spontaneous or induced derepression (release of a suppressor gene) of a latent specific viral gene. The viral gene contained the genes coding for the transformation of a normal cell to a cancer cell; it was named by Huebner and Todaro as "oncogene" (Greek: onco, tumor). Chemical, radiation, or genetic events might trigger the derepression of the viral gene, thereby releasing the oncogene to stimulate the proliferation of cells.

RNA Oncogenic Viruses (Retroviruses)

Of the many classes of RNA viruses only one group has been shown to have oncogenic action, the retroviruses (Table 15-1) (20,45). Retroviruses are found in a large number of animals and man. One retrovirus, human T-cell lymphocyte virus I (HTLV-I) causes human T-cell leukemia, a rare form of leukemia found in the northern and northeastern islands of Japan (66), the coastal regions of Central Africa, and less frequently, in Taiwan, the Caribbean basin (12), and in aborigines of Papua, New Guinea.

Another virus, human T-cell lymphocyte virus II (HTLV-II), is believed to cause a few cases of the rare "hairy cell" leukemia in humans (Table 15-2) (38,45).

The third, human T-cell lymphocyte virus III (HTLV-III), better known as the HIV (human immunodeficiency virus), is the agent causing the clinical disease AIDS (2,10). The HIV virus does not transform cells but infects T4 lymphocytes that are important in protecting the body against infections. With the infection and death of T4 lymphocytes and the loss of their immune response there is not only an increased risk for developing infections but an added complication occurs, the risk of malignant neoplasms. Kaposi's sarcoma and a malignant lymphoma are the neoplasms most commonly associated with AIDS (45).

THE VIRUS AS A SIGNIFICANT FACTOR IN CARCINOGENESIS

Epstein-Barr Virus and Hodgkin's Lymphoma

One of the cancers of the lymphatic system, the malignant lymphomas, is the well known Hodgkin's disease which was thought for some time to be an infectious disease but is now known to be a malignant neoplasm. Associated with it has been the presence of the Epstein-Barr virus (EBV) in many cases. The virus is present in the characteristic cell of the disease, the Reed-Sternberg cell, and in from 30 to 70 percent of its morphologic subtypes. A confounding factor is that a very high percentage of individuals throughout the world have been exposed to the EBV virus, usually in childhood or adolescence.

Patients with Hodgkin's disease often have a high serum titer of anti-EBV antigens. The virus can be demonstrated in the Reed-Sternberg cell by use of the LNP-1 antigen or by the in situ hybridization of EBER-1 antigen. There is a variable percentage distribution of the EBV virus in the different morphologic subtypes of Hodgkin's disease, with the highest frequency (62 percent) in the mixed cell group (22).

The *bcl*-2 oncogene is able to prevent the death of cells from apoptosis (programmed death of cells) (see chapter 17) by conferring a longer half life to the cell, which then permits cell repair. The EBV virus encodes the late membrane protein (LMP-1) which can up-regulate the bcl-2 protein and prevent death. The majority of Hodgkin's disease cells express abundant bcl-2 mRNA (34).

There are two strains of EBV, type A and B, that can be distinguished at three divergent gene loci. Fifteen EBV infected cell lines showed that EBV DNA was detected in about 70 percent of patients with Hodgkin's disease (47). The vast majority of Hodgkin's cells demonstrated high levels of bcl-2 mRNA and a protein pattern that suggests the possibility that a type of Hodgkin's disease originates in a germinal center of the lymph node (45).

A study of Hodgkin's disease in Mexico showed that EBV was detected in the nuclei of 42 percent of the Reed-Sternberg cells and that EBV encoded the late membrane protein (LMP-1) expression in 34 percent of cases (69). The authors believed that this corroborates a role for EBV in Hodgkin's disease, at least in some cases.

In a study of 116 cases of EBV-related Hodgkin's disease, overexpression of the *p53* gene occurred in 32 percent of the cases. EBV was noted in all cases, even in those that were *p53* negative. Overexpression of *p53* was heterogenous and there was no simple correlation between EBV infection and *p53* overexpression (51).

In a semiquantitative analysis of viral DNA in Swiss patients with Hodgkin's disease, Knecht et al. found an absence of EBV DNA in three cases with numerous Reed-Sternberg cells and the presence of only a few viral copies in four cases with numerous Reed-Sternberg cells (42). They concluded that the virus is a modulating rather than a causal factor.

Brousset et al. detected EBV mRNA in 30 percent of neoplastic cells from lymph node biopsies (11). The virus was demonstrated in the Reed-Sternberg and similar cells. The authors believed that there was a direct role for EBV in the pathogenesis of Hodgkin's disease. Normal and reactive lymph nodes were negative for EBV in 39 cases.

Does the presence of EBV in Reed-Sternberg cells in from about 30 to 70 percent of cases of Hodgkin's disease indicate a relationship that is incidental, modulating, or causal? With the present evidence it would appear that the presence of EBV is incidental.

Herpes Virus 8 and Kaposi's Sarcoma

The most common tumor complication of the AIDS disease is Kaposi's sarcoma which is 300 times more frequent in patients with AIDS than in

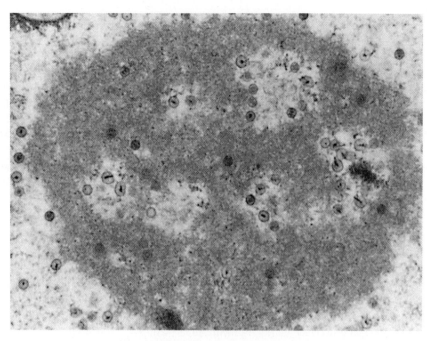

Figure 15-10
VIRUSES IN KAPOSI'S
SARCOMA IN AIDS
Electron micrograph of a nucleus in a cell of Kaposi's sarcoma in a patient with AIDS. Viral nucleocapsids (small circles) are present in the nucleus and cytoplasm. (Fig. 2a from Orenstein JM, Alkan S, Blauvelt A, et al. Visualization of human herpesvirus type 8 in Kaposi's sarcoma by light and transmission electron microscopy. AIDS 1997;11:39.)

those with other immunosuppressive diseases. Berel and colleagues of the Centers for Disease Control, Atlanta, Georgia, found that of 89,000 patients with AIDS, over 13,000 (15 percent) had Kaposi's sarcoma (6). Earlier, Knowles et al. of Columbia University pointed out the presence of a herpes-like DNA sequence in patients with AIDS-associated Kaposi's sarcoma (13).

Seroepidemiological studies by Lennette of Virolab, Berkeley, and associates of the University of California, San Francisco, showed that all patients with AIDS-associated Kaposi's sarcoma and 96 percent of American HIV-infected homosexual men were positive for the lytic antigen of human herpes virus 8 (HHV-8). In the American general population, 18 to 28 percent of older men were positive for HHV-8 antibodies (44).

Starkus et al. of the University of Minnesota investigated the possible link between HHV-8 and Kaposi's sarcoma at different stages of the disease. Kaposi's sarcoma-associated herpes virus (KSHV) was expressed by every tumor, from the earliest histologically recognized stage to the advanced stage. In situ hybridization with a mRNA-specific probe was used to demonstrate that the KSHV was present in the spindle-shaped tumor cells, which also stained with the immunochemical CD34 antigen known to be present in many Kaposi sarcoma cells (61).

Jan M. Orenstein of George Washington University and colleagues have demonstrated HHV-8 in tissues from three patients with AIDS-related Kaposi's sarcoma (53). EBV and cytomegalic (CMV) virus tested negative. Electron microscopy revealed herpes virus in spindle cells as well as mononucleated cells. A mRNA probe specific for HHV-8 RNA (T1.1) was used in an in situ hybridization test to identify the HHV-8 virus (fig. 15-10).

KSHV-encoded chemokines (chemoattractant cytokines) have been shown to have the potential to directly induce angiogenesis. The latter is an important feature of Kaposi's sarcoma (9).

These and other studies indicate that HHV-8 has to be considered to be more than a passenger virus and is a significant causal factor in the carcinogenesis of Kaposi's sarcoma.

THE CANCER CRUSADE

In 1971 the United States Congress and President Richard Nixon passed legislation which made available a relatively large amount of funds for cancer research in the hope that a cure of, or vaccine against, cancer might be more quickly achieved by this massive assault against the disease. The analogy was the successful mobilization of government, industry, and science to put a man on the moon and return him safely to earth.

R. A. Rettig has published a detailed study of the origin of the National Cancer Act (55). The strong influence of powerful citizens, political figures, and prominent scientists and physicians is discussed. The opposing views of basic scientists and clinical scientists are considered. The problems with the National Cancer Institute and its relation to cancer research and the other institutions at National Institutes of Health were examined. The book is a primer of the complex interplay of social, political, scientific, and public opinion influences involved in the progress of legislation from its inception to final resolution. It is an intriguing story of an important landmark in the funding of cancer research.

VIRUSES AS CAUSATIVE AGENTS IN CARCINOGENESIS

Viruses have been demonstrated to cause cancer in animals and to be involved in the genesis of some human cancers. Present evidence does not indicate that viruses play a causal role in most human cancers, but in some cases they appear to be the transforming agent.

REFERENCES

1. Baltimore D. RNA-dependant DNA polymerase in virions of RNA tumor viruses. Nature 1970;226:1209–11.
2. Barre-Sinoussi F, Chermann JC, Rey F, et al. Isolation of a T-lymphotropic retrovirus from a patient at risk for acquired immune deficiency syndrome (AIDS). Science 1983;220:868–71.
3. Bean WB. Walter Reed: a biography. Charlottesville: Univ. VA Press, 1982.
4. Behbehani AJ. The smallpox story: in words and pictures. Kansas City, KA: Univ. Kansas Med Ctr, 1988.
5. Beijerinck MW. Bemerkung zu dem Aufsatz von Herren Ivanowski über die Mosaikkrankheit der Tabakspflanze. Centralbl. f Bakt., Abt II, 1899;5:310–311.
6. Beral V, Peterman TA, Berkelman R, Jaffe HW. Kaposi's sarcoma among persons with AIDS: a sexually transmitted infection. Lancet 1990;335:123–6.
7. Bittner JJ. Some enigmas associated with the genesis of mammary cancer in mice. Cancer Res 1948;88:625–39.
8. Bittner JJ. Some possible effects of nursing on the mammary gland tumor incidence in mice. Science 1936;84:162.
9. Boshoff C, Endo Y, Collins PD, et al. Angiogenic and HIV-inhibitory functions of KSHV-encoded chemokines. Science 1997;278:290–4.
10. Broder S, Gallo RC. A pathogenic retrovirus (HTLV-III) linked to AIDS. N Engl J Med 1984;311:1292–7.
11. Brousset P, Chittal S, Schlaifer D, et al. Detection of Epstein-Barr virus messenger RNA in Reed-Sternberg cells of Hodgkin's disease by in situ hybridization with biotinylated probes on specially processed modified acetone methyl benzoate xylene (ModAMeX) section (see comments). Blood 1991;77:1781–6.
12. Catovsky D, Greaves MF, Rose M, et al. Adult T-cell lymphoma-leukemia in blacks from the West Indies. Lancet 1982;1:639–43.
13. Chang Y, Cesarman E, Pessin MS, et al. Identification of herpesvirus-like DNA sequence in AIDS-associated Kaposi's sarcoma. Science 1994;266:1865–9.
14. Cook PJ, Burkitt DP. Cancer in Africa. Br Med Bull 1971;27:14–20.
15. Cooper, G.M. Oncogenes. Boston: Jones & Bartlett, 1990:52.
16. Davis BD. The background: from classical to molecular genetics. In: Davis BD, ed. The genetic revolution. Baltimore: Johns Hopkins Univ. Press, 1991:8–27.
17. D'Herelle F. Sur an microbe invisible antagoniste des bacilles dysénteriques, Compt. rendus hebdomadaires des seances de la academis des sciences 1917;165:373–5.
18. Dulbecco R. The nature of viruses. In: Dulbecco R, Ginsberg HS, eds. Virology, 2nd ed. Philadelphia: JB Lippincott, 1988:1–26.
19. Dulbecco R. Oncogenic viruses: I, DNA-containing viruses. In: Dulbecco R, Ginsberg HS, eds. Virology. Philadelphia: JB Lippincott, 1988:335–54.
20. Dulbecco R. Oncogenic viruses: II, RNA-containing viruses (retrovirus). In: Dulbecco R, Ginsberg HS, eds. Virology. Philadelphia: JB Lippincott, 1988:355–83.
21. Elleman V, Bang, O. Experimentelle leukämia bei hühnern. Zentbl Bakt Parasitkde Orig Abt I 1908;46:595–609.
22. Enblad G, Sandvej K, Lennette E, et al. Lack of correlation between EBV serology and presence of EBV in the Hodgkin and Reed-Sternberg cells of patients with Hodgkin's disease. Int J Cancer 1997;72:394–7.
23. Epstein MA, Achong BG, Barry YM. Virus particles in cultured lymphoblasts from Burkitt's lymphoma. Lancet 1964;1:702–3.
24. Ewing J. Neoplastic diseases. A treatise on tumours, 2nd ed. Philadelphia: WB Saunders, 1922:119,133–4.
25. Finkel MP, Reilly CA. Observations suggesting the viral etiology of radiation-induced tumors, particularly osteogenic sarcoma. In: Sanders CL, Brusch RM, Ballon JE, Mahlum DD, eds. Radionuclide carcinogenesis. Oak Ridge, TN: U.S. Atomic Energy Comm, 1973:278–88.
26. Friedewald WF, Rous P. The initiating and promoting elements in tumor production. J Exp Med 1944;80:101–26.
27. Ginsberg HS. EB (Epstein-Barr) viruses and infectious mononucleosis. In: Dulbecco R, Ginsberg HS, eds. Virology. Philadelphia: JB Lippincott, 1988:174–7.

28. Ginsberg HS. Hepatitis viruses. In: Dulbecco R, Ginsberg HS, eds. Virology. Philadelphia: JB Lippincott, 1988:321–34.

29. Gross L. Attempt to recover a filterable agent from an x-ray-induced leukemia. Acta Haematol 1958;19:353–61.

30. Gross L. Oncogenic viruses. 3rd ed, vols 1, 2. Oxford: Pergamon Press, 1983:490–570.

31. Gross L. "Spontaneous" leukemia developing in C3H mice following inoculation in infancy with AK-leukemic extracts of AK-embryos. Proc Soc Exp Biol Med 1951;76:27–32.

32. Hadziyannis SJ, Giannoulis G, Hadziyannis E, et al. Hepatitis C virus infection in Greece and its role in chronic liver disease and hepatocellular carcinoma. J Hepatology 1933;17:S72–77.

33. Harvey JJ. An unidentified virus which causes the rapid production of tumors in mice. Nature 1964;204:1104–5.

34. Hell K, Lorenzen J, Fischer, R, Hansmann JL. Hodgkin cells accumulate mRNA for bcl-2. Lab Invest 1995;73:492–6.

35. Henle G, Henle W, Diehl V. Relation of Burkitt's tumor-associated herpes-type virus to infectious mononucleosis. Proc Natl Acad Sci USA 1968;59:94–101.

36. Huebner RJ, Todaro GJ. Oncogenes of RNA tumor viruses as determinants of cancer. Proc Natl Acad Sci USA 1969;64:1087–94.

37. Ivanowski DA.Über die Mosaikkrankheit der Tabakspflanze, 1894. Quoted by Shimkin MB. In: Contrary to Nature: being an illustrated commentary on some persons and events of historical importance of knowledge concerning cancer. Bethesda: U.S. Department of Health, Education, & Welfare, 1977:181–2.

38. Kalyanaraman VS, Sarngadharan MB, Robert-Guroff M, Miyoshi I, Golde D, Gallo RC. A new subtype of human T-cell leukemia virus (HTLV-II) associated with a T-cell variant of hairy cell leukemia. Science 1982;218:571–3.

39. Kirsten WH, Mayer LA. Morphologic responses to a murine erythroblastosis. JNCI 1967;39:311–35.

40. Klein G. Immunological studies on Burkitt's lymphoma. Postgrad Med J 1971;47:151–5.

41. Klein G. The role of gene dosage and genetic transpositions in carcinogenesis. Nature 1981;294:313–8.

42. Knecht H, Odermatt BF, Bachmann E, et al. Frequent detection of Epstein-Barr virus DNA by the polymerase chain reaction in lymph node biopsies from patients with Hodgkin's disease without genomic evidence of B- or T-cell clonality. Blood 1991;78:760–7.

43. Lederberg J. Genetic recombination in bacteria: a discovery account. Annu Rev Genet 1987;21:23–46.

44. Lennette ET, Blackbourn DJ, Levy JA. Antibodies to herpesvirus type 8 in the general population and in Kaposi's sarcoma. Lancet 1996;348:858–61.

45. Levine AJ. Viruses. New York: Scientific American Library, 1992:2, 7, 21, 24–45, 57–85, 88–103, 113–72, 176–93, 207–9.

46. Lieberman M, Kaplan H. Leukemogenic activity of filtrates from radiation-induced lymphoid tumors of mice. Science 1959;130:387–8.

47. Lin JC, Lin SC, De BK, Chan WC, Evatt BL, Chan WC. Precision of genotyping of Epstein-Barr virus by polymerase chain reaction predominance of type A virus associated with Hodgkin's disease. Blood 1993;81:3372–81.

48. Lucké B. Carcinoma in the leopard frog: its probable causation by a virus. J Exper Med 1938;68:457–68.

49. Moloney JB. A virus-induced rhabdomyosarcoma of mice. Natl Cancer Inst Monogr 1966;22:139–42.

50. Murphy EL, Bryzman S, Williams AE, et al. Demographic determinants of hepatitis C virus seroprevalence among blood donors. JAMA 1996;275:995–1000.

51. Niedobitek G, Rowlands DC, Young LS, et al. Overexpression of p53 in Hodgkin's disease: lack of correlation with Epstein-Barr virus infection. J Pathol 1993;169:207–12.

52. Old LJ, Boyse EA, Oettgen HJ, et al. Precipitating antibody in human serum to an antigen present in cultured Burkitt's lymphoma cells. Proc Natl Acad Sci USA 1966;56:1699–704.

53. Orenstein JM, Aikan S, Blauvelt A, et al. Visualization of human herpesvirus type 8 in Kaposi's sarcoma by light and transmission electron microscopy. AIDS 1997;11:F35–F45.

54. Reed W, Carroll J, Agramonte A, Lazear JW. The etiology of yellow fever. A preliminary note. Phil Med J 1900;6:790–6.

55. Rettig RA. Cancer crusade: the story of the National Cancer Act of 1971. Princeton: Princeton Univ. Press, 1977.

56. Rous P. A sarcoma of the fowl transmissible by an agent separable from the tumor cells. J Exp Med 1911;13:397–411.

57. Rous P. Transmission of a malignant new growth by means of a cell-free filtrate. JAMA 1911;56:198.

58. Rous P. The virus tumors and the tumor problem. Harvey Lectures 1935–1936;31:74–115.

59. Rous P, Beard JW. The progression to carcinomas of virus-induced rabbit papilloma (Shope). J Exp Med 62:523–48.

60. Shope RE. A filtrable virus causing a tumor-like condition in rabbits and its relationship to virus myxomatosum. J Exp Med 1932;56:803–22.

61. Starkus KA, Zhong W, Gebhard K, et al. Kaposi's sarcoma-associated herpesvirus gene expression in endothelial (spindle) tumor cells. J Virol 1997;71:715–9.

62. Stewart SE, Eddy BE, Gochenour AM, Borgese G, Grubbs GE. The induction of neoplasms with a substance released from mouse tumors by tissue culture. Virology 1957;3:380–400.

63. Temin H, Mizutani S. RNA-dependant DNA polymerase in virions of Rous sarcoma virus. Nature 1970;226:1211–3.

64. Timmermans A, Bentvel zen P, Hagerman PC, Calafat J. Activation of a mammary tumor virus in 020 strain mice by irradiation and urethane. J Gen Vir 1969;104:619–21.

65. Twort FW. An investigation of the nature of ultra-microscopic viruses. Lancet 1915;2:1241–3.

66. Uuhiyama T, Yodoi J, Sagawa J, Takatsuki K, Uchino H. Adult T-cell leukemia: clinical and hematological features of 16 cases. Blood 1977;50:481–92.

67. Vogt P, Dulbecco R. Virus-cell interaction with a tumor producing virus. Proc Natl Acad Sci USA 1960;46:365–70.

68. Wold WS, Green M. Historic milestones in cancer virology. Semin Oncol 1979;6:461–78.

69. Zarate-Osorno A, Roman LN, Kingma, DW, Meneses-Garcia A, Jaffe ES. Hodgkin's disease in Mexico. Prevalence of Epstein-Barr virus sequences and correlations with histologic subtype. Cancer 1995;75:1360–6.

70. Zinder ND, Lederberg J. Genetic exchange in Salmonella. J Bacteriol 1952;64:679–99.

71. zur Hausen H. Molecular pathogenesis of cancer of the cervix and its causation by specific human papilloma virus types. Curr Top Microbiol Immunol 1994;186:131–56.

It was recognized early in man's history that he could recover from some infectious diseases but that the disease might recur, once or several times (69). A few diseases, smallpox (3), plague, and measles, when not fatal gave rise to immunity from subsequent attacks. The mechanism of immunity was not known. Since the body could develop lifelong resistance to some diseases and temporary resistance to others, was there a comparable resistance to cancer? Could the body build up an immunity, temporary or permanent, to cancer just as it did to some infectious diseases?

TRANSPLANTATION OF CANCER

Human to Human

At various periods in history it was believed by many that cancer was a contagious disease (see chapter 12). In the late 18th century and beginning 19th century attempts were made to test whether cancer could be passed from one person to another.

James Nooth, an English surgeon, ". . . conveyed a minute portion" of a tumor of the female breast into ". . . a small incision on my arm." In 1777 he repeatedly performed the same experiment with the same result: there was only a local inflammatory reaction which soon ". . . perfectly healed" (54).

In 1808, Jean Louis Alibert, a leading French dermatologist and physician to Louis XVIII, allowed himself to be injected with breast cancer tissue from a patient to determine whether cancer was a contagious disease (2). A medical student and two other men also underwent the same procedure. After a temporary local inflammatory reaction at the site of the injection there were no subsequent reactions. A week later Alibert and a colleague repeated the same procedure. Alibert had the same slight inflammatory reaction at the injection site and his colleague developed a more severe response which involved the axillary and cervical lymph nodes. This was before the germ theory of disease was conceived and the response may have been a septic infection of the wound caused by bacteria. Alibert concluded that cancer was not contagious.

C.M. Southam and colleagues of the Sloan-Kettering Institute subcutaneously transplanted human cancer cells into 20 healthy male human volunteers: the result was transient growth of the transplants followed by complete regression in 3 or 4 weeks (35). Injection of a suspension of human epidermoid cancer cells into healthy volunteers resulted in the growth of a nodule of cancer cells in the subcutaneous tissue of the thigh in about three quarters of the volunteers. All nodules regressed, usually within 7 weeks. In patients with advanced cancer, the regression of the nodule, produced under similar circumstances, was delayed in the majority of cases (71).

Melanoma, a cancer, has been transplanted in a few cases from a pregnant mother through the placenta to her child, resulting in the death of the child within months after birth (12).

Human or Animal to Animal

Many attempts in the 19th century to transplant cancers from humans to animals failed (56,67). Transplantation of cancer from one animal to another was also unsuccessful until 1875 when N. A. Novinsky, a Russian veterinary student, transplanted small fragments of an invasive cancer of the nose of a female dog to 1-month-old puppy. The transplant grew and 2 months later fragments of the tumor were transplanted into three puppies. One transplant metastasized to a lymph node (56).

Novinsky also transplanted a sarcoma of the uterus from a 6-year-old female dog into two puppies. Two months later a tumor the size of a hazel nut appeared in each of the puppies. The histology of the transplanted tumor was similar to that of the original tumor. A decade after Novinsky, A. N. Hanau, a German pathologist, successfully transplanted a metastatic cancer of the vulva from one rat into another rat (31).

A. E. Moore and A. C. Caparo of the Sloan-Kettering Institute injected filtrates and tissue culture preparations of human cancers, benign lesions, and normal tissues into about 4,000 newborn mice. About 10 percent of the animals given inoculations of malignant lymphoma developed tumors compared to about 4 percent of uninoculated controls. Preparations of other malignant lesions did not show an increase of tumors over control mice. It was believed that the increase of tumors from inoculated malignant lymphoma material was caused by the activation of tumor viruses already present in the mice (53).

Animal to Animal

Leo Loeb, a pioneer oncologist at Washington University, St. Louis, had shown in 1901 that it was possible to transplant the cancers of animals into other animals of the same species and strain. He transplanted a sarcoma through 40 generations in rats of the same strain and a thyroid cancer through seven generations of the same strain (47,48).

Loeb also investigated a strain of waltzing mice that had been bred in Japan for centuries. He found a tumor that could be transplanted to successive generations of these mice but which failed to grow when injected into mice of a different strain. When the Japanese waltzing mice were bred with mice of another strain, however, the progeny were found to be susceptible to a transplant of the tumor from the waltzing mice, indicating that the susceptibility to transplantation was inherited in the progeny (46). E. E. Tyzzer, an early cancer investigator from the United States, concluded that susceptibility to transplantation of the tumor was a dominant inherited characteristic (78).

As a result of many investigations it was concluded that: transplantation of tumors into a foreign species invariably failed; transplantation into unrelated members of the same species usually failed; and autografts (grafts into animals of the same strain) almost invariably were successful. The closer the "blood relationship" between donor and recipient the more likely the graft would be successful. It was also recognized that a period of days occurred between the primary engraftment and its eventual rejection. A second graft was rejected in a shorter period of time than the first (65,69).

IMMUNE MECHANISMS

The mechanism behind the immune process was first considered in regard to humoral factors because of the Humoral Doctrine (8). Later, in the 1850s Virchow focused attention on the cell as the site of disease response but the details of the immune process were not known.

Cellular Immunity

After the epochal discoveries of Pasteur, Koch, and others which gave rise to the germ theory of disease, humoral factors became important. It was found that some cells were present in inflammatory reactions, and because bacteria often could be seen within these cells, it was believed that they might be a factor in the body's defense system (8,68). Ely Metchnikoff, a Russian zoologist working at the Pasteur Institute in Paris, suggested in 1884 that a blood cell, the monocyte, was important in the immune response (51). He also believed that the pus formed in response to bacterial infections was a protective response of the body; the pus contained a number of white blood cells, including phagocytes (Greek: eating cells). Metchnikoff discovered phagocytic action of cells in transparent starfish larvae when they surrounded little thorns from a tangerine tree that he placed within the larvae. The cells that could move freely throughout the larvae were massed about the thorns. Metchnikoff proposed that the phagocytes in the pus constituted the first line of defense against disease because of their ability to ingest and destroy bacteria.

Humoral Immunity

In 1888, a few years after Metchnikoff's suggestion, von Behring and Kitasato in Germany found a powerful toxin in filtrates of the diphtheria bacillus which when injected into rabbits killed them. However, if the toxin were given in smaller repeated doses over a period of time, an immunity developed which could protect the immunized rabbits against a dose of diphtheria toxin that would kill nonimmunized rabbits. The immunity could be passed on to nonimmunized rabbits by injecting them with serum from the blood of the immunized rabbits. The serum from the immunized rabbits contained something, named an antitoxin, that protected the nonimmunized rabbits; it was called diphtheria antitoxin (4).

Soon protection was provided against other infectious diseases by injecting killed bacteria into animals and humans so that protective substances against the bacteria, called antibodies, would be formed by the immune system. These antibodies could be demonstrated in the serum of the protected individuals. The immune serum from patients or animals containing these antibodies could be injected into other humans or animals, respectively, to give them the same immunity against the disease.

At the end of the 19th century the serum antitoxins and antibodies were considered to be the main defensive weapons against infectious agents (69). The cellular response was considered to be less important.

Antigen-Antibody Relationships

Agents that provoked a host to respond to its presence by producing antibodies in the serum of a human or animal were called antigens. The antibodies produced by the antigens were highly specific, i.e., the antigens reacted with antibodies that they induced or to antibodies closely related to them, and antibodies reacted only with the antigens that instigated them. A serum with protective antibodies against one disease did not protect the animal or patient against other diseases.

Antigens might be bacteria, parasites, foreign bodies, proteins, polysaccharides, nucleoproteins, lipoproteins, polypeptides, or small molecules linked to protein. Antibodies were globular proteins called immunoglobulins.

If the body could normally develop antibodies that counteracted the effects of some bacteria, parasites, and a host of chemical compounds, could it develop, in similar fashion, antibodies or antitoxins against cancer? To answer this question it is important to know how the body killed or rebuffed infectious agents in those diseases that were successfully combated.

Ehrlich's Side Chain Hypothesis. Paul Ehrlich (1854–1915), a German investigator and a pioneer in the field of immunology (fig. 16-1), had studied with the famous German chemist Emil Fischer and had maintained an interest in the relationship between chemical structure and biological function. To explain the immune response to infectious agents he proposed a hypothesis explaining how an antigen caused the formation of an antibody.

Since antibodies were specific for some antigens and not for others, Ehrlich reasoned that the cells of the body that made the antibody must have receptors on their surface that permitted recognition of the antigen. The chemical binding of the antigen and antibody then occurred on the surface of the cell. He suggested that immunologic specificity was caused by a unique stereochemical relationship wherein the active sites on the antigen and the antibody fitted together like a lock and key (15). This was the "side chain" hypothesis (fig. 16-2).

By the 1930s it was known that antibodies were proteins but it was not known how antibodies to the millions of possible antigens that conceivably might impinge on a cell could be synthesized. The vertebrate animals did not seem to possess enough genes, if one gene were required for one antibody as

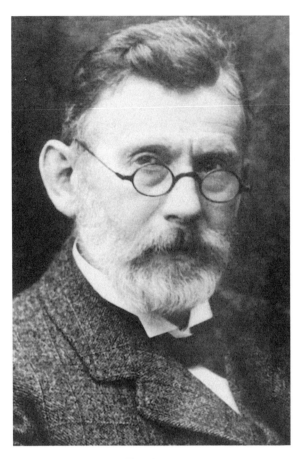

Figure 16-1
PAUL EHRLICH

German investigator who formulated an early hypothesis to explain antibody formation; he also used chemotherapy to treat syphilis. (Fig. 1.1 from Ada G, Nossal G. The clonal-selection theory. In: Paul WE, ed. Immunology, recognition and response. Readings from Scientific American magazine. New York: WH Feeman, 1991:5.)

then thought, to give rise to the millions of different antibodies that might be required for the number of potential antigens to which cells might be exposed.

The Clonal Theory of Immunity. A concept espoused by F. M. Burnet, an Australian pathologist (9), W. K. Jerne, a Danish scientist (36), and D. W. Talmadge, a microbiologist in Colorado (75), offered what appeared to be the best explanation for the process. It was called the clonal theory of immunity.

The theory postulated that one type of antibody was present normally on the surface of each cell of the immune system that generated that antibody. Cells had developed antibodies and stored them on the surface of the lymphocytes over the long period of evolution. A presenting antigen selected the cell

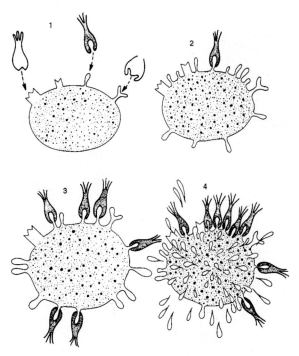

Figure 16-2
SIDE CHAIN HYPOTHESIS
Ehrlich's side chain theory suggested that antibodies existed with specific receptors resting on cell surfaces. Antigens with specific shapes (black bodies) that fitted the specific receptor of the antibodies interlocked with them (key and lock analogy). (Fig. 1.2 from Ada G, Nossal G. The clonal-selection theory. In: Paul WE, ed. Immunology, recognition and response. Readings from Scientific American Magazine. New York: WH Freeman, 1991:6.)

with the matching antibody receptor (the key and lock metaphor), became bound to the cell surface, and caused that cell to multiply. The cell proliferated into a clone of cells with the same antigen specificity as the original parent cell (fig. 16-3). It differentiated into a plasma cell which then synthesized the specific antibody matching the antigen.

Immunoglobulins

Gerald Edelman of Rockefeller University (13) and Rodney Porter then of Cambridge University (58), discovered independently that the immunoglobulins were composed of four units, called chains. Each antibody possessed two identical heavy chains and two identical light chains. All the subunits of immunoglobulins are divided into variable (V), constant (C), diverse (D), and joining (J) segments. A light chain and a heavy chain form an active site for recognition of the antibody, thereby increasing the diversity of response because of the number of possible pair combinations. The further division of the antibody into different parts of the light and heavy chains increased the possible combinations of types of antibodies that could be synthesized.

Families of Genes

An intricate mechanism by which the genome was able to increase further the number of different antibodies that could be produced was discovered

Figure 16-3
CLONAL HYPOTHESIS
SELECTION
Each cell makes one type of antibody; antigen (red dot) recognizes the corresponding receptor (Y-shaped body) and combines with it, setting cell into division, and secreting receptors (Y-shaped figures). (Fig. 1.3 from Ada G, Nossal G. The clonal-selection theory. In: Paul WE, ed. Immunology, recognition and response. Readings from Scientific American magazine. New York: WH Freeman, 1991:8.)

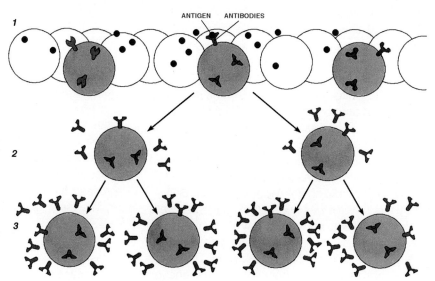

by S. Tonegawa, a Japanese investigator at the Basel Institute of Immunology (77). Tonegawa found that the immunoglobulin was encoded by four different sets or families of mini-genes located in widely separated genes in the genome. These coded for different parts of the immunoglobulin. Almost two million combinations of the mini-gene were possible. Other factors further increased this number (55).

Following World War II there was an explosive growth of immunological studies and attention was focused on the role of cells in the immune response. The immune system's response to disease is complicated and involves many types of host blood cells and cells of the immune system. The most important cells reacting to the antigen of a foreign substance were the white cells of the blood, particularly the lymphocyte, the plasma cell, and the macrophages (phagocytes). The lymphocyte played a predominant role (19,44).

Cellular Immunity

The Lymphocyte. The pioneer studies of Paul Ehrlich, a German investigator, in which he introduced the differential staining of the different types of white cells (leukocytes) of blood smeared on a glass slide, initiated studies of hematopoiesis (Greek: generation of blood). The ability to differentiate the various types of white blood cells, i.e., polymorphonuclear leukocytes, lymphocytes, monocytes, phagocytes, eosinophiles, and basophiles, led to the understanding of many diseases (14).

The lymphocyte was shown to comprise two major classes of cells: the T cell and the B cell (44,61). Subsequently, it was discovered that cells involved in the immune response secreted a group of low molecular weight proteins that were involved in cell-to-cell communication. They were called cytokines. Those secreted by lymphocytes were called lymphokines.

The discovery of monoclonal antibodies (MoAb) (see below) has allowed the different stages in the maturation of the leukocytes to be identified by markers. Cancers arising from different stages of development may present clinically different behavior and laboratory findings (42,45).

B- and T-Cell Lymphocytes. It has been estimated that there are about 10^{12} (a thousand billion) lymphocytes in the adult human body, about 5 to 10 percent of all the cells in the body. The lymphocytes arise from stem cells in the bone marrow and thymus, migrate through the body via the blood and lymph, and are most prevalent in the lymph nodes, spleen, and thymus. Lymphocytes continuously circulate through the blood and lymphatic systems (61).

As mentioned above, there are two major types of lymphocytes: the T-cell lymphocytes which originate from stem cells in the thymus gland and the B-cell lymphocytes which, in man, arise from stem cells in the bone marrow (fig. 16-4). The B cell lymphocytes, lymphocytes primarily involved in the cellular immune response, circulate for a short while in the blood and then home into lymphoid organs. They represent the humoral phase of the immune response. Later, they enter the blood again, recirculate, and migrate to secondary lymphoid organs. When the B cell encounters an antigen it begins to divide into two types of cells: plasma cells and memory cells. The plasma cell is a nonreplicating cell which synthesizes an antibody, an immunoglobulin specific for the antigen encountered.

The T cell lymphocytes deal with intracellular agents such as viruses and bacteria and are involved primarily in the cellular phase of the immune response. The lymphokine compounds that they secrete regulate cellular responses and activities of B-cell lymphocytes and other lymphocytes. They are involved in other aspects of the immune response. In some functions both B and T lymphocytes are involved.

There are two major subgroups of T-cell lymphocytes: T helper (T_H) cells and T cytotoxic (T_C) cells. Generally, the T helper (T_H) and cytotoxic (T_C) lymphocytes display the CD8 marker (see below). The cells are effector cells which secrete various lymphokines. The T_C lymphocytes differentiate into an effector cell called a cytotoxic T lymphocyte (CTL) which is involved in the elimination of virus-infected cells, tumor cells (fig. 16-5), and cells of a foreign tissue graft.

In the antigen-antibody immune response, the antigen of a foreign substance reacts with the macrophages whose enzymes break down the antigen into a sequence of amino acids and then present the fragments to a T-cell or B-cell lymphocyte.

Some T cells have receptors which bind to major histocompatibility complex (MHC) class II molecules (see below) and are known as killer T-cell lymphocytes (T_K). Another subset of lymphocytes is known as the natural killer (NK) lymphocytes and function in the rejection of grafts, immunity against tumors, and the regulation of hematopoiesis (blood cell growth

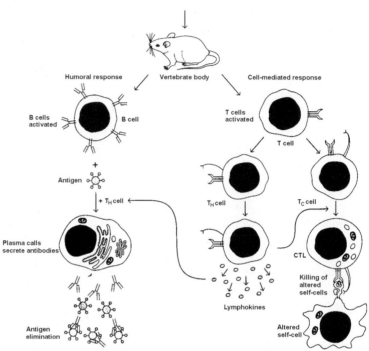

Figure 16-4

PATHWAYS OF DEVELOPMENT OF
DIFFERENT TYPES OF LYMPHOCYTES

B-cell and T-cell lymphocytes, and plasma
cells in the humoral and cell-mediated response system. (Fig. 1.7 from Kuby J. Immunology. New York: WH Freeman, 1992:11.)

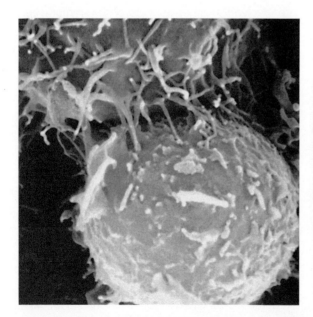

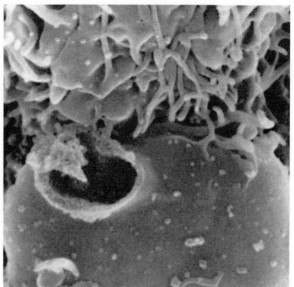

Figure 16-5

A LYMPHOCYTE ATTACKING A TUMOR CELL

Left: A cytotoxic killer cell lymphocyte (upper cell) attacking a tumor cell (bottom cell). The pseudopods of the killer lymphocyte
attach to the tumor cell and secrete a protein which has opened up pores in the tumor cell membrane.

Right: The tumor cell has lost its villi and has a large hole in its cell membrane. Holes permit the entrance of fluids which cause the cell
to swell and this is soon followed by the death of the tumor cell. (Fig. 7.1 from Young JD, Cohn ZA. How killer cells kill. In: Paul WE, ed.
Immunology, recognition and response. Readings from Scientific American Magazine. New York: WH Freeman, 1991:84,85.)

and maturity). The NK lymphocytes, neither T nor B cells, may act directly against cells containing foreign antigens on their surface (18).

There are a variety of substances, interferons and interleukins, which enhance the action of the NK lymphocytes. Mice lacking NK lymphocytes have more extensive metastatic growth of some transplanted tumors than do mice that have NK lymphocytes (55).

There is also a subset of lymphocytes called suppressor T-cell lymphocytes (Ts) which may modulate both T and B lymphocytes by suppressing the replication, maturation, and/or functions of these cells (44).

Macrophages, in collaboration with T- and B-cell lymphocytes and in the presence of antigens of cancer cells, may be activated by nonspecific cytokines (see below).

Cytokines. The complex interactions between the cells of the immune system are mediated by a group of secreted, low molecular weight proteins called cytokines (44). Cytokines regulate and modify the actions of the cells of the immune system. They were discovered when the supernatant of the culture media in which lymphocytes were growing was found to contain factors that could regulate proliferation, differentiation, and maturation of many types of lymphoid and accessory cells. Among these factors were T-cell growth factor, B-cell growth factor, B-cell differentiation factor, mitogenic protein, and many other proteins. When the factors were finally defined chemically a standardized nomenclature designated most of them as "interleukins" because of their cellular communication among leukocytes. Interleukin 1 had been previously ascribed under the names of at least eight factors and interleukin 2 accounted for the activities ascribed to four factors. For example, a cell line of helper T (TH) cells is dependent on interleukin 2 (IL-2) for continuous growth; IL-2 also enhances the activity of some NK and TC cells. Interleukin 1 (IL-1) originally was obtained from culture medium in which activated macrophages were growing. The list of numbered interleukins comprises at least ten and several other cytokines have been named for their biologic activity.

Some abnormalities in cytokine function are related to neoplasia. A beta (β) cell myeloma secretes IL-6 which serves as a stimulator of its own growth (autocrine secretion) (44). A cytokine tumor necrosis factor, alpha (TNFα), has been isolated and chemically defined as a protein by Lloyd Olds, S. Green, and colleagues of Sloan Kettering Institute (44). It was later further defined as a polypeptide that is produced by macrophages. It can kill some cancer cells and affects vascular endothelium, giving rise to hemorrhagic necrosis of tumors. It is important in the process of inflammation and acts in conjunction with other cytokines to produce its effects (57).

Histocompatibility Systems. Skin grafts and organ transplants are rejected by animals of a strain different than the donor animal. The mechanisms involved in such rejection were studied by G. D. Snell of the Jackson Laboratory, Bar Harbor, Maine and Peter Gorer of London (28,70). The rejection or acceptance of a transplanted organ, such as skin, from one strain of mice to a different strain is regulated by a set of genes called the major histocompatibility complex (MHC). A comparable set of genes in the human is called the human lymphocyte antigen (HLA) complex. The gene complexes encode cell surface glycoproteins on donor cells that act as antigens. These are important for cellular interactions concerning the recognition of "self" (like) and "non-self" (non-like) cells and tissues. One group, called the class I genes, includes a self-recognition system and is present on all somatic cells. These genes are involved in the immune response to cell-bound antigens and permit the recognition of similar "self" cells and dissimilar "non-self" foreign cells as well as cells altered by viruses or chemicals.

When a tissue such as skin from one human is grafted onto the skin of another human it is the recognition by the host's lymphocytes of the HLA system that indicates that the donor graft is foreign and sets in motion the well known transplantation rejection response. The skin graft dies in a matter of days and is sloughed off (Note 1). Cells of the same strain of mice which had the proper glycoprotein antigens on their surface were recognized as "self" by the MHC lymphocytes, were not attacked, and the graft was accepted by the host's cells (70).

Note 1: There are about 32 different genes in the class I mouse MHC system. Each genetically distinct inbred strain expresses a distinctive set of MCH glycoprotein antigens on the surface of its cells. These antigens are the target antigens for signaling an attack by a special class of lymphocytes, the cytolytic T-cell lymphocytes (CTL). When the lymphocytes attack unlike or "non-self" cells, the latter are lysed and killed (28,70).

TUMOR REJECTION

Some tumors in animals are recognized as "foreign" to a strain and are rejected because of incompatibility with the MHC system. Loss or decreased expression of class I MHC antigens has been found in some animal and human cancers. With tumor progression, the recognition markers of some tumor cells are altered or lost. A mouse leukemia strain (AKR) that did not express a MCH antigen on its surface was relatively resistant to killing by T_K lymphocytes and when injected into the rodents grew into a tumor. In contrast, an AKR leukemia cell strain whose cells expressed an MHC antigen that was regarded as foreign required a thousandfold greater number of cells to produce a tumor when injected into the mice (44). Many known human epithelial cancers express little or no class I antigens on their surface—mammary carcinomas, choriocarcinomas, epidermoid carcinomas, and colorectal carcinomas—and they are not rejected by the MHC system (44).

Paradoxically, attempts to protect animals against tumor growth by active immunization with tumor antigens or by passive immunization with antitumor antibodies resulted in enhancing the growth of the tumors. Blocking agents of various types have been suggested to cause these effects (44).

Another set of histocompatibility genes, those of class II, is concerned with the response to soluble antigens and communications between cells involved in the regulation of the immune response. Class II genes are active in regulating antibody response to certain foreign antigens. Activation of lymphocytes by a foreign antigen requires the presentation of the foreign antigen in conjunction with MHC class II cell surface markers.

A third set of histocompatibility genes, class III, controls the expansion of certain components of the complement system involved in the clotting of blood (29,45).

With the advent of highly inbred strains of mice and the recognition of the histocompatibility system (MHC) it was thought that the rejection of tumor transplants was the result of a different system in the tissues of mice of a different strain. Many concluded that tumor cells had no distinct immunological features other than the MHC antigens (40).

In 1943, Ludwig Gross showed that an inbred line of mice could be immunized against its "own" tumor, independently of the MHC system. He used a methylcholanthrene (MCA)-produced sarcoma in C3H mice and immunized against the tumor by repeated intradermal injection of a relatively small number of tumor cells. Later, the transplantation of a much larger tumor inoculum was rejected (30).

E. J. Foley of the Harvard Dana-Farber research group reported on his studies of a chemically-induced sarcoma in C3H mice that could be transplanted to mice of the same strain. The tumor was surgically ligated after it had grown in mice; necrosis of the tumor followed. A subsequent transplantation of a second chemically-induced sarcoma to the mice whose first tumor was ligated resulted in its rejection. It was assumed that the product of the necrosis of the ligated tumor acted as an antigen on the mouse's immune system so that an immune response was instigated which caused the rejection of the second tumor graft (23).

The strain of mice on which the sarcomas were grafted was one in which mammary carcinomas arose spontaneously. When a spontaneously arising mammary carcinoma was transplanted to the mice that had been pregrafted with the chemically-induced sarcoma and the sarcoma was subsequently ligated, the mammary carcinoma did not cause an immune response and grew without difficulty. This showed that the rejection of the sarcoma as a second graft in the animals with the ligated sarcoma was not the result of histocompatibility differences since the sarcoma and mammary cancer were from mice of the same highly inbred strain. The antigen which produced the immunity must have resided in the sarcoma that was ligated; the immunity was against the sarcoma antigen and not against a breast carcinoma antigen.

TUMOR-SPECIFIC
TRANSPLANTATION ANTIGENS

Tumor-specific transplantation antigens (TSTA) had been shown by the work of Foley (23), Prehn and Main (59), and George and Eva Klein (41) to occur in chemically-induced tumors. The antigens were individually specific for a tumor cell line and did not recognize other tumor cell lines induced in the same animal strain by the same chemical carcinogen. TSTAs were demonstrated on the surface of tumor cells but occasionally they were cytoplasmic proteins which were processed to peptides and presented with class I MHC molecules on the surface of the tumor cell (44). In contrast, virus-induced tumors expressed antigens common to all tumors induced by the same virus. If mice were injected with killer cells from a polyoma-produced tumor they developed an immunity and were protected against subsequent challenge from live cells from a polyoma-induced tumor (44).

Hewitt and colleagues, British investigators, reported that none of 27 murine tumors of spontaneous origin exhibited any TSTA immunogenicity (33). Regression or rejection of tumor was never observed when transplants of spontaneous tumors were used in the same strain of animal. These results were the opposite of the immune response to chemical- and viral-induced tumors (52). There was also no cross-reactivity rejections in many virally-induced cancers. Hewitt's findings seemed to reduce the possibility that antigens might be found in human tumors.

The animal host response to TSTA was found to be analogous to transplantation immunity in that lymphocytes played a prominent role in both types of reaction. Serum in reactive animals was not cytotoxic to the tumor cells nor could it confer passive immunity.

Viral antigens have not generally been found in human cancers but the nuclei of the Burkitt lymphoma cells of children have been shown to possess an antigen of the Epstein-Barr virus (EBV). The squamous cancer cells of the nasopharynx tumors of patients in India also contain the EBV nuclear antigen (20).

IMMUNE SURVEILLANCE HYPOTHESIS

One of the early prominent hypotheses concerning the cause of cancer was reintroduced in the 1960s and 1970s when spectacular advances were being made in the field of immunology. Since the immune system could develop an offense against some bacteria, parasites, viruses, and other foreign agents, it was believed that it might also have in its armamentarium a method for dealing with abnormal cells such as cancer cells. There was postulated the existence of an immune system that surveyed the cells in the body and that would remove or destroy abnormal ones; it was called the immune surveillance mechanism. Failure of this protective mechanism would result in cancer (44).

The hypothesis of immune surveillance was first suggested in 1909 by Paul Ehrlich (16). It was revived in 1959 by Lewis Thomas, a medical scientist and biology watcher in the United States (76)

and by F. M. Burnet of Australia (10) who developed the hypothesis in more detail. Evidence supporting the hypothesis was the observation by R.A. Gatti and R.A. Good of the University of Minnesota, of the high frequency of malignant neoplasms in children with inherited immune deficiency (26). Patients who received kidney transplants and were given immunosuppressive drugs later had a high incidence of cancers (72). George Klein of Stockholm has indicated that there is little evidence for the existence of such a mechanism in some cases but that there is evidence in other cases (39). O. Stuttman from Sloan-Kettering Institute has found little evidence in favor of such a concept except possibly under special circumstances, i.e., with polyoma oncogenesis, other DNA viruses, and feline leukemia virus (74). With regard to why tumor-associated antigens occur in experimentally produced animal tumors and not in spontaneous tumors of animals and humans, George Klein suggested that spontaneous tumors develop over a longer period of time thereby permitting a small number of aberrant cells to avoid the host immune system, to be favored in growth, and then evolve into a clone of cancer cells (39).

ATTEMPTS TO INCREASE HOST RESPONSE

There have been attempts to increase immune reactions by treating animals or humans with a nonspecific immune stimulant such as the bacillus Calmette-Guerin (BCG) (17) which had been used as an antituberculosis vaccine. The results with BCG were generally not successful (24).

A lymphokine, interleukin 2 (IL-2), turned a poorly immunogenic tumor into a strongly immunogenic one when introduced into the poorly immunogenic murine colon cancer line of cells (21). Cytokine gene therapy has been attempted in the laboratory and in human cell lines. Gene transfection of tumor cells by the IL-2 genes stimulated a histocompatibility (MHC) class I restricted–cytolytic T lymphocyte (CTL) response against the parental tumor (25). IL-2 and interferon gamma (IFN-gamma) are produced following the antigen-induced activation of helper lymphocytes. The cytokines are formed in the engineered tumor cells after the transduction of the cytokine genes and the induction of a generation of cytotoxic T lymphocytes. They have been used against human melanoma cell lines (22). It is not known whether poorly immunogenic or nonimmunogenic tumors can have their immunogenic responses activated or increased (50).

More recently, IL-2 has been used in humans in the attempt to stimulate host immune response against metastatic cancers. S. Rosenberg et al. of the National Institutes of Health have used concentrations of lymphokine-activated killer lymphocytes (LAK) in association with IL-2 in therapy against some cancers, but with mixed results (62–64). IL-2 seems to have no direct effect on cancer cells but as a cytokine produced by lymphocytes it can stimulate the growth of activated lymphocytes, the killer lymphocytes, that can lyse tumor cells. In addition, antitumor effects occurred after IL-2 expanded the number of T cells with specific MHC-restricted recognition of human tumor antigens, which resulted in the death of target cells. Dramatic regression of the tumors has been reported in a small percentage of patients with metastatic melanoma and renal cell cancers. These results establish the fact that regression can be brought about in selected cases for some months (62–64). However, as pointed out by E. Kedar of the Hebrew University-Hadassah Medical School of Jerusalem and Eva Klein of the Karolinska Institute of Stockholm, in an extensive survey of clinical and experimental immunotherapy of cancer (37), there are major problems with the immunologic approach that must be solved before any significant lasting therapeutic results can be expected in the treatment of human cancer.

HUMAN CANCER ANTIGENS

Carcinoembryonic Antigen

P. Gold and S.O. Freedman of Montreal, Canada, isolated a substance from a human colon cancer, injected it into the rabbit, and produced antibodies against the substance (27). The rabbit antibodies were used to test the serum of the colon cancer patients to see if there was a specific antigen-antibody reaction between them: if the antigen-antibody reaction occurred it would indicate that there was an antigen specific for that cancer, which would have shed into the bloodstream.

Results showed that many patients with cancer of the gastrointestinal tract shed an antigen into the bloodstream; this antigen could be detected and measured by its reaction with rabbit antibodies produced against the human cancer. The antigen

is called the carcinoma embryonic antigen (CEA). CEA is present in the gastrointestinal tract of the human embryo but as cells of this organ differentiate into mature cells the genes expressing the antigen are thought to be repressed and the CEA level in the serum of normal patients thereby decreased to a very low level.

When a patient develops a cancer of the gastrointestinal tract, the genes producing the CEA which had been repressed during the cancer-free period are de-repressed and cause the secretion of an increased amount of CEA into the serum. Unfortunately, some noncancerous diseases can also elevate serum CEA, other types of cancer elevate CEA, and some cancers of the gastrointestinal tract do not elevate CEA (66).

G.I. Abelev, of Moscow State University, had earlier described an alpha-fetoprotein (AFP) which led to a test for hepatocellular carcinoma (1). As with the CEA test it has its limitations.

MONOCLONAL ANTIBODIES AND IMMUNOCYTOCHEMICAL TECHNIQUES

One of the significant developments of the great advances in immunology after World War II was a technique whereby large amounts of specific antibodies could be produced. This was achieved by the use of cell fusion techniques (see chapter 21) which made use of a hybrid cell formed from a B-cell lymphocyte primed for a specific antibody and a malignant plasma cell of a myeloma. The hybridization of these cells produced the monoclonal growth of immortal cells (from the myeloma) which secreted a prescribed specific antibody (from the B-cell lymphocyte) (43).

Monoclonal antibodies (MoAb) can be used to purify antigens, to identify subpopulations of cells, to detect and kill tumor cells, and in many diagnostic tests. Catalytic monoclonal antibodies (abzymes) have been identified. T-cell hybridomas have been developed by fusing primed T cells with T-cell thymomas; the cytokines secreted by the T-cells have been isolated and purified (44).

Monoclonal antibodies have been used to localize antigens in histologic sections of tissues and cells (43). Antigens can be measured in cells and parts of cells as well as in the blood of humans and animals. One of the most successful applications has been the identification of polypeptide hormones in pancreatic islet cell tumors (fig. 16-6) (32).

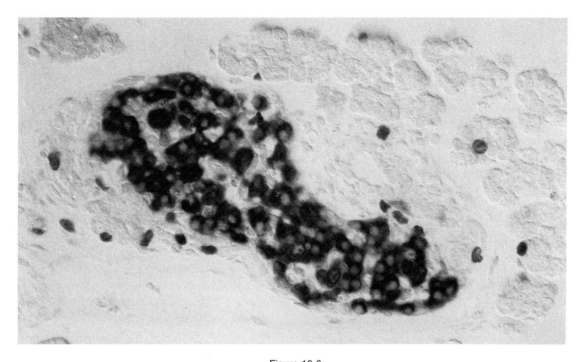

Figure 16-6
MONOCLONAL ANTIBODY IDENTIFYING INSULIN IN THE ISLET CELLS OF THE PANCREAS OF A YOUNG RAT
The red stain indicates the presence of antibodies to insulin in the beta cells of the islet. The light brown nuclei indicate, by the bromo-deoxuridine reaction, that the nuclei were proliferating. (Courtesy of Professor Gunther Klöppel, the University of Kiel, Germany.)

MoAb Markers and Hematopoietic Neoplasms

The malignant lymphomas and leukemias form a special class of neoplasms that arise from cells in the bone marrow (leukemias) or the lymphatic system (malignant lymphomas) (24,45). The recent systematic delineation of the many cellular markers of the cells of the hematopoietic and immunopoietic systems and their tumors (42) has clarified understanding of the cell of origin, stage of development of the cell of origin, and the pathogenesis of these neoplasms. Cultures of cells in different stages of development and the neoplasms arising from them have provided pure lines of various tumors of the bone marrow and lymphatic systems for study.

Cluster of Differentiation Markers

During the process of cell differentiation many changes take place in the surface antigens, and the antibodies against them may be used to identify these various stages. There is considerable overlap of antigens, so to lessen the confusion about terminology closely associated antigens are gath-

ered together and given a single number, a CD (cluster of differentiation) number. Some antigens are more activation antigens than specific stage markers. For the malignant lymphomas, heterogeneity of markers in the T-cell lymphomas is not as common as with the B-cell lymphomas. A few typical CD markers are listed below (42).

CD45. This marker represents all cells of the hematopoietic system, except erythrocytes and platelets. It is also known as the leukocyte common antigen (LCA). Most B-cell and T-cell non-Hodgkin's lymphomas and lymphatic leukemias are positive for this antigen. Some Hodgkin's tumors and practically all carcinomas and sarcomas are negative for the antigen.

CD10. The common acute lymphoblastic leukemia antigen (CALLA), represented by several MoAbs, is expressed by about 75 percent of precursor B-cell acute lymphoblastic leukemias (ALL) and by more than 90 percent of chronic myeloid leukemias (CML) in lymphoblastic crisis.

CD2. About 95 percent of thymocytes and mature peripheral blood and lymphoid cells are positive for CD2, as are natural killer (NK) cells. CD2 is a pan-T-cell lymphocyte antigen which identifies all normal T cells and the majority of lymphoid malignancies, precursor and post-thymic non-Hodgkin's lymphomas, and lymphatic leukemias.

CD4/CD8 Ratio. The T-cell lymphocyte population contains two mutually exclusive and functionally distinct subpopulations: CD4-positive cells which are helper/inducer T-cell lymphocytes and CD8-positive lymphocytes known as suppressor/cytotoxic T-cell lymphocytes. CD4 and CD8 are glycoproteins that belong to the immunoglobulin (Ig) gene superfamily that is expressed on the surface membrane of functionally distinct T-cell populations.

A lymphoid proliferation in which 80 percent or more cells are CD4 positive (+) CD8 negative (–), or CD4–CD8+ raises the possibility of a T-cell neoplasm. A double positive (CD4+CD8+) subset or a double negative subset (CD4–CD8–) is distinctively abnormal and highly suggestive of a malignant T-cell tumor.

THE RECOGNITION OF TUMOR-SPECIFIC ANTIGENS BY CYTOLYTIC T CELLS

A startling change has occurred concerning tumor cell antigens. T. Boon and colleagues at the Ludwig Institute for Cancer Research, Brussels, have introduced new techniques by which it has been shown that many tumors, in animals and humans, have antigens that can be recognized by certain cytolytic T cells (CTL) (5,6,79,80). Early studies indicated that cytolytic T lymphocytic cells of the mouse could kill (lyse) virus-infected cells and cells of tumors induced by chemicals or by ultraviolet radiation. Attempts to find specific target antigens on spontaneous animal and human tumor cancer cells that would make them susceptible to destruction by CTLs had not been previously successful. No antigens had been found on the cancer cells of spontaneous tumors in aging mice (33). Boon's group, however, found that certain CTLs recognized antigens on spontaneous mouse tumor cells, including CBA/H$_1$ leukemias, and destroyed them (80).

In vitro stimulation of T lymphocytes of human cancer patients to produce CTLs resulted in specific action against antigens of autologous tumor cells. By the use of complicated culture techniques, Boon et al. found that clones of CTL cells, mostly CD8+ T lymphocytes that recognized a complex of tumor antigens and their associated HLA class 1 molecules, could be produced and then used in antitumor studies (80). Antitumor CTL lymphocytes have been generated against the human melanoma tumor (80).

The use of CTL lymphocytic clones has revealed the presence of six distinct CTL-defined antigens expressed by melanoma cells (MZ2) (79). The first human tumor antigen identified was antigen MZ2-E, expressed by the MZ2-MEL melanoma cell line. By following a gene transfection approach, the gene coding the antigen MZ2-E was isolated. The gene, located on chromosome X, was named MAGE-1 and it is a member of a family of at least 12 genes. Other tumor antigens recognized by autologous CTL lymphocytes were also encoded by members of the MAGE gene family. The MZ2-E antigen was found to be processed by the class 1 HLA gene, specifically the HLA-A1 allele which is present in 26 percent of Caucasian individuals.

BAGE and GAGE families of genes were recognized to code for highly specific tumor antigens in patients with a wide range of tumor types. More than 60 percent of Caucasian patients with melanoma bear one of the antigens encoded by MAGE, BAGE, or GAGE. From 20 to 40 percent of patients with neck or bladder cancers have at least one such antigen.

Boon and van den Brugger believe that tumor cells that express antigens that are specific for CTL lymphocytes can be eliminated by the immune action of the T lymphocytes and that this approach might be an effective form of antitumor therapy (6). Chemically-induced mouse and rat tumors were found some years ago to generate tumor-specific tumor antigens (TSTA) (see above) (40). The TSTAs had individually distinct antigenic specificity in contrast to the virus-induced tumors which carried group-specific antigens common to all tumors induced by the same virus. The virus-induced TSTAs were found to be associated with a histocompatibility complex of class 1 molecules and peptides derived from virally-induced proteins. Ikeda et al. reported that in a panel of methylcholanthrene-induced sarcomas of mice, one sarcoma (CMS5) elicited a strong cytotoxic cell response of CTL lymphocytes with a high specificity for the tumor (34). The cloned CTL line (C18) recognized an antigen in the tumor cells whose gene was identified as one which encoded mutated protein kinase (MAPK). The target peptide had a mutant substitution of a single amino acid (34). Klein pointed out the importance of the findings of Ikeda et al. and raised fundamental questions regarding the immunosuppression of methylcholanthrene and the emergence of tumors (38). The discovery of TSATs by the Boon technique has revived the long hope of immunologists that antigens that are present on cancer cells, and not on normal cells, might allow T lymphocytes to destroy the cancer cells.

Recent stereochemical studies by Wiley and colleagues at Harvard University on the structure of the major histocompatibility (MHC) proteins associated with immunogenic peptides have been most informative (49,73). The MHC proteins are glycoproteins consisting of a heavy chain and a light chain that are bound to specific peptides. A groove in the complex holds peptides in an extended conformation in the MHC residues. These advances greatly add to our understanding of the function of the human MHC (7,49). Rammansee of the German Cancer Research Center at Heidelberg has reviewed in detail the association between peptides and MHC molecules and described the motifs required for allele-specific peptide–MHC complex interactions (60).

Because neither an adoptive transfer of melanoma-specific CTLs nor specific active immunotherapy with whole melanoma cells or cell-derived preparations has led to the eradication of melanoma or to the long-term survival of most patients, Cox et al. of the University of Virginia have focused upon epitope peptides. They isolated one that is recognized by high affinity CTLs from five different patients with melanoma. They suggest that this may be a promising approach for use in peptide-based vaccines against the melanoma tumor (11).

The turn-around in the matter of the presence of specific tumor antigens on cancer cells that could be detected by the CTL lymphocytes using the Boon techniques (6) has given new impetus toward the employment of the host immune system as a possible agent for therapy against cancer. High hopes are now held that the immune system can be employed to develop vaccines, antibodies, or other immunologic responses to destroy or modify cancer cells. Success has obtained in some animal but not human cancers.

REFERENCES

1. Abelev GI. Alpha-fetoprotein in oncogenesis and its association with malignant tumors. Adv Cancer Res 1977;14:295–358.
2. Alibert JL. Description des Maladies de la Peau observeés à l'Hôpital St.-Louis, Paris: Chez Barrois l'âiné et fils, 1806–14:118.
3. Behbehani AM. The smallpox story: in words and pictures. Kansas City: Univ. Kansas Med Ctr, 1988.
4. Behring E, Kitasato S. Ueber das Zustandekommen der diptherie-immutat. und der tetanus-immunitat bei thieren. Dtsch Med Wochenschr 1890;16:1113.
5. Boon T, Coulie P, Marchand M, Wolfel T, Brichard V. Genes coding for tumor rejection antigens: perspectives for specific immunotherapy, In: Devita VD, Hellman S, Rosenberg SA, eds. Important advances in oncology. Philadelphia: JB Lippincott, 1994:53–69.
6. Boon T, van den Bruggen P. Human tumor antigens recognized by T-lymphocytes. J Exp Med 1996;183:725–9.
7. Brown JH, Jardetsky TS, Gorga JD, et al. Three-dimensional structure of the human class II histocompatibility antigen HLA-DRI. Nature 1993;364:33–9.
8. Bulloch W. History of doctrines of immunity. In: The history of bacteriology. London: Oxford Univ. Press, 1938:255–83.
9. Burnet FM. The clonal selection theory of acquired immunity. London: Cambridge Univ. Press, 1959.
10. Burnet FM. The concept of immunological surveillance. Prog Exp Tumor Res 1970;13:1–27.
11. Cox, AL, Skipper J, Chen Y, et al. Identification of a peptide recognized by five melanoma-specific human cytotoxic T cell lines. Science 1994;264:716–9.
12. Dargeon HW, Eversole JW, DelDuca V. Malignant melanoma in an infant. Cancer 1950;3:299–306.
13. Edelman GM, Cunningham BA, Gall WE, Gottlieb PD, Rutisha U, Watdal MJ. The covalent structure of an entire YG immunoglobulin molecule. Proc Natl Acad Sci USA 1969;63:78–85.
14. Ehrlich P. Farbenanalytische Untersuchungen zur Histologie und Klinik des Bluts. Berlin: A Hirschwald, 1891.
15. Ehrlich P. On immunity with special reference to cell life. Proc Roy Soc London 1900;66:424–48.
16. Ehrlich P. Uber den jetzigen Stand der Karzinomforschung. In: Himmelweit P, ed. The collected papers of Paul Ehrlich London: Pergamon Press, 1957:550.
17. Eilber FR, Morton DL, Holmes EC, Sporks FL, Ramming KP. Adjuvant immunotherapy with BCG in treatment of regional-lymph node metastases from malignant melanoma. N Engl J Med 1976;294:237–40.
18. Eisen HN. Cell-mediated immunity. In: Davis BD, Dulbecco R, Eisen HN, Ginsberg HS, eds. Microbiology. Philadelphia: JB Lippincott, 1990:445.
19. Eisen HN. Immunology. In: Davis BD, Dulbecco R, Eisen HN, Ginsberg HS, eds. Microbiology, 4th ed. Philadelphia: JB Lippincott, 1990:237–47.
20. Fahraeus R, Rymo L, Rhim JS, Klein G. Morphologic transformation of human keratinocytes expressing the LMP gene of Epstein-Barr virus. Nature 1990:345:447–9.
21. Fearon ER, Pardoll DM, Itaya T, et al. Interleukin-2 production by tumor cells bypasses T helper function in the generation of an antitumor response. Cell 1990;60:397–403.

22. Foa R, Guarini A, Cignetti A, Cronin K, Rosenthal F, Gansbacher B. Cytokine gene therapy: a new strategy for the management of cancer. Nat Imm 1994;13:65–75.

23. Foley EJ. Antigenic properties of methylcholanthrene-induced tumors in mice of the strain of origin. Cancer Res 1953;13:835–7.

24. Freireich EJ, Lemek NA. Milestones in leukemia research and therapy. Baltimore: Johns Hopkins Univ. Press, 1991:120–4.

25. Gansbacher B, Zier K, Cronin K, et al. Retroviral gene transfer induced constitutive expression of interleukin-2 or interferon-gamma in irradiated human melanoma cells. Blood 1992;80:2817–25.

26. Gatti RA, Good RA. Occurrence of malignancy and immunodeficiency diseases. A literature review. Cancer 1971;28:89–98.

27. Gold P, Freedman SO. Demonstration of tumor-specific antigens in human colonic carcinomata by immunological tolerance and absorption tests. J Exp Med 1963;121:434.

28. Gorer PA. The antigenic structure of tumors. Adv Immunol 1961;1:345–93.

29. Götze D. The major histocompatibility system in man and animals. Berlin: Springer-Verlag, 1977.

30. Gross L. Intradermal immunization of C3H mice against a sarcoma that originated in an animal of the same line. Cancer Research 1943;3:326–33.

31. Hanau A. Erfolgreiche experimentelle Uebertragung von Carcinom. Fortschr Med 1889;7:321–39.

32. Heitz PU, Kasper M, Polak JM, Klöppel G. Pancreatic endocrine tumors: immunocytochemical analysis of 125 tumors. Hum Path 1982;13:263–71.

33. Hewlitt HB, Blake ER, Walder AS. A critique of the evidence for active host defense against cancer based on personal studies of 27 murine tumors of spontaneous origin. Br J Cancer 1976;33:241–59.

34. Ikeda H, Ohta N, Forukawa K, et al. Mutated nitrogen-activated protein kinase: a tumor rejection antigen of mouse sarcoma 2. Proc Natl Acad Sci 1997;94:6375–9.

35. Itoh T, Southam CM. Isoantibodies to human cancer cells in healthy recipients of cancer hemotransplants. J Immunology 1963;91:469–83.

36. Jerne NK. The natural selective theory of antibody formation. Proc Natl Acad Sci USA 1955;41:849–57.

37. Kedar E, Klein E. Cancer immunotherapy: are the results discouraging? Can they be improved? Adv Cancer Res 1992;59:245–322.

38. Klein G. Commentary. Rejection antigens in chemically induced tumors. Proc Natl Acad Sci 1997;94:5991–2.

39. Klein G. Immunological surveillance against neoplasia. Harvey Lect 1973;69:71–102.

40. Klein G. Tumor-specific transplantation antigens. G.H.A. Clowes Memorial Lecture. Cancer Res 1968;28:625–35.

41. Klein G, Sjögren HO, Klein E, Hellstrom KE. Demonstration of resistance against methylcholanthrene-induced sarcomas in the primary autochthonous host. Cancer Res 1960;20:1561–72.

42. Knowles DM, Chadburn A, Inghirami G. Immunophenotypic markers useful in the diagnosis and classification of hematopoietic neoplasms. In: Knowles DM, ed. Neoplastic hematopathology. Baltimore: Williams & Wilkins, 1992:73–167.

43. Kohler G, Milstein C. Continuous cultures of fused cells secreting antibody of predefined specificity. Nature 1975;256:495–7.

44. Kuby J. Immunology. New York: WH Freeman, 1992:9–19, 39–72, 141–56, 245–70, 516–9, 522–5.

45. Lee GR. Wintrobe's clinical hematology, 10th ed. Baltimore: Williams & Wilkins, 1998.

46. Loeb L. The biological basis of individuality. Springfield, IL: Univ. Chicago Press, 1945.

47. Loeb L. Further investigations in transplantation of tumors. J Med Res 1902;8:44–73.

48. Loeb L. On transplantation of tumors. J Med Res 1901;6: 28–39.

49. Madden DR, Garboczi DN, Wiley DC. The antigenic identity of peptide-MHC complexes: a comparison of the conformations of five viral peptides presented by HLA-A2. Cell 1993;75:693–708.

50. Melief CJ. Tumor eradication by adoptive transfer of cytotoxic T lymphocytes. Adv Cancer Res 1992;58:143–75.

51. Metchnikoff O. Life of Eli Metchnikoff 1845–1916. Boston: Houghton Mifflin, 1921.

52. Middle JG, Embleton MJ. Naturally arising tumors of the inbred WAB/NoF rat strain. II. Immunogenicity of transplanted tumors. JNCI 1981;67:637–43.

53. Moore AE, Caparo AC. Tumors occurring in newborn mice after injection of human cancer material. Cancer Res 1964;24:765–9.

54. Nooth J. Observations on the treatment of scirrhous tumors of the breast, 2nd ed. London: J Johnson, 1806:13.

55. Nossal GJ. Life, death and the immune system. Sci Am 1993;269:52–62.

56. Novinsky MA. On the question of inoculation of malignant neoplasms (thesis). Quoted by Shimkin MB, Novinsky MA. In: A note on the history of transplantation of tumors. Cancer 1955;8:653–5.

57. Old L. Tumor necrosis factor. Sci Am 1988;258:59–75.

58. Porter RH. Structural studies of immunoglobulins. Science 1973;180:713–6.

59. Prehn RT, Main JM. Immunity to methylcholanthrene-induced sarcomas. JNCI 1957;8:769–78.

60. Rammensee HG. Chemistry of peptides associated with MHC class and class II molecules. Curr Opin Immunol 1995;7:85–96.

61. Rauler DH, Eisen HN. Cellular basis for immune responses. In: Davis, BD, Dulbecco R, Eisen HN, Ginsberg HS, eds. Microbiology. Philadelphia: JB Lippincott, 1990:319–62.

62. Rosenberg SA, Aebersold P, Cornetta K, et al. Gene transfer into humans—immunotherapy of patients with advanced melanoma, using tumor-infiltrating lymphocytes modified by retroviral gene transduction. N Engl J Med 1990;323:570–8.

63. Rosenberg SA, Barry JM. The transformed cell: unlocking the mysteries of cancer. New York: Putnam, 1992.

64. Rosenberg SA, Yang JL, Topalian SL, et al. Treatment of 283 consecutive patients with metastatic melanoma or renal cell cancer using high-dose bolus interleukin 2. JAMA 1990;27A:907–13.

65. Schöne G. Die heteroplastische und homöoplastische transplantation. Berlin: Springer-Verlag, 1912.

66. Sell S, ed. Serological cancer markers. Totowa, NJ: Humana Press, 1992.

67. Shimkin MB, Novinsky MA. A note on the history of transplantation of tumors. Cancer 1955;8:653–5.

68. Silverstein AM. Cellular versus humoral immunity: determinants and causes of an epic nineteenth century battle. In: Silverstein AM, ed. A history of immunology. New York: Academic Press, 1989:38–58.

69. Silverstein AM. A history of immunology. New York: Academic Press, 1989:1–23, 279, 281–2.

70. Snell GD. The genetics of transplantation. JNCI 1953;14: 691–700.
71. Southam CM. Host defense mechanisms and human cancer. Paris: Ann Inst Pasteur, 1964;107:585–97.
72. Starzl TE, Penn I. Iatrogenic alterations of immunogenic surveillance in man and their influence on malignancy. Trans Rev 1971;7:112–45.
73. Stern LJ, Brown JH, Jardetzky TS, et al. Crystal structure of the human class 11 MHC protein HLA-DR1 complexed with an influenza virus peptide. Nature 1994;368:215–21.
74. Stutman O. Immunological surveillance. In: Hiatt HH, Watson JD, Winsten JA, eds. Origins of human cancer. Book B. Cold Spring Harbor: Cold Spring Harbor Laboratory Press, 1977:729–50.
75. Talmage DW. The acceptance and rejection of immunological concepts. Ann Rev Immun 1986;4:1–11.
76. Thomas L. On immunosurveillance in human cancer. Yale J Biol Med 1982;55:329–33.
77. Tonegawa S. The molecules of the immune system. Sci Am 1985;253:122–31.
78. Tyzzer EE. A series of spontaneous tumors in mice with observations on the influence of heredity on the frequency of their occurrence. J Med Res 1909;21:479–518.
79. Van Pel A, van der Bruggen P, Coulie PG, et al. Genes coding for tumor antigens recognized by cytolytic T-lymphocytes. Immunol Rev 1995;145:229–50.
80. Van Pel A, Vessiere F, Boon T. Protection against two spontaneous mouse leukemias by immunogenic variants obtained by mutagenesis. J Exp Med 1983;157:1992–2001.

✻ ✻ ✻

EPIDEMIOLOGY AND THE DETECTION OF CAUSE(S) OF CANCER

HISTORICAL ASPECTS

The earliest associations of cancer and possible causative agents were made by astute observers, usually physicians and surgeons practicing medicine. Important correlations were made in the 18th century when Bernardino Ramazzini (1633–1714), a physician of Medina, Italy, collected information about artisans and the diseases associated with their occupations. He noted that nuns had a higher incidence of breast cancer than other women, which he attributed to the former's celibacy (95).

The London surgeon, Percival Pott, reported in 1775 that scrotal cancer in young men occurred in those who had been employed as chimney sweeps earlier in life (93). Later, von Volkmann, a German surgeon, reported three patients with tumors of the skin of the scrotum who had continual contact with tar or soot (122). In 1879, F. H. Härting and A. F. Hesse, Austrian physicians, noted the increased incidence of cancer of the lung in coal miners of Schneeberg and Joachimstal (37); later this was ascribed to the radioactive ores. In 1895, Ludwig Rehn, a German surgeon of Frankfort a Main, found bladder tumors in 3 of 45 aniline dye workers (96). In 1911, A.R. Ferguson, a British pathologist, postulated that the Bilharzia parasite caused cancer of the bladder in Egyptians (29). Many observers noted that farmers and sailors, with their more extensive exposure to sunlight, had more skin cancers than persons not so exposed to the actinic rays of the sun (108,120).

From the study of epidemics of infectious diseases there evolved a discipline called epidemiology (Greek: study of diseases of epidemics). It has been defined recently as being ". . . concerned with the patterns of disease occurrence in human populations and of the factors that influence the patterns.

The epidemiologist is primarily interested in the occurrence of disease by time, place and persons" (64). Most of the known causes of human cancer have been discovered by use of the epidemiological approach, in its broadest sense (66,75,78,88,103).

N. L. Petrakis, of the University of California, San Francisco, has given a historical account of the epidemiological approach to cancer, which emphasized its early relationship to the development of statistics (88) (Note 1). With the decline in deaths from infectious diseases in the late 19th and early 20th centuries, there arose a debate as to whether the incidence of cancer was increasing. It was soon realized that cancer statistics of the day were incomplete and many were not accurate. The age factor in cancer deaths was pointed out in 1893 by King and Newsholme of England who noted that there was a higher incidence of cancer in older age groups (54).

By the 1920s, cancer mortality statistics in the United States were becoming more reliable (102) and it soon became evident that there was an increased incidence of lung cancer (88). Population-based cancer surveys began in the United States in the 1920s and 1930s and cancer registries were founded about a decade later (109). In the 1930s, H. F. Dorn and S. J. Cutler of the National Cancer Institute began the series of National Cancer Surveys which indicated the magnitude of the morbidity from cancer and gave an evaluation of the results of treatment (25). By the 1960s a large number of population-based cancer registries were established throughout the world (88).

After World War II, the techniques of epidemiology that had been used by A. Bradford Hill, Richard Doll (fig. 17-1), and colleagues in the study of infectious diseases began to be employed in the study of cancer, particularly the use of a control group chosen by randomization techniques (21,22) (Note 2).

Note 1: Graunt, in 1622, made a fundamental approach to epidemiology with his count of mortality in a population. Other advances in statistical methods were Pierre Louis' "numerical method," Quetelet's "average man," the correlation coefficient of Francis Galton, the chi square test of Karl Pearson, the student "t" test of Gossett, and the randomization methods of R.A. Fisher (88).

Note 2: Hill's contributions have been assessed by Doll (21) and a delightful vignette concerning the personality of Hill has been written by Benedict Duffy (26).

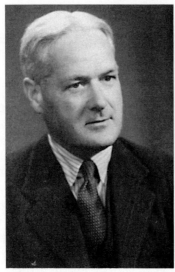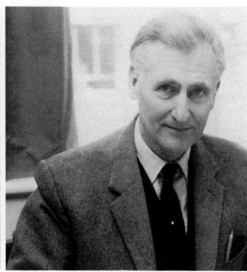

Figure 17-1
AUSTIN BRADFORD
AND RICHARD DOLL
Austin Bradford Hill (left) and Richard Doll (right), British epidemiologists, applied clinical trials previously used in infectious diseases to clinical trials in cancer. Both have been knighted. (From Shimkin MB. Contrary to nature. Washington D.C.: U.S. Department of Health, Education, and Welfare, 1977:153.)

METHODOLOGY

Case-Control Studies

This approach was used to determine whether patients with a specific type of cancer had a higher or lower percentage of a certain factor(s)—social, physical, occupation, or other—than a control group who did not have cancer.

Breast Cancer. In a study in 1924, Janet E. Lane-Claypon of England, reported data on the personal attributes of a large number of women with breast cancer and compared them with the attributes of similar women who did not have cancer (56). She concluded that the incidence of breast cancer was greater in single women than in married women and in less fertile women than in more fertile women. There was some suggestion that parents of women with breast cancer had more cancer than parents of the control group, but the data was too unreliable to substantiate such a conclusion. Injury to the breast and chronic mastitis were more common in the cancer group.

Cigarette Smoking and Lung Cancer. One of the most important cancer associations found in epidemiological studies was that of tobacco smoking and lung cancer. In 1929, F. Lickint of Küchwald, Chemnitz, Germany, suggested that tobacco was related to lung cancer (61). In 1939, F. H. Müller examined the autopsy records at the University of Koln, Germany, and discovered a rise in the percentage of cases of lung cancer from 1918 to 1937 (76). Examination of the smoking habits of 86 patients with

primary lung cancer indicated that the use of tobacco (cigars, cigarettes, or pipe smoking) was extreme in 29 percent, very heavy in 21 percent, heavy in 15 percent, moderate in 31 percent, and only 3.5 percent were nonsmokers. The comparable figures in a control group without cancer were extreme, 4.9 percent; very heavy, 6 percent; heavy, 25.6 percent; moderate, 47 percent; and nonsmoker, 47.7 percent. The amount in grams of tobacco smoked was estimated to be more than twice as much in the lung cancer patients than in the control group (76). This was a significant study, but it was not until 1950 that the relationship between cigarette smoking and lung cancer was verified by other investigators.

In 1950 it was reported by five groups of investigators, four from the United States and one from England, that there was a causal relationship between cigarette smoking and lung cancer (24,57, 71,104,127). The report from Washington University, St. Louis, by Ernst Wynder and Evarts Graham, probably had the most impact, principally because of the prominence of Graham, a pioneer thoracic surgeon who had previously denied the relationship of cigarette smoking and lung cancer. Wynder and Graham studied 605 patients with lung cancer and 780 patients with other diseases. They found a stronger association between heavy, prolonged cigarette smoking and lung cancer than between nonsmokers and lung cancer. They pointed out that lung cancer was very rare in nonsmokers (127) (Note 3). Levin et al. reported that lung cancer occurred more than twice as frequently in long-term smokers as in nonsmokers of the same age (57). Schreck et al. (104) and Mills and Porter (71) found a higher percentage of smokers in the lung cancer groups than in controls. Doll and Hill, from England (fig. 17-1), published the results of their exemplary case-control study of over 1,465 patients with and 1,465 persons without cancer of the lung. The two groups were matched for sex, age, geographic region, smoking history, and some other characteristics (24). Their findings were similar to those of the other four groups.

These studies were most important because cigarette smoking today is recognized as the single most important known cause of a major cancer. About 30 percent of all cancer deaths are said to be linked to cigarette smoking (121). The histologic findings in 150 autopsied patients of O. Auerbach of the U.S. Veterans Association and A. P. Stout of Columbia University, revealed that hyperplastic changes in the epithelium of the lung mucosa were greater in cigarette smokers than in nonsmokers. The changes became more marked as the smoking increased. The incidence of carcinoma in situ of the lung occurred in 1 percent of patients who did not smoke, in 4 percent of those who smoked less than a pack of cigarettes per day, and in 6 percent in those who smoked more than a pack of cigarettes per day for years. All 34 patients who died of bronchial carcinoma were smokers (4).

Asbestos and Lung Cancer

Case-control methods were used to examine the effect of cigarette smoking and exposure to asbestos on the incidence of cancers of the respiratory tract. Asbestos had been shown in retrospective studies to be associated with an increased incidence of cancer of the lung by Merewether of London (70). Wagner and associates of South Africa linked asbestos with a rare tumor, mesothelioma of the pleura of the lungs (123). I. J. Selikoff, J. Churg, and E. C. Hammond of the Mt. Sinai Medical School in New York City, in a prospective study of asbestos insulator union members, found a higher number of deaths caused by lung cancer than expected. Mesothelioma caused the death of 37 of 198 (19 percent) asbestos workers, a relatively very high incidence of this rare tumor (105).

Selikoff and colleagues discovered dual factors operating in cancers of the lung in patients exposed to asbestos (106). Asbestos and cigarette smoking were independently capable of increasing the risk of lung cancer, but when combined they increased the risk greatly. Nonsmoking asbestos workers had a 4- to 5-fold increased risk of lung cancer compared to nonsmoking, nonasbestos-exposed workers. The risk of lung cancer in a cigarette-smoking worker exposed to asbestos has been estimated to be from 17 to 92 times greater than that of a nonsmoking, nonasbestos-exposed man in the general population (79).

Relative Risk

Another epidemiological parameter, the relative risk (RR), has been used to indicate the association of possible causative factors in carcinogenesis. This is designated by the relationship:

$$RR = \frac{\text{Number of observed cases of cancer}}{\text{Number of expected cases of cancer from a control group}}$$

The RR may vary greatly.

At what level an increased relative risk should be considered significant is debatable. Some experts believe that a relative risk of three or four times that of a control group is significant; others would accept a 50 percent increase (RR=1.5) as significant if confirmed by well-controlled studies (27,118).

Odds Ratio

In the early studies of the association of cigarette smoking and lung cancer it became apparent that the proportion of smokers was different in the test and control groups, and simple comparison between groups could not give a quantitative figure as to how much the risk of lung cancer really was increased by smoking. In 1951, Cornfield suggested a simple method of estimating the odds ratio by

---

Note 3: A possibly apocryphal story was told about Graham who was to perform for the first time a pneumonectomy, removal of an entire lung, as treatment for lung cancer in a young obstetrician. The latter requested a 2-week interlude to arrange his affairs, telling Graham that he wanted some dental work performed. The long operation was a success and the obstetrician outlived Graham by many years. What he did not tell Graham was that in the granted interlude he also bought a lot in a cemetery.

Table 17-1

ODDS RATIO*

	Male Lung Cancer Patients	Male Patients with Non-Lung Cancer
Smokers	647 (99.7%)	622 (95.8)
Nonsmokers	2	27
Total	**649**	**649**

*Stolley and Lasky, using data from Doll and Hill, illustrated the calculation of the odds ratio (116). The odds ratio of the cross product by this method was calculated:

$$OR = \frac{(647) \times (27)}{(622) \times (2)} = 14.04$$

A ratio of 14 indicates a clear risk of smoking.

employing a two-by-two table and using the cross products as a ratio, the odds ratio (OR), as an estimate of the risk (Table 17-1) (17,116).

Interpreting Relative Risk

In his discussion of the recent spate of contradictory epidemiological studies in the press, Gary Taubes pointed out some of the reasons for the increasing public skepticism of such studies (118). Among the factors involved are the tendency of the mass media to emphasize the novel and spectacular and the tendency of public news releases by some journals and scientists to overemphasize the significance of the findings. One of the chief reasons for confusion is a lack of understanding by the public of the inherent defects of the methodology itself, that in many studies there are built-in biases and confounding factors that may lead to wrong conclusions. Even with controlled studies there is the possibility of hidden bias in the choice of the controls. A healthy skepticism is needed in evaluating epidemiologic studies in humans, particularly those with a low relative risk ratio.

Absolute Risk

It has long been recognized in oncology that certain "cancer families" (125) exist, e.g., the increased frequency of breast cancer in women who have first degree relatives (mother, sister, or aunt) with breast cancer. The relative risk of a woman with such a family history of getting breast cancer was thought, from the anecdotal experience of

oncologists, to be greater than that of a woman who had no such relatives. There was an inability to distinguish clearly between genetic and environmental causative factors (81). The relative risk was not related to age and this deficiency was highlighted by a tongue-in-cheek statement that a woman's chance of developing breast cancer before the age of 25 years was the same as the actuarial risk of drowning in 1 year (10).

An absolute risk assessment, explained as the cumulative risk of developing a breast cancer during a specified time interval, has been developed. It takes into consideration many clinical factors of significance such as the relative's age when her breast cancer appeared and other data (81).

The need for more accurate risk estimates for the genetic counseling of members of families which appear to have a greater risk of breast cancer than the population at large has given rise to different sets of control data that might be used (81). The sets differ in the populations of women from which the data were obtained: from women with at least one sister with breast cancer; from a study of over 117,000 women monitored since 1976; from white women, examined yearly in a large government-sponsored study, who had an affected mother and maternal aunt; and from another government-sponsored agency studying the incidence rates of breast cancer for all groups under the age of 70 years. In general the sets agree fairly well where comparable but there are different figures on risk assessment in the different groups (81).

Risk assessment in breast cancer has become even more important recently because of the discovery that there are gene mutations associated with a small percentage of breast cancer patients. The patients carry one or more mutated genes that are associated with a higher risk for the cancer process (see chapter 21).

Change in Incidence and Mortality

Richard Doll of Oxford has used epidemiological techniques to evaluate the change in incidence and mortality for different types of cancer in two different time periods, 1970–74 and 1985–87 (22). In some cancers there has been an increase and in others a decrease in incidence from the earlier to the latter period. Cancers of the uterine cervix, colon, rectum, ovary, and endometrium in women and lung cancer in males have shown a decreased incidence.

Cohort Studies

This method follows for some years a group of subjects, similar in all known aspects, except for the factor to be studied, to determine whether there is a significantly different incidence of disease between a subgroup with the factor of interest, e.g., cigarette smoking, and another subgroup of the cohort who are nonsmokers. The study may be prospective or retrospective. Doll and Hill reported a 10-year follow-up cohort study of British physicians (smokers and nonsmokers) which showed that cigarette smoking was significantly related to the incidence of lung cancer. In addition, they also showed a decreased incidence of lung cancer in those physicians who stopped smoking (23).

Migrant Populations and Change in Incidence of Cancer

The study of migrant populations has documented the effect of changes in lifestyle and cultural or environmental factors on the incidence of cancer. W. Haenszel et al. of the National Institutes of Health reported that the risk for cancer of the colon in Japanese who have emigrated to Hawaii or California increased from the relatively low rates that prevailed in Japan. The risk in emigrants approximated the relatively higher risk of the population in Hawaii or the mainland. The increased risk occurred after a generation of residence in the country to which the Japanese emigrated, suggesting that age at migration was important. If the migration occurred after 20 years of age, the incidence of gastric cancer resembled that of the country of origin, suggesting that initiation of the cancer process probably occurred within the first two decades of life (35).

HORMONES AND CANCER

Hormones (Greek: to arouse) are chemical compounds synthesized and stored in a gland, secreted into the bloodstream, and carried to a different target tissue, organ, or cell. Bayliss and Sterling, physiologists at University College, London, gave the name "hormone" to an active principle which they extracted from the duodenum and jejunum of the dog. When the extract was injected into a dog or other animal it caused the secretion from the pancreas of a juice containing digestive enzymes (5). The hormone was named "secretin."

It is formed by the epithelial lining cells of the duodenum after they are activated by the stimulus of acid contents from the stomach.

Insulin, a hormone secreted by the beta cells of the islets of the pancreas into the blood, is involved in the metabolism of carbohydrates; prolactin from the pituitary gland controls the secretion of milk in the female; and thyroxine, secreted by the thyroid gland, controls metabolic rates of cells. Other hormones involving the central nervous system act through the propagation of an electrical charge from the neuron which exerts its effect by means of a chemical liberated from a nerve ending; the chemical is called a neurotransmitter. Acetylcholine is a classic neurotransmitter.

Estrogens and Breast Cancer

The relatively high incidence of cancer of the breast in women and its relative rarity in men has long suggested to oncologists that the female sex hormones play a role in carcinogenesis of the female breast. In 1896, Beatson, a British surgeon, removed the ovaries in women with advanced breast cancer and believed that in some women there was temporary suspension of growth of the tumor caused by the removal of the estrogen-secreting organ (7).

The significance of estrogens in carcinogenesis was emphasized in 1932 by Lacassagne, a French scientist, who gave the female hormone, estrogen, to male mice and produced cancers of the breast (55). Later it was shown that mouse mammary viruses and genetic factors were associated with carcinogenesis (see chapter 15).

Estrogens, the feminizing hormones, affect a variety of tissues, particularly those of the female reproductive system. They are involved in the synthesis and accumulation of fat in adipose tissue. Estrogens stimulate genetic transcription, the introduction of ribonucleic acid (RNA) polymerase, and the increase of phospholipid and protein synthesis (74). Estradiol (an estrogen) binds to a receptor protein in the nucleus of the cell and changes the action of the receptor, which then acts with the responsive elements of the DNA of the cell genome to affect genetic expression (52).

The clinical aspects of estrogen were emphasized by Brian MacMahon and colleagues of the Harvard School of Public Health who found that women having a first child after 35 years of age were three times more likely to develop breast cancer than women who were first-time mothers before the age of 20 years. It was suggested that the longer period of exposure to estrogens of the women having their first baby late in the reproductive period might be a factor in their development of breast cancer (65).

With the advent of contraceptives there began a long debate as to whether oral contraceptives increased the incidence of cancers of the uterus and breast. A large number of New Zealand women who had cancer of the breast were studied by the case-control method to determine the relationship of the use of contraceptives and the incidence of breast cancer. There was no increase in the risk of breast cancer in those who used contraceptives compared to the control group (85); however, the follow-up period was relatively short. Estrogens given for years to women as replacement therapy for the relief of menopausal signs and symptoms have been associated with a higher incidence of cancer of the endometrium of the uterus. The later addition of progesterone and the decrease of estrogen in the medication lowered the risk of uterine cancer (87).

Oral Contraceptives

It has been estimated that 40 to 60 percent of human cancers are associated with exposure to sex hormones, endogenous or exogenous (59). Oral estrogenic and progestational hormones are used by tens of millions of women in the United States (39,73).

Early oral sequential contraceptives, particularly Oracon, were associated with an increased incidence of cancer of the endometrium of the uterus (46,111). A nonsequential combination of oral contraceptives decreased the risk for endometrial cancer to about half that of women who had used sequential contraceptives (53).

About 46,000 married women of the United Kingdom were divided into two groups: those who had used oral contraceptives (ever users) and those who never used contraceptives (never users); both were followed for 25 years (8). The oral contraceptive was a combined one containing 50 mg of estrogen. After 25 years there was no difference in the risk of mortality in the two groups. However, in current and recent users the risk of colorectal and ovarian cancer decreased, the risk of uterine cervical cancer increased, and there was an increase in cardiovascular diseases. Breast

cancer incidence was increased slightly during use and for 10 years after cessation of the contraceptive. In women who had stopped contraceptive use for 10 years or longer there were no significant changes in the risk of any overall or specific cause of death; adverse effects were not present 10 years or more after the use of a contraceptive ceased.

Diethylstilbestrol and Cancer

Some women who were treated with diethylstilbestrol (DES), an exogenous sex sterol, during pregnancy to stop bleeding gave birth to daughters who, years later in puberty or adulthood, presented with adenosis (increased formation of glands) and tumors of the vagina. A few developed clear cell adenocarcinomas of the vagina, a very rare tumor in this age group (41,42). From 1 to 5 percent of daughters whose mothers were exposed to DES in pregnancy showed a 2- to 4-fold increase of vaginal and cervical dysplasias and carcinoma in situ (CIS) of the uterine cervix (97). The transplacental transmission from the mother to the baby of a carcinogenic factor was demonstrated by these results.

Some sons born to these mothers had congenital defects: maldescent of testicles, meatal stenosis of the penis, and decreased development of the penis (18). In elderly males given DES for prostate cancer, a breast carcinoma (82) and a papillomatosis of the nipple of the breast have been reported (124).

Androgens and Prostate Cancer

The male hormone, testosterone, an androgen, is important in the development of normal male sexuality. Pioneer studies on cancer of the prostate were performed by Charles Huggins, a surgeon at the University of Chicago. He used orchiectomy (excision of the testicles) as a method of treatment for cancer of the prostate (48,49). Experimental findings had shown that castration of dogs caused shrinkage of the prostate.

Prolonged administration of testosterone to rats caused grossly recognizable enlargement of the prostate which was thought to be cancer of the prostate (80). Testosterone acted as a promoter of cancer of the prostate in Lobund-Wistar rats previously given the carcinogen MNU (N-methylnitrosourea) (91).

Metastasizing cancer of the prostate has been produced by prolonged administration of testosterone and a carcinogen (90). It has been prevented by administration of retinamide (16,92) (Note 4). A few men receiving anabolic androgens for body muscle building purposes have developed adenoma or cancer of the liver (46).

Pituitary Gland and Organ Hormones

The complex relationship of hormones and organs was illustrated by the studies of Jacob Furth, an experimental pathologist of the Rosewell Park Institute. Furth postulated a cybernetic feedback relationship between the pituitary gland and other organs such as the hypothalamus, thyroid gland, sex organs, adrenal gland, kidney, and breast (33). Disruption of this relationship has resulted in tumors of the pituitary.

Administration of estrogen to rodents of some strains gave rise to a pituitary tumor, a prolactinoma, that promoted milk production in the rodent breast (60). Pituitary hormones may be involved in carcinogenesis since hypophysectomy (removal of the pituitary gland) prevents or decreases the action of estrogens in producing breast tumors in some strains of rats (33).

Mechanism of Action of Hormones

Hormones elicit the process of tumorigenesis by epigenetic mechanisms, generally by inducing cell proliferation (58). The binding of a hormone to a receptor brings about an allosteric change in the confirmation of the receptor, which triggers a series of molecular events, interaction of the hormone-receptor complex with genetic material, or a cascade of enzymatic events. Steroid and thyroid hormones diffuse freely through the plasma membrane of the cell and can act with specific receptors, primarily in the nucleus. Amine peptide-protein hormones cannot enter the cell and must interact with specific receptors present in the cell membrane. The nuclear receptor hormone complex acts directly with DNA; the membrane receptor-hormone complex triggers the synthesis/transport of a soluble intracellular "second messenger" (cAMP) which transports the information to the cell machinery (signal transduction) resulting in a biological response.

Nandi et al. from the University of California at Berkeley have reported that the estrogens that

produce breast cancer in mice and rats do not induce mitosis or act as direct carcinogens, although their presence is required for growth and carcinogenesis. Progesterone, a hormone produced by the ovary, may be directly involved in growth and carcinogenesis of the mammary cells in the presence of exogenous carcinogens. Estrogen's role may be that of an inducer of progesterone receptors. The synthesis and release of the hormone prolactin from the pituitary gland is also required for the growth of the mammary gland cells. It is believed that hormones are the upstream regulators of breast cancer cell proliferation by stimulating different parts of the ductal and stromal systems to produce different growth factors in the carcinogenesis process (77).

In regard to testosterone and prostatic cancer, it is uncertain whether testosterone alone can produce the cancer. S. M. Ho and colleagues of Tufts University showed that in rats combined androgenic-estrogenic (testosterone or dehydrotestosterone and free 17β-estradiol [E_2]) action is a necessary factor in the genesis of the dysplastic process, the initiation of a preneoplastic lesion. It was speculated that E_2 acting in concert with an androgen elevated a receptor (type II ER) to levels that directly conferred a higher proliferative potential to the prostate tissue (45).

The mechanism(s) of action of most hormones has not been delineated in detail. It is believed that they may modify target tissues by promotional or co-carcinogenic means through an effect on the immune system, activation of viruses, modification of receptors, or regulation of the growth factors involved in the growth of tumor cells (60).

DIET AND CANCER

"You are what you eat" is an ancient dictum and most individuals and cultures have believed that dietary factors play a major role in the maintenance of health and the prevention of disease (fig. 17-2).

Epidemiologic studies have shown significant differences in the incidence of cancer from country to country, in different ethnic groups, or in various cultures (15). Among the possible factors causing such differences are dietary habits. The incidence

Note 4: A recent report states that the cancer produced by the experimental animal model of prostate cancer (90) actually is a cancer of the seminal vesicle, an organ adjacent to the prostate (16). It has been suggested that since the seminal vesicle and the prostate arise from the same embryonic area, their action should be similar. However, it remains to be demonstrated that a chemotherapeutic drug that affects seminal vesicle cancer necessarily affects prostatic cancer similarly.

Figure 17-2
DIET AND DISEASE
The common concept that diet is all important as a cause of cancer and many other diseases has been with mankind probably throughout its history. Many chemicals fed to animals cause cancer. Many of these carcinogens are suspected of causing cancer in man but the conclusive evidence for this relationship is still lacking. (Author's cartoon, by Richard Larocco.)

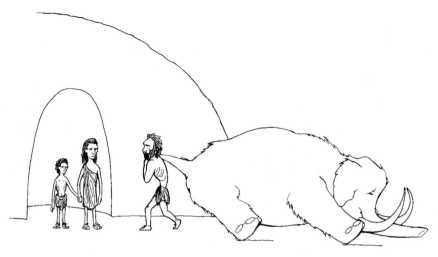

You are what you eat

of cancers have been examined to determine if there are significant associations between specific cancers and foods or culinary practices.

There has been a relatively low incidence of gastric cancer in Japan (1 per 100,000 inhabitants) compared to a much higher incidence in the United States (100 per 100,000 inhabitants) (44). This was thought to be caused by an average low caloric intake or the low percentage composition of meat in the Japanese diet (35). It has been reported that there is a lower incidence of colon cancer in Africans than Americans and this has been postulated as related to the larger, bulkier stools of the African due to a higher percentage of fiber in the food intake (12).

Carcinogens and Mutagens in Food

Many animal carcinogens have been found in the foods of humans. Among them are nitrosamines, polycyclic hydrocarbons, amines, heterocyclic aromatic amines, and mycotoxins. Some of these have been suspected of being causal factors in the carcinogenesis of human neoplasms.

Nitrosamines. One of the most important classes of carcinogens, the N-nitrosamines, was

discovered by two British scientists investigating an epidemic of deaths in turkey molts. Peter Magee and J.M. Barnes found that the turkey feed was contaminated by the compound dimethylnitrosamine (NDMA). When NDMA was fed to rats, it severely damaged the liver. Subsequent studies revealed that NDMA caused cancer of the liver in rats (69). Over 300 different N-nitroso compounds have been demonstrated to produce cancers experimentally in more than 40 species of animals, including some primates (67,68,119).

The significance of the nitrosamines resides in the fact that certain oxides of nitrogen, formed during food preparation and preservation, can react with amino compounds and other nucleophiles in the diet to produce nitrogen, carbon, oxygen, and sulfur nitroso-compounds (72) (Note 5). Major sources of oxides of nitrogen are the nitrate and nitrite additions to foods, e.g., the well-known custom of adding nitrate or nitrite to fresh meat to give it a red appearance.

In the experimental animal, endogenous formation of nitrosamines resulted from the synthesis from precursor compounds in the bowel (72). It has been

Note 5: Foodstuffs containing N-nitroso compounds have been classified into six groups (119): those preserved by the addition of nitrate or nitrite, such as meat products (bacon) and cheese; those prepared by smoking (fish and meat); those subjected to drying by combustion gases containing oxides of nitrogen (malt for beer or whiskey, low fat dried milk products, and spices); pickled and salt-preserved food (pickled vegetables in which microbial reduction of nitrate to nitrite occurs); food stored under humid conditions favoring the growth of fungi; and migration of, or formation of, nitrosamines from materials in contact with food (nitrosamines in rubber used for rubber pacifiers or rubber nipples in baby feeding bottles).

established that N-nitroso compounds can be found in many foodstuffs (67,68,72,101,119). Volatile nitrosamines in the diet may also be a hazard (Note 6).

Because of their route of entry, the nitrosamines and nitrosamides are involved in carcinomas of the esophagus, stomach, and nasopharyngeal regions. In an area of China, the Linxian, where there is a high incidence of esophageal cancer, foods have been shown to have a high concentration, about 1μg/kg, of a nitroso compound, NMAMBA (N-nitroso-N-[1 methyl-acetonyl]-3-methylbutylamine) (112). It has been suggested that in Kashmir, India, an area with a high incidence of esophageal cancer, the increased risk of the cancer may be caused by the dietary exposure to N-nitroso compounds.

Nasal cavity tumors have been developed in rats fed Cantonese salted fish from Hong Kong. High concentrations of volatile nitrosamines occur in salted fish from the Hong Kong area (129). John Weisburger, then at the National Institute of Health, and colleagues, showed that extracts from nitrite-treated fish from Japan induced adenocarcinomas of the stomach in rats (126).

R.M. Hicks, a British pathologist, and colleagues, in clinical and experimental studies have concluded that the N-nitroso compounds seen in the urine of Egyptians with bladders infected with the parasitic fluke *Schistosoma hematobium* may act as an initiating agent; the parasite could then function as an accelerating cause in bladder cancer (43) (Note 7).

Polynuclear Aromatic Hydrocarbons. Polynuclear aromatic hydrocarbons are formed from the heating of organic compounds at high temperatures or from the incomplete combustion of organic matter. They are also present in the atmosphere from the exhausts of engines, the burning of fuels, and the emissions from factories. Some of these compounds are potent mutagenic and carcinogenic agents in animals, but most are not (62). The compounds have to be activated to the dihydrodiol epoxide metabolite to be carcinogenic (see chapter 13).

Examples of polynuclear aromatic hydrocarbons are benzo[α]pyrene (the tar cancer carcinogen), 7,12-dimethylbenz[α]anthracene, and dibenz[α,h]anthracene. There is a correlation between the extent of covalent binding of the carcinogen to DNA and the carcinogenic activity on the skin of animals (11).

These carcinogens can also be formed in the cooking of food. Wood smoke and smoked foods contain benzo[α]pyrene at levels of about 1 ppb (1 part per billion). Charcoal broiled steaks have a benzo[α]pyrene concentration up to 50 ppb. Sausage cooked over burning logs have as much as 200 ppb of benzo[α]pyrene. It was suggested that benzo[α]pyrene forms when the rendered fat of the meat drips into the hot charcoal, is pyrolized (decomposed by heat), and forms compounds that rise with the smoke and are deposited on the meat. Oven cooking, cooking with the heat source above the meat, or segregation of the meat from the smoke results in food with negligible amounts of benzo[α]pyrene (63).

Mycotoxins. *Aflatoxin B1.* Some molds may contain toxic substances that are carcinogens. One of the most potent of carcinogens has been found as a contaminant in animal and human food. It is a mycotoxin, a metabolite of the mold (fungus) *Aspergillus flavus,* which grows in contaminated human and animal feeds. The mycotoxin is aflatoxin B1 (AFB$_1$), which is found in stored agricultural

---

Note 6: Volatile nitrosamines are also a possible source of concern. In Germany, attention to the nitrosamine NDMA has resulted in a drop from a daily beer consumption of 0.74 mg/day in 1979–80 to 0.10 mg/day in 1987. In most Western countries the exposure to volatile nitrosamines is generally of the order of 0.3 to 1.0 mg/day; it is considerably higher in China (119).

Note 7: Bladder cancer in Egyptians is usually associated with the presence in the bladder of the parasitic worm *Schistosoma haematobium.* The female worm migrates to the bladder and deposits thousands of eggs which result in infection of the bladder.

Hicks and colleagues had shown that in an area prevalent with parasitic infections, young Egyptian men had increased bacterial infections of the bladder and increased levels of N-nitroso compounds in the urine compared to controls in an area of low risk for the infection. The increased presence of nitrate-reducing bacteria in the urine of those with infected bladders was related to the higher levels of N-nitroso compounds in the urine.

The bladder of baboons previously infected with *Schistosoma haematobium* and then given an experimental bladder carcinogen, BEN (N-butyl-N-[4-hydroxybutyl] nitrosamine) was compared to bladders of control animals given a different type of noninfectious worm (43). Only the bladders of the baboons infected with the parasite and injected with the nitrosamine showed neoplastic changes: one papillary carcinoma and three early adenocarcinomas; none was noted in the control animals. Hicks concluded that the N-nitroso compounds in the urine of infected bladders acted as an initiating agent for bladder cancer; the parasite could then accelerate the carcinogenesis.

commodities such as peanuts, cotton seed, corn, and tree nuts (13). When fed a diet containing one part in a million of AFB_1 over a period of 2 years 10 percent of male rats developed liver cancer. Many animal species are susceptible to AFB_1. It may be found in milk from cows eating feed contaminated with the mold (13).

The importance of AFB_1 in causing human liver cancer has been a matter of debate. In some studies there is a positive correlation between the AFB_1 levels in the diet and the development of human liver cancer (47,107). In Fusai, China, a region with one of the highest incidences of liver cancer in the world, there was almost a linear relationship between the concentration of AFB_1 level in the diet and the liver cancer mortality (128). There is a similar correlation with the infectious hepatitis B virus (HBV) (6). In areas of Swaziland where there is a high incidence of liver cancer, there is little correlation with HBV but in the subregions where there is less exposure to HBV, there is a strong association of liver cancer with the exposure to AFB (86). It has also been suggested that the two postulated carcinogens of liver cancer, HBV and AFB_1, may act in concert (36).

Many other mutagens and carcinogens that have been demonstrated to cause cancer in animals have been shown to be present in the diet of man (1,20,28,30,51,62,83,94,115,130).

Fat and Fiber Content, Caloric Intake, and Dietary Protein. Roberfroid has summarized the conflicting results on the influence of fat, fiber, and caloric intake on experimental carcinogenesis of the breast in female animals (98). The animal investigations of the type of fat in the diet and the incidence of cancers have given controversial data (100). Fat per se seems to have had no modulating effect on chemically induced carcinogenesis (114). However, a diet rich in lipids might cause a breakdown in metabolism and lead to carcinogenic metabolites. Birt and colleagues showed that a high fat diet, with controlled caloric intake, produced an increase in the number of intraductal cancers of the pancreas in the hamster after the administration of a nitrosamine (9).

In classic experiments, Alfred Tannenbaum and colleagues of the University of Illinois found that a restriction of caloric intake in animals resulted in a decreased incidence of tumors as well as a delay in the time of appearance of tumors (117). Some carcinogens often caused decreased appetite in animals and a decrease in the incidence, or delay in the appear-

ance, of tumors. This may have been interpreted as an anticarcinogenic effect in some studies rather than the result of decreased dietary intake.

A high content of fiber in the diet did not protect against the risk of colon cancer or adenoma in a Nurses Health Study of 88,000 women over a follow-up period of 16 years (32).

E. J. Hawrylewicz, of the College of Medicine, University of Illinois, Chicago, has reviewed the effect of proteins and amino acids as modulators of carcinogenesis. Most studies show an increased risk for breast cancer associated with high protein and fat consumption. Colon cancer also appears to have a positive correlation with high protein consumption. High protein diets increase pancreatic and pituitary tumors but decrease the number of kidney tumors. Liver cancer increases with a high protein diet during the tumor promotion phase in aflatoxin-treated rats. Methionine is necessary for tumor growth; dietary methionine and tryptophan can affect initiation and progression of tumors. Leucine and isoleucine can function as promotors of bladder carcinogenesis (38).

Alcohol

Excessive intake of alcohol is a known causal factor in cancer of the liver, mouth, pharynx, larynx, and esophagus (99). The consumption of alcohol has been reported to increase the risk of female breast cancer. A similar association between male beer drinkers and rectal cancer has been suggested (100).

Vitamins and Cancer

Claims have been made at various times that one or more vitamins have had an anticancer effect. Vitamins A, B, C, D, E, and K in some experimental studies in animals have shown protective effects against cancer, but many other studies have found a lack of protection, and even an enhancing, of tumor production (89).

Vitamin A and Derivatives. An important advance toward the prevention of cancer has been the discovery by Michael Sporn of the National Institutes of Health that retinoids, metabolites of vitamin A, may prevent some cancers (113). Vitamin A and several retinoids (related to vitamin A) have been shown to be anticarcinogenic in experimental cancers of the skin, mammary gland, urinary bladder, and other organs of animals. They may also have an opposite effect, enhancing carcinogenesis in some organs, i.e., lung, skin, liver, and others. A deficiency of vitamin A may increase the number of cancers of the bladder and colon. Excessive amounts of vitamin A decreased skin cancers in animals caused by DMBA (dimethylnitrosamine) but was associated with a reduction in body weight, a possible confounding factor (100).

Beta carotene, a metabolite of vitamin A, reduced tumorigenesis in skin cancers of the mouse produced by ultraviolet light or polycyclic aromatic hydrocarbons. Dietary administration of retinoids or vitamin A was less effective than local application (100). The mortality in rats with metastasizing cancer of the prostate has been reported as greatly reduced by retinoids (92) (Note 4).

High concentrations of dietary vitamin A did not protect against colon or liver cancer in rats given DMH or AFB_1, respectively, or against bladder tumorigenesis in rats given N-[4-5-2 furyl-2-thiazolyl] formamide (100).

Cigarette smokers in Finland were given beta carotene and vitamin E dietary supplements and their incidence of lung cancer was compared to cigarette smokers without such supplements (Alpha-Tocopherol, Beta Carotene [ATBC] Cancer Prevention Study [2]). The group given the vitamin supplements, surprisingly, had a significantly higher incidence of lung cancer than those who did not receive either beta carotene, vitamin E, or a combination of both. This study has been criticized because the subjects smoked heavily and the dosage of the vitamins was considered inadequate by some investigators.

Other clinical trials of vitamin A and/or beta carotene have been reported. In the Beta Carotene and Retinol Efficacy Trial (CARET) over 18,000 persons were involved (84). One group comprised men who had been occupationally exposed to asbestos for at least 15 years and were also cigarette smokers, persons with a high risk for lung cancer. Half of the subjects were given 30 mg of beta carotene and 25,000 IU of vitamin A daily. The comparable control group was given a placebo. Four years later, again a surprising effect: 25 percent more lung cancers were diagnosed and 17 percent more deaths from lung cancer occurred in the group given the vitamin and beta carotene than in the control group (84). The study was stopped because of possible further harmful effects.

In another clinical trial, The Physicians Health Study (PHS), over 22,000 male physicians were

studied for a period of 12 years (40). The test group received 50 mg of beta carotene every other day; the control group received a placebo. At the end of the trial there was no difference in the overall incidence of cancer between the groups and the number of cases of lung cancer deaths was not statistically significantly different. The incidence of lung cancer was relatively low in both groups because of the low percentage of smokers. The results of beta carotene and vitamin A ingestion in humans did not match the results in some animal experiments, illustrating the problem of extrapolating results in one species to those of another species.

Minerals

Metals have been implicated in carcinogenesis, particularly, low levels of selenium (50). Studies of the selenium concentration in the toenail clippings of over 62,000 female nurses who were followed for 41 months did not indicate that selenium protected them from breast cancer or other cancers (14,34).

A more detailed description of the role of minerals in epidemiology is given by Fraumeni and colleagues (31).

Carcinogens: Mechanism of Action

It is obvious from the multistage complex process of carcinogenesis that any one of the stages might be affected by various chemical, immunological, or other substances. A detailed definition of the individual clinical stages is needed in order to determine in which stages, if any, dietary factors may act.

In a recent book edited by Joseph C. Arcos and colleagues (3), carcinogenesis has been considered to be the result of various combinations of carcinogenic factors acting through intricate networks of metabolism to produce cancer (20). They believe that the classic concept that a given carcinogen is the sole etiologic agent causing cancer is outdated, except in controlled laboratory demonstrations and clinically recognized occupational or lifestyle exposures. They give many examples of factors or parameters that can modify chemical carcinogenesis. Emphasis, in addition to the well-known genotoxic factors, is placed on epigenetic changes that may modify DNA conformation, chromatin proteins, and, possibly, nucleic matrix proteins (3).

The many different factors affecting the initiation or promotion of cancer present a bewildering array of agents that appear to have no common agent or mechanism of action. This wide spectrum of carcinogens suggests that there are many pathways for the cancer transformation process. It throws some doubt on the likelihood that a single final common causal pathway, yet undiscovered, underlies all carcinogenesis.

The balance in the cell between transformation and nontransformation to cancer appears to be a fragile one, at least in older persons, a balance that may be upset by many agents that may give the coup de grace that decides the issue. It is likely that many factors have to be operative before the final action is successful in producing transformation. At present, it is not known whether a definite sequence of processes or a definite number of nonsequential events is needed to set the stage for transformation.

REFERENCES

1. Aeschbacher HU, Turesky RJ. Mammalian cell mutagenicity and metabolism of heterocyclic aromatic amines. Mutat Res 1991;259:235–50.
2. Alpha-tocopherol, Beta carotene Cancer Prevention Study Group. The effect of vitamin E and beta carotene on the incidence of lung cancer and other changes in male smokers. N Engl J Med 1994;330:1029–35.
3. Arcos JC, Argus MF. Multifactor interaction network of carcinogenesis—a "tour guide." In: Arcos JC, Argus MF, Woo YT, eds. Chemical induction of cancer. Boston: Birkhäuser, 1995:1–20.
4. Auerbach O, Gere JB, Forman JB, et al. Changes in the bronchial epithelium in relation to smoking and cancer of the lung. N Engl J Med 1957;256:97–104.
5. Bayliss WM, Starling EH. The mechanism of pancreatic secretion. J Physiol 1902;28:325–53.
6. Beasley RP, Hwang LY Epidemiology of hepatocellular carcinoma. In: Vyas GN, Dienstag J, Hoffnagel JH, eds. Viral hepatitis and liver disease. New York: Grune and Stratton, 1984;209–24.
7. Beatson GE. On the treatment of inoperable cases of carcinoma of the mamma: suggestions for a new method of treatment. Lancet 1896;2:104–7, 162–5.
8. Beral V, Hermon C, Kay C, Hannaford P, Darby S, Reeves G. Mortality associated with oral contraceptive use: 25 year follow up of a cohort of 46,000 women from Royal College of General Practitioners' oral contraception study. Br Med J 1999;318:96–100.
9. Birt DF, Julius AD, White LT, Pour PM. Enhancement of pancreatic carcinogenesis in hamsters fed a high-fat diet ad libitum and at a controlled calorie intake. Cancer Res 1989;49:5848–51.
10. Blakeslee S. Faulty math heightens fears of breast cancer. Week in review, New York Times, March 1992;14:1.
11. Brookes P, Lawley PD. Evidence for the binding of polynuclear aromatic hydrocarbons to the nucleic acids of mouse skin: relation between carcinogenic power of hydrocarbons and their binding to deoxynucleic acid. Nature 1964;202:781–4.
12. Burkitt D. Colonic-rectal cancer: fiber and other dietary factors. Am J Clin Nutr 1978;31:S58–64.
13. Chu FS. Mycotoxins: food contamination, mechanism, carcinogenic potential and preventive measures. Mutat Res 1991;259:291–306.
14. Clark LC, Alberts DS. Selenium and cancer: risk or protection? JNCI 1995;87:473–5.
15. Clemmesen J, ed. Symposium on geographical pathology and demography of cancer. Held at Regent's Park College, Oxford, England. Council for the Coordination of International Congresses of Medical Sciences, World Health Organization, United Nations Educational, Scientific and Cultural Organization, 1950.
16. Cohen MB, Heidger PM, Lubaroff DM. Gross and microscopic pathology of induced prostatic complex tumors arising in Lobund-Wistar rats. Cancer Res 1994;54:626–8.
17. Cornfield J. Cited by Stolley CO, Lasky T. Investigating disease patterns: the science of epidemiology. New York: Scientific American Library, 1995.
18. Cosgrove MD, Benton B, Henderson BE. Male genitourinary abnormalities and maternal diethylstilbestrol. J Urol 1977;117:220–2.
19. DeVita VT Jr, Hellman S, Rosenberg SA, eds. Cancer principles and practice of oncology. 2nd ed. Philadelphia: JB Lippincott, 1985.
20. Dipple A, Bigger CA. Mechanism of action of food-associated polycyclic aromatic hydrocarbon carcinogens. Mutat Res 1991;259:263–76.
21. Doll R. Clinical trials: retrospect and prospect. Stat Med 1982;1:337–4.
22. Doll R. Progress against cancer: an epidemiologic assessment. Am J Epidemiol 1991;134:675–88.
23. Doll R, Hill AB. Mortality in relation to smoking: ten years' observation of British doctors. Br Med J 1964;1:1399–410.
24. Doll R, Hill AB. Smoking and carcinoma of the lung. Br Med J 1950;2:739–48.
25. Dorn HF, Cutler SJ. Morbidity from cancer in the United States. Public Health Monograph No. 56. Washington, D.C.: GPO, 1959.
26. Duffy BJ. Austin Bradford Hill–young at heart. Stat Med 1982;1:305–9.
27. Falk H, Herbert J, Crowley S, et al. Epidemiology of hepatic angiosarcoma in the United States 1964–1974. Environ Health Perspect (US) 1981;41:107–3.
28. Felton JS, Knize MG. Occurrence, identification and bacterial mutagenicity of heterocyclic amines in cooked food. Mutat Res 1991;259:205–17.

29. Ferguson AR. Associated bilharziasis and primary malignant disease of the urinary bladder, with observations on a series of forty cases. J Path 1911;16:76–94.

30. Feron VJ, Til HP, de Vrijer F, Woutersen RA, Cassee FR, van Bladeren PJ. Aldehydes: occurrence, carcinogenic potential, mechanism of action and risk assessment. Mutat Res 1991;259:363–85.

31. Fraumeni JF Jr, Devesa SS, Hoover RN, Kinlen LJ. Epidemiology of cancer. In: DeVita VT Jr, Hellman S, Rosenberg SA, eds. Cancer principles and practice of oncology, 4th ed. Philadelphia: JB Lippincott, 1997:150–81.

32. Fuchs CS, Giovannuco EL, Colditz GA, et al. Dietary fiber and the risk of colorectal cancer and adenoma in women. N Engl J Med 1999;340:169–76.

33. Furth J. Hormones as etiologic agents in neoplasia. In: Becker FF, ed. Cancer—a comprehensive treatise, vol 1. New York: Plenum Press, 1975:75–120.

34. Garland M, Morris JS, Stampfer MJ, et al. Prospective study of toenail selenium levels and cancer among women. JNCI 1995;87:497–505.

35. Haenszel W, Berg JW, Segi M, et al. Large bowel cancer in Hawaiian Japanese. JNCI 1973;51:1765–79.

36. Harris CC, Sun TT. Interactive effects of chemical carcinogens and hepatitis B virus in the pathogenesis of hepatocellular carcinoma. Cancer Surv 1986;5:765–80.

37. Härting FH, Hesse W. Der Lungenkrebs, die Bergkrankheit in den Schneeberger Gruben. Vertlischr gerlichtl Med 1879;30:296–309, 31:102–32.

38. Hawrylewicz EJ. Modulation by protein and individual amino acids. In: Aeros JC, Argus MF, Woo YT, eds. Chemical induction of cancer: modulation and combination effects: an inventory of the many factors which influence carcinogenesis. Boston: Birkhäuser, 1995:284–315.

39. Hemminki E, Kennedy DL, Baum D, McKinlay SM. Prescribing noncontraceptive estrogens and progestrins in the United States, 1974–1986. Am J Pub Health 1988;78:1479–81.

40. Hennekens CH, Buring JE, Manson JE, et al. Lack of effect of long-term supplementation with beta carotene on the incidence of malignant neoplasms and cardiovascular disease. N Engl J Med 1996;334:1145–9.

41. Herbst AL, Scully RE. Adenocarcinoma of the vagina in adolescence. A report of seven cases including 6 clear-cell carcinomas (so-called mesonephromas). Cancer 1970; 25:745–57.

42. Herbst AL, Ulfelder H, Proskanzer DC. Adenocarcinoma of the vagina: association of maternal stilbestrol therapy with tumor appearance in young women. N Engl J Med 284:878–81.

43. Hicks RM. Nitrosamines as possible etiological agents in bilharzial bladder cancer. In: Magee PN, ed. Nitrosamines and human cancer. Cold Spring Harbor, NY: Cold Spring Harbor Laboratory, 1982.

44. Higginson J, Muir CS, Muñoz N. Stomach. Human cancer: epidemiology and environmental causes. Cambridge: Cambridge Univ. Press, 1992:273–82.

45. Ho SM, Yu M, Leav I, Viccione T. The conjoint actions of androgens and estrogens in the induction of proliferative lesions in the rat prostate. In: Li JJ, Nandi S, Li SA, eds. Hormonal carcinogenesis. Proceedings of the First International Symposium. New York: Springer-Verlag, 1992:18–26.

46. Hoover RM. Sex hormones and human carcinogenesis epidemiology. In: Becker KL, ed. Principles and practice of endocrinology and metabolism. Philadelphia: JB Lippincott, 1990:1647–54.

47. Hsieh DP. Potential human health hazards of mycotoxins. In: Natori S, Hashimoto K, Ueno Y, eds. Mycotoxins and phycotoxins '88: a collection of invited papers presented at the Seventh International IUPAC Symposium on mycotoxins and phycotoxins. Amsterdam: Elsevier, 1989:69–80.

48. Huggins CB, Hodges CV. Studies of prostatic cancer: effect of castration, of estrogen and of androgen injection of serum phosphatases in metastatic carcinoma of prostate. Cancer Res 1941;1:293–7.

49. Huggins CB, Stevens RE Jr, Hodges CV. Studies of prostatic cancer: effects of castration on advanced carcinoma of the prostate gland. Arch Surg 1941;43:209–23.

50. Jacobs MM, Pienta RJ. Modulation by minerals. In: Arcos JC, Argus MF, Woo YT, eds. Chemical induction of cancer. Boston: Birkhäuser, 1995:335–56.

51. Jägerstad M, Skog K, Grivas S, Olsson K. Formation of heterocyclic amines using model systems. Mutat Res 1991;259:219–33.

52. Jensen EV. Current concepts of sex hormones action (an overview). In: Li JJ, Nandi S, Li SA, eds. Hormonal carcinogenesis. New York: Springer-Verlag, 1992:43–50.

53. Kaufman DW, Shapiro S, Slone D, et al. Decreased risk of endometrial cancer among oral contraceptive users. N Engl J Med 1980;303:1045–7.

54. King G, Newsholme A. On the alleged increase of cancer. Proc R Soc London, 1893;53:405–7.

55. Lacassagne A. Apparition de cancers de la mammelle chez la souris màle, soumise à des injections de folliculine. Compt Rend Acad Sci 1932;195:630–2.

56. Lane-Claypon JE. A further report on cancer of the breast with special reference to its associated antecedent conditions. Reports on the public health and medical subjects, No. 32. Ministry of health, His Majesty's Stationery Office, London, 1926.

57. Levin ML, Goldstein H, Gerhardt PR. Cancer and tobacco smoking. A preliminary report. JAMA 1950;143:336–8.

58. Li JJ, Li SA. The effect of hormones on tumor induction. In: Arcos JC, Argus MF, Woo YT, eds. Chemical induction of cancer: modulation and combination effects: an inventory of the many factors which influence carcinogenesis. Boston: Birkhäuser, 1995:397–449.

59. Li JJ, Mueller GC, Sekely LI. Workshop report, division of cancer etiology, National Cancer Institute. Current perspectives and future trends in hormonal carcinogenesis. Cancer Res 1991;51:3626–9.

60. Li JJ, Nandi S. Hormones and carcinogenesis: laboratory studies. In: Becker KL, ed. Principles and practice of endocrinology and metabolism. Philadelphia: Lippincott, 1990:1643–7.

61. Lickint F. Tabak und Tabakrauch als aetiologischer Factor des carcinoms. Z Krebsforsch 1929;30:349–65.

62. Lijinsky W. The formation and occurrence of polynuclear aromatic hydrocarbons associated with food. Mutat Res 1991;259:251–61.

63. Lijinsky W, Shubik P. Benzo[a]pyrene and other polynuclear hydrocarbons in charcoal-broiled meat. Science 1964;145:53–55.

64. Lilienfeld AM, Lilienfeld DE. Foundations of epidemiology, 2nd ed. New York: Oxford Univ. Press, 1980:3.

65. MacMahon B, Cole P, Brown J. Etiology of human breast cancer: a review. JNCI 1973;50:21–42.

66. MacMahon B, Pugh TF. Epidemiology: principles and methods. Boston: Little, Brown, 1970.

67. Magee PN. Nitrosamines and human cancer. Banbury report 12. Cold Spring Harbor, NY: Cold Spring Harbor Laboratory, 1982.

68. Magee PN, Barnes JM. Carcinogenic nitroso compounds. Adv Cancer Res 1967;10:163–246.

69. Magee PN, Barnes JM. The production of malignant primary hepatic tumors in the rat by feeding dimethylnitrosamine. Br J Cancer 1956;10:114–22.

70. Merewether ER. Annual report of the chief inspector of factories for the year 1947. London: His Majesty's Stationery Office, 1949.

71. Mills DA, Porter MM. Tobacco smoking habits and cancer of the mouth and respiratory system. Cancer Res 1950;10:539–42.

72. Mirvish SS. Role of N-nitroso compounds (NOC) and N-nitrosation in etiology of gastric, esophageal, nasopharyngeal and bladder cancer and contribution to cancer of known exposures to NOC. Cancer Lett 1995;93:17–48.

73. Mosher WD, Pratt WF. Contraceptive use in the United States, 1973–1988. Advance data from vital health statistics, No. 182. Hyattsville, MD: National Center for Health Statistics, 1990.

74. Mueller G. Estrogen action: a study of the influence of steroid hormones on genetic expression. In: Smellie RM, ed. The biochemistry of steroid hormone action. London: Academic Press, 1971:1–29.

75. Muir CS. Epidemiology, basic science and the prevention of cancer: implications for the future. Cancer Res 1990;50:6441–8.

76. Müller FH. Tabakmissbrauch und lungencarcinom. Z Krebsforsch 1939;49:57–85.

77. Nandi N, Guzman RC, Miyamoto S. Hormones, cell proliferation and mammary carcinogenesis. In: Li JJ, Li SN, Li SA, eds. Hormonal carcinogenesis. Proceeding of the First International Symposium. New York: Springer-Verlag, 1991:73–7.

78. Newell GR. Epidemiology of cancer. In: DeVita VT Jr, Hellman S, Rosenberg SA, eds. Cancer: principles and practice of oncology. 2nd ed. Philadelphia: JB Lippincott, 1985:151–95.

79. Newhouse M. Epidemiology of asbestos-related tumors. Semin Oncol 1981;8:250–7.

80. Noble RL. The development of prostate adenocarcinoma in Nb rats following prolonged sex hormone administration. Cancer Res 1977;37:1929–33.

81. Offit K, Brown K. Quantitating familiar cancer risk: a resource for clinical oncologists. J Clin Oncol 1994;121:1724–36.

82. O'Grady WP, McDivitt RW. Breast cancer in a man treated with diethylstilbestrol. Arch Pathol 1969;88:162–5.

83. Ohgaki H, Takayama S, Sugimura T. Carcinogenicities of heterocyclic amines in cooked food. Mutat Res 1991;259:399–410.

84. Omenn GS, Goodman GE, Thornquist MD, et al. Risk factors for lung cancer and for intervention effects in CARET, the beta-carotene and retinol efficacy trial. JNCI 1996;88:1550–9.

85. Paul C, Skegg DC, Spears GF. Oral contraceptives and risk of breast cancer. Int J Cancer 1990;46:366–73.

86. Peers F, Bosch X, Kaldor J, Linsell A, Pluijiman M. Aflatoxin exposure, hepatitis B virus infection and liver cancer in Swaziland. Int J Cancer 1987;39:545–53.

87. Persson I, Adami HO, Bergkvist L, et al. Risk of endometrial cancer after treatment with estrogens alone or in conjunction with progestogens: results of a prospective study. Br Med J 1989;298:147–51.

88. Petrakis NL. Historic milestones in cancer epidemiology. Semin Oncol 1979;6:433–45.

89. Petru E, Woo YT, Berger MR. Modulation by vitamins. In: Arcos JC, Argus MF, Woo YT, eds. Chemical induction of cancer. Boston: Birkhäuser, 1995:316–34.

90. Pollard M, Luckert PH. Production of autochthonous prostate cancer in Lobund-Wistar rats by treatments with N-nitroso-N-methylurea and testosterone. JNCI 1986;77:583–7.

91. Pollard M, Luckert PH, Snyder DL. The promotional effect of testosterone on induction of prostate cancer in MNU-sensitized L-W rats [Letter]. Cancer 1989;45:209–12.

92. Pollard M, Luckert PH, Sporn MB. Prevention of primary prostate cancer in Lobund-Wistar rats by N-(4-hydroxyphenyl) retinamide. Cancer Res 1991;51:3610–1.

93. Pott P. Chirurgical observations relative to the cataract, the polypus of the nose, the cancer of the scrotum, the different kinds of ruptures, and the mortification of toes and feet. London: TJ Carnegy, 1775.

94. Povey AC, Schiffman M, Taffe BG, Harris CC. Laboratory and epidemiologic studies of fecapentaenes. Mutat Res 1991;259:387–97.

95. Ramazzini B; Wright WC, trans. De morbis Artificum. Chicago: Univ. Chicago Press, 1940.

96. Rehn L. Blasengeschwülste bei Fuchsin-Arbeitern. Arch Fur Klin Chir 1895;1:588–600.

97. Robboy SJ, Noller KL, O'Brien P, et al. Increased incidence of cervical and vaginal dysplasia in 3980 diethylstilbestrol-exposed young women. JAMA 1984;252:2979–83.

98. Roberfroid MB. Dietary modulation of experimental neoplastic development: role of fat and fiber content and calorie intake. Mutat Res 1991;259:351–62.

99. Rogers AE, Conner MW. Alcohol and cancer. In: Poirier LA, Newberne PM, Pariza MW, eds. Symposium on the role of essential nutrients in carcinogenesis. New York: Plenum Press, 1986:473–95.

100. Rogers AE, Longnecker MP. Dietary and nutritional influences on cancer: a review of epidemiologic and experimental data. Lab Invest 1988;59:729–59.

101. Sander J. Kann Nitrit under menschlichen Narung ursache einer Krebsentstehung durch Nitrosaminbildung sein? Arch Hygien und Bacteriologie 1967;151:22–8.

102. Schereschewsky JW. The course of cancer mortality in the ten original registration states. AS Public Health Service, Public Health Bulletin No. 155. Washington, D.C.: GPO, 1926.

103. Schottenfeld D, Fraumeni JF. Cancer epidemiology and prevention. Philadelphia: WB Saunders, 1982.

104. Schreck R, Baker LA, Ballard GP, Dolgof S. Tobacco smoking as an etiological factor in disease. I. Cancer. Cancer Res 1950;10:49–58.

105. Selikoff IJ, Churg J, Hammond EC. Relation between exposure to asbestos and mesothelioma. N Engl J Med 1965;272:560–5.

106. Selikoff IJ, Hammond EC, Churg J. Asbestos exposure, smoking and neoplasia. JAMA 1968;204:106–12.

107. Shank RC. Environmental toxicoses in humans. In: Shank RC, ed. Mycotoxins and N-nitroso compounds, environmental risks, Vol. I. Boca Raton, FL: CRS Press, 1981;107–53.

108. Shield AM. A remarkable case of multiple growth of the skin caused by exposure to the sun. Lancet 1899;1:22–3.

109. Shimkin MB. Contrary to nature: being an illustrated commentary on some persons and events of historical importance of knowledge concerning cancer, Washington, D.C.: Department of Health Education and Welfare, Public Health Service, National Institutes of Health, 1977:__.

110. Siddiqi M, Preusmann R. Esophageal cancer in Kashmir—an assessment. J Cancer Res Clin Oncol 1989;115:111–7.

111. Silverberg SG, Makowski EL. Endometrial carcinoma in young women taking oral contraceptive agents. Obstet Gynecol 1975;6:503–6.

112. Singer GM, Chuan J, Roman J, Min-Hsin L, Lijinsky W. Nitrosamine and nitrosamine precursors in foods from Linxian China, a high incidence area for esophageal cancer. Carcinogenesis 1986;7:733–6.

113. Sporn MB. Carcinogenesis and cancer: different perspectives on the same disease. Cancer Res 1991;51:6215–8.

114. Stemmermann GN, Nomura AM, Heilbrun LK. Dietary fat and the risk of colorectal cancer. Cancer Res 1984;44:4633–7.

115. Stich HF. The beneficial and hazardous effects of simple phenolic compounds. Mutat Res 1991;259:307–24.

116. Stolley PD, Lasky T. Investigating disease patterns: the science of epidemiology. New York, Scientific American Library, 1995:61, 62.

117. Tannenbaum A. The dependence of tumor formation on the degree of caloric restriction. Cancer Res 1945;5:609–25.

118. Taubes G. Epidemiology faces its limits. Science 1995;269:164–9.

119. Tricker AR, Preussman R. Carcinogenic N-nitrosamines in the diet: occurrence, formation, mechanisms and carcinogenic potential. Mutat Res 1991;259:277–89.

120. Unna PG. Die Histopathologie der Hautkrankheiten. Berlin: Hirschwald, 1894.

121. U.S. Department of Health and Human Services, Public Health Services. Strategies to Control Tobacco Use in the United States. Smoking and tobacco Control Monographs, Vol. 1 (No. 90–3316). Bethesda, MD: National Institute of Health, 1991.

122. Volkmann, R. Ueber Theer und Russkrebs. Archiv Für Klinische Chirurgie 1874;1:3–5.

123. Wagner JC, Sleggs CA, Marchand P. Diffuse pleural mesothelioma and asbestos exposure in North Western Cape Province. Br J Ind Med 1960;17:260–71.

124. Waldo ED, Sidhu GS, Hu AW. Florid papillomatosis of the male nipple after diethylstilbestrol therapy. Arch Pathol 1975;99:364–6.

125. Warthin AS. Heredity with reference to carcinoma as shown by the study of the cases examined in the pathological laboratory of the University of Michigan, 1895–1913. Arch Intern Med 1913;12:546–55.

126. Weisburger JH, Marquardt H, Hirota N, Mori H, Williams GH. Induction of cancer of the glandular stomach in rats by an extract of nitrite-treated fish. JNPI 1980;64:163–7.

127. Wynder EL, Graham EA. Tobacco smoking as a possible etiologic factor in bronchiogenic carcinoma. A study of six hundred and eighty four proved cases. JAMA 1950;143:329–36.

128. Yeh FS, Yu M, Mo CC, Luo S, Tong MJ, Henderson BE. Hepatitis B virus, aflatoxins and hepatocellular carcinoma in southern Guangxi, China. Cancer Res 1989;49:2506–9.

129. Yu MC, Nichols PW, Zou XN, Estes J, Henderson BE. Induction of malignant nasal cavity tumors in Wistar rats fed Chinese salted fish. Br J Cancer 1989;60:198–201.

130. Zimmerli B, Schlatter J. Ethyl carbamate: analytical methodology, occurrence, formation, biological activity and risk assessment. Mutat Res 1991;259:325–50.

✳ ✳ ✳

PART IV
DNA, MOLECULAR BIOLOGY,
AND THE GENE
(WORLD WAR II TO END OF 20TH CENTURY)

MOLECULAR BIOLOGY

There have been astounding advances made in the biological sciences during the 20th century, particularly since World War II. One of the most spectacular disciplines, a new field and one in which so many advances in areas such as biochemistry, virology, genetics, and oncology depended for their recent successes, is that of "molecular biology." The focus of this field of study was upon large molecules, macromolecules such as DNA (deoxyribonucleic acid), RNA (ribonucleic acid), proteins, and polymers. Interest in molecular biology has opened up many lines of investigation and from these have come new concepts concerning carcinogenesis. It has led to a better understanding of the cell and its function.

The following is a summary of some of those developments pertinent to a study of the etiology of neoplasia.

In 1938 Warren Weaver, director of the Rockefeller Foundation, wrote, "Among the studies to which the Foundation is giving support is a series in a relatively new field, which may be called molecular biology, in which delicate modern techniques are being used to investigate even more minute details of certain life processes" (85). The term may have been used by others (10,14,43), but Weaver is often given the credit for it (Note 1).

One Gene, One Enzyme

In 1941 an important event occurred which linked genetics and biochemistry. George Beedle and Edward Tatum of the Rockefeller Institute while studying a red mould, *Neurospora crassica,* a yeast that grew on bread, proposed that a gene controlled the activity of a single enzyme, the "one gene, one enzyme" hypothesis. The concept and its apt phraseology sparked much interest in the subject of the genetic control of biochemical processes although the hypothesis had to be modified later (5). It directed much thought and energy to the subject of the genetic control of biological systems.

DNA as a Genetic Transforming Factor in Bacteria

In the 1920s and 1930s, F. Griffith, a bacteriologist in the British Ministry of Health pathology laboratory, showed that some strains of the *Pneumococcus* bacillus were lethal when injected into mice while other strains were avirulent (36). The lethal strains grew out in smooth surface colonies, called the smooth (S) type; the avirulent *Pneumococcus* grew out in culture media as irregular, granular, flat colonies called the rough (R) type. Griffith found that when he injected the smooth colony bacteria into mice they died; injection of the strains which formed rough colonies were not lethal to the mice.

The *Pneumococcus* bacterial strains could also be divided by the type of polysaccharide present in the capsule of the bacterium. A type I polysaccharide was characteristic of the avirulent strain; type II polysaccharide was characteristic of the smooth strain. The polysaccharides were consistently representative of each type.

In an experiment, mice were injected with nonvirulent type I (R) bacteria to which was added heat-killed smooth (S) bacteria with a type II polysaccharide capsule. This led to the death of the mice and the *Pneumococcus* cultured from the blood and lungs of the dead mice contained the S type bacteria with the type II polysaccharide. The avirulent type I polysaccharide had been transformed into the type II polysaccharide of virulent pneumococci by the injected killed smooth (S) strain of bacteria (36).

In 1944, Oswald Avery and his colleagues, Colin McCleod and Maclyn McCarty of the Rockefeller Institute, confirmed Griffith's findings in mice and investigated the phenomenon further (fig. 18-1).

Note 1: Among the investigators being supported by the Rockefeller Foundation were Max Perutz of the Cavendish Laboratory of Cambridge University, William Astbury of Manchester, England, and Linus Pauling of California Institute of Technology, all of whom were studying the atomic structure of biologic substances using X ray diffraction techniques and laying the foundation for advances in molecular biology. In addition, biochemists such as Erwin Chargaff of Columbia University were employing new techniques of chromatography to study nucleotides and nucleic acids (14,43).

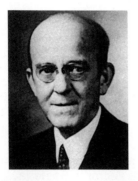

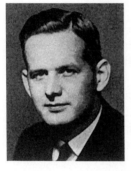
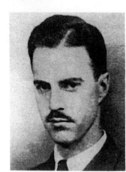

Figure 18-1
OSWALD T. AVERY, COLIN MCLEOD,
AND MACLYN MCCARTY

Drs. Oswald T. Avery (top), Colin McLeod (bottom right) and Maclyn McCarty (bottom left) of the Rockefeller Institute who, in 1944, discovered that the transforming hereditary factor in pneumococcal bacteria was deoxyribonucleic acid (DNA). (Modified from Shimkin MB. Contrary to nature. Washington D.C.: U.S. Department of Health, Education, & Welfare, 1977:441, 442.)

They showed that the transformation of type I bacterial polysaccharide to type II could be carried out not only by injection of the killed (S) bacteria into a growing culture of type I (R) bacteria but also by an injection of a soluble factor prepared from the (S) pneumococcus type II capsule. A precipitate of the soluble fraction of the capsule of the type II bacterium changed the type I into a type II bacterium; it was called the transforming factor.

When used in a dilution of less than 1 in 100 million the transforming factor could still transform the bacterial polysaccharide of type I. The newly transformed S type II pneumococci retained their specificity from generation to generation without the addition of further transforming factor and the

change was therefore a hereditary one. Avery, MacLeod, and McCarty analyzed the transforming factor and found that it was not a protein, as expected, but that it was DNA (2).

Most biologists at the time assumed that genes were composed of protein because it was believed that only such a large chemical compound as a protein, with its thousands of polypeptides, could contain all the genetic information necessary to give rise to the countless proteins and other compounds that made up biological systems. DNA, a nucleic acid, at that time was believed to be composed of a relatively simple structure: four nucleotides, a pentose sugar, and phosphate groups. It did not appear to have the biochemical capacity to encode all the genetic information necessary for the function of even such a relatively small organism as a bacterium. It was suggested by skeptics that a small amount of protein could remain in the alleged protein-free transforming substance. The findings of Avery and colleagues remained relatively neglected for some years (24) (Note 2).

The Phage Group

Max Delbrück, a physicist at the Kaiser Wilhelm Institute in Berlin who had a varied background in theoretical physics, left Germany in 1937 to study viral genetics at the California Institute of Technology in Berkeley (fig. 18-2) (30). He later transferred to Vanderbilt University in Tennessee.

By studying a relatively simple, rapidly multiplying organism such as the bacteriophage, Delbrück believed that one might learn fundamental information about inheritance. In a challenging 1946 Harvey Society lecture, Delbrück indicated his approach to a biological problem:

"... when a physicist is shown an experiment in which a virus particle enters a bacterial cell and twenty minutes later the bacterial cell is lysed, ruptured and destroyed, and one hundred virus particles are liberated, he will say: How come one particle has become one hundred particles of the same kind in twenty minutes? ... Let us find out how it happens ... This is so simple a phenomenon that the answers cannot be hard to find." (21)

Note 2: An authoritative, interesting biography of Avery, his colleagues, the Rockefeller Institute, and the discovery of the importance of DNA in inheritance, was described in *The Professor, The Institute and DNA,* by Rene Dubos. Dubos was a distinguished scientist, author, a member of the Rockefeller Institute, and a colleague of Avery (24).

The answers to Delbrück's question were not easy to obtain and it took longer to find them than Delbrück implied, but only a few years longer. The direct, intellectually rigorous, physicist's approach to problems using a relatively simple system but with new techniques and imaginative experiments paid off with amazing results over the next few decades (43) (Note 4).

Microbial Genetics

By the 1940s the study of bacteriophages had begun to yield important information (25). Just as bacteria infected humans, so did a smaller organism, the bacteriophage, infect bacteria, some killing the host bacterium others not injuring the host but setting up a "live in" arrangement whereby the bacteriophage seemed to coexist in harmony with the bacterium (see chapter 15). If, as in some cases, the host bacterium was killed after infection by the phage, a much greater number of bacteriophage particles was released than the original number of infecting particles. It was believed that what must have happened was that the bacteriophage, which did not have a mechanism by which it could replicate itself, must have multiplied in the bacterium by using the bacterium's own genetic mechanism to synthesize the nucleic acids and protein needed for its own multiplication.

In 1946, Joshua Lederberg, then at Columbia University, discovered conjugation, the joining of bacteria so that a connection between them was formed through which DNA could flow from one bacterium to another (49). This was followed by the demonstration by Zinder and Lederberg (90) of transduction, wherein a bacterial virus (a bacteriophage), acting as a vector, picked up from its host cell a fragment of DNA and transmitted the DNA to the cell that it infected. This was proof that genetic information could be transmitted from bacterium to bacterium by a virus.

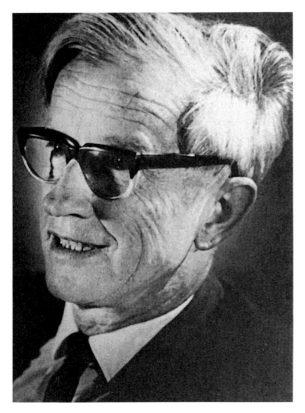

Figure 18-2
MAX DELBRÜCK
Dr. Max Delbrück, leader of the phage group, was a dynamic investigator and early pioneer in molecular biology. (Courtesy of National Library of Medicine.)

Delbrück gathered together a group of investigators who became known as the "phage group" because of their use of bacteriophages (see chapter 15) as a model organism by which they would explore genetic factors. Delbrück, Salvador Luria from Italy, and Alfred Hershey of the Cold Spring Laboratory in New York, were the founders of the group which grew to include many distinguished scientists (10) (Note 3).

Note 3: Since Delbrück was born in Germany, Luria in Italy, and Hersey's goal in life was to devote as much time as possible to experiments, Delbrück, facetiously, referred to the threesome as "two enemy aliens and another misfit in society." They shared a Nobel prize in 1969.

Note 4: It has been said that two leading theoretical physicists were responsible for some other physicists becoming interested in biology. The lecture by Niels Bohr, "Light and Life," in 1923 and the book, *What Is Life?* by Erwin Schrodinger in 1944 played significant roles in focusing the interest of physicists on biology. Max Delbrück, for example, was influenced by Bohr's lecture; he became involved in a study of genes and proposed in 1935 that the gene was a physical unit. Delbrück's later work with the phage group confirmed his prediction that the resolution of the problem of how bacteriophages are processed by bacteria would give fundamental information of importance to biology (21). Watson also stated that Schrodinger's book aroused his interest in "finding out the secret of the gene" (81).

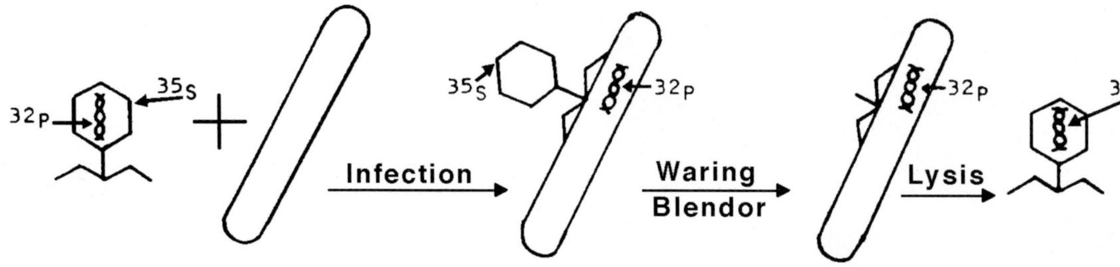

Figure 18-3

SCHEMATIC SUMMARY OF EXPERIMENTS OF A. HERSHEY AND M. CHASE

Schematic summary of experiments of Drs. A. Hershey and M. Chase of the Cold Spring Laboratory (39) who showed that a bacteriophage whose DNA was labeled with radioactive phosphorus (^{32}P) infected bacteria and gave rise to progeny bacteriophage whose DNA was labeled with ^{32}P. Protein of the bacteriophage labeled with ^{35}S was not incorporated into the DNA of the progeny bacteriophage. The genome of the bacteria, therefore, used the DNA of the bacteriophage to synthesize the DNA of the progeny bacteriophage. (Fig. 8.10 from Portugal FH, Cohen JS. A century of DNA: a history of the discovery of the structure and function of the genetic substance. Cambridge, MA: The MIT Press, 1977:182.)

Synthesis of Bacteriophage

Alfred Hershey and Martha Chase of the Phage Group used isotopic labeling to test whether protein or DNA was the carrier of the genetic material of bacteriophage. They used two radioactive labels: sulfur (^{35}S) which would become incorporated into protein because of the presence of two amino acids containing sulfur (methionine and cysteine) in protein and phosphorus (^{32}P) which would become incorporated mostly into nucleic acids (fig. 18-3).

Working with the bacteriophage that infected the common bacterium, *Escherichia coli,* Hershey and Chase showed that bacteria synthesized more bacteriophage by using the DNA (labeled with ^{32}P) of the original bacteriophage as its precursor for the synthesis of the DNA of the new bacteriophage than by employing the protein of the bacteriophage labeled with radioactive sulfur (^{35}S) (39).

This was evidence favoring the hypothesis that the DNA of the bacteriophage contained the genetic information that was used as a template for the synthesis of the new bacteriophage.

NUCLEIC ACIDS AND THE CELL

DNA

In 1869, Friedrick Miescher, a Swiss physiologist and physician-biochemist, working in Hoppe-Seyler's laboratory in Tubingen, was studying lymphoid cells. To obtain these cells he collected discarded bandages containing pus from a nearby surgical clinic, extracted cells from the bandages, and isolated nuclei from the cells. From the nuclei he extracted a substance which he called "nuclein." The same substance was found in the nuclei of yeast cells; kidney, liver, and testicular cells; and nucleated red blood cells. It was not a protein and was later identified as a nucleic acid, deoxyribonucleic acid (DNA) (56,57,69).

Because the sperm of the plentiful salmon of the Rhine river had relatively large nuclei, Miescher used the fish for further studies. He discovered not only nuclein but another compound, which he called protamine, in the cell nuclei (69). A. Kossel, a Swiss physician-biochemist, showed that Miescher's protamine was a protein that was also present in goose nucleated red blood cells. He named the protein "histone" (45). Derivatives of the nuclei of yeast cells yielded the nucleotides adenine, guanine, xanthene, and hypoxanthine. Later, two more nucleotides, thymine and cytosine, and a carbohydrate were identified in the nuclei. By 1900, three pyrimidine bases (thymine, cytosine, and uracil) and two carbohydrates (ribose and deoxyribose) were identified in the nucleic acids (fig. 18-4) (1). Ribonucleic acid (RNA) was similar to DNA except that its sugar was a ribose instead of the 2' deoxyribose in DNA. The

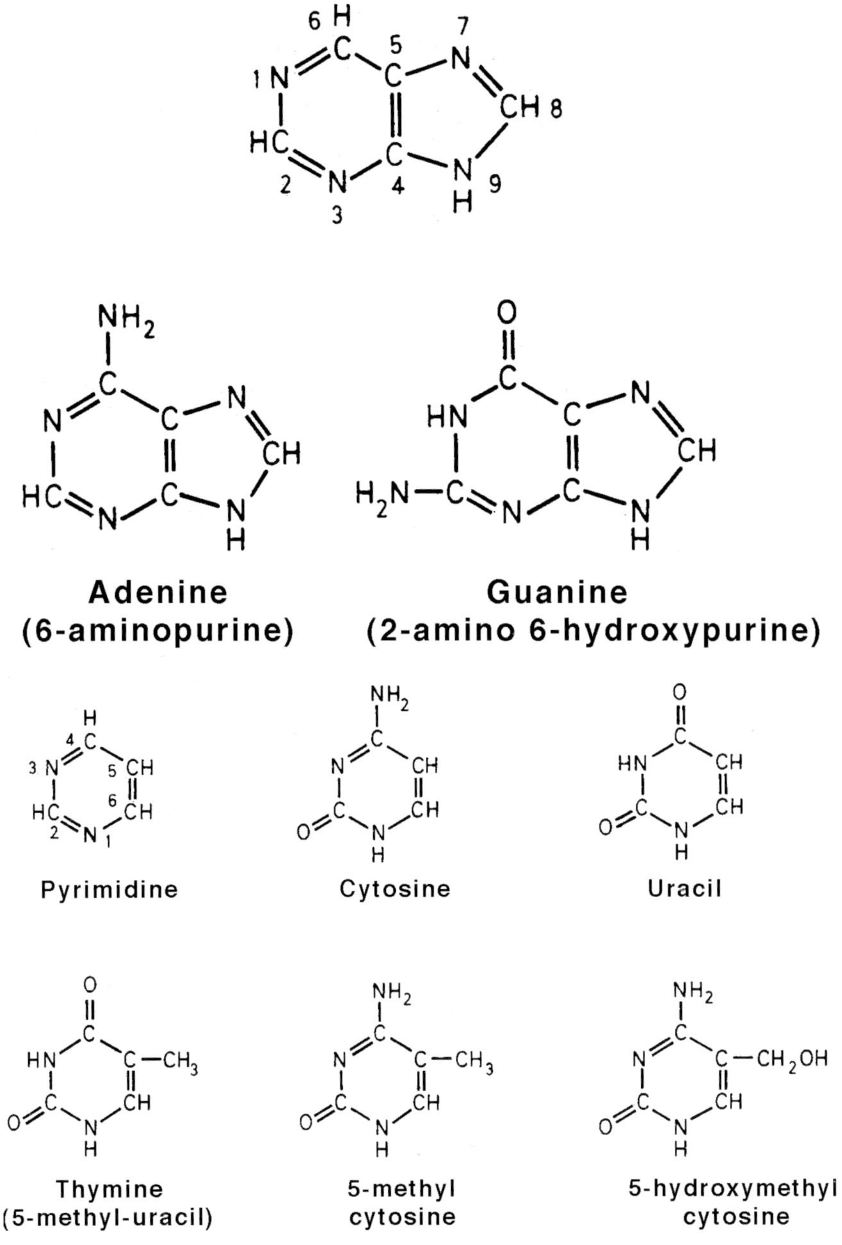

**Adenine
(6-aminopurine)**

**Guanine
(2-amino 6-hydroxypurine)**

Pyrimidine

Cytosine

Uracil

**Thymine
(5-methyl-uracil)**

5-methyl
cytosine

5-hydroxymethyl
cytosine

Figure 18-4
CHEMICAL STRUCTURE
OF THE BUILDING BLOCKS
OF THE NUCLEIC ACIDS
Adenine, guanine, thymine, cytosine, and uracil are the bases of DNA. In RNA, uracil replaces thymine. Upper panel represents purines. Lower panel represents pyrimidines. 5' methyl cytosine and 5' hydroxymethyl cytosine are minor bases sometimes found in RNA. (Figs. 2.3 and 2.1, from Adams RL, Knowler JT, Leader DP. The biochemistry of the nucleic acids, 11th ed. London: Chapman & Hall, 1992:6.)

pyrimidine nucleotide uracil (U) paired with adenine (A) in RNA in contrast to thymine (T) pairing with adenine (A) in DNA.

P. Levene at the Rockefeller Institute concluded that in yeasts the four bases—adenine, guanine, cytosine, and thymine—were present in equal amounts in nucleic acid and suggested a simple tetranucleotide configuration for the molecule (51). A distinction was made between the nucleic acids of plants and animals but eventually it was shown that DNA and RNA occurred in both plant and animal cells (22,69).

Cellular Distribution of Nucleic Acids

Torbjörn Caspersson of the Karolinska Institute in Stockholm, a biologist-geneticist (fig. 18-5), devised in the 1930s an ultraviolet (UV) microscope to demonstrate the presence and amount of nucleic acids in parts of the cell. Ultraviolet light of a specific wave length (2570Å) was absorbed to a greater extent by nucleic acids than by protein and this difference could be used to indicate the relative distribution of nucleic acids and protein in the nucleus

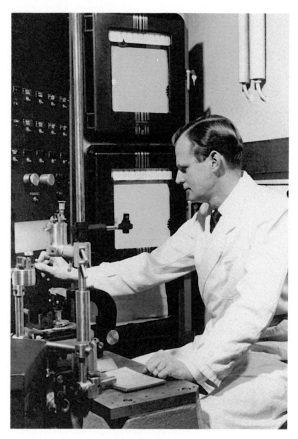

Figure 18-5
TORBJÖRN CASPERSSON

Torbjörn Caspersson, a Swedish cytologist-geneticist, with his ultraviolet microscope that he used to measure the location and amount of nucleic acids in components of cells during different normal functions of the cell, and in cancer (12,13). He later discovered that individual bands of chromosomes were recognizable when the chromosome was stained with quinacrine mustard and exposed to ultraviolet radiation (see chapter 19). (Photograph courtesy of the author.)

the Rockefeller Institute and others had noted particles containing RNA in the cytoplasm (17) but the complex mechanism by which information from DNA was relayed from the nucleus to the RNA of the cytoplasm was not clarified until later.

The Cell Cycle

In early studies of the cell in the final quarter of the 19th century and early 20th century, much attention was devoted to the process of mitosis, a means by which the cell divided into two daughter cells. Cytologists had designated two stages in the life of the cell: 1) Mitosis, recognized by the condensation of the DNA of the nucleus into thread-like bodies, the chromosomes, which were visible under the light microscope and were seen to split into sister chromatids. The chromatids were aligned on a metaphase plate, became attracted to opposite poles of the mitotic spindle, and separated at anaphase to become part of daughter cells (fig. 18-6) (69); and 2) Interphase, in which the cell resumed its usual appearance, a nucleolus became visible, and the DNA was clumped and dispersed irregularly throughout the nucleus. Relatively little was known about the interphase period.

In 1952 in England, Stephan Pelc, a physicist, and Alma Howard, a cytologist, collaborated in a classic study of dividing cells (40). Since each cell divided in half to give rise to two daughter cells and each daughter cell contained the same amount of DNA as its parent cell, there would have to be a doubling of the amount of DNA in the parent cell before division. It was not known in which part of the cell cycle the DNA was synthesized.

Howard and Pelc employed *Vicia faba,* an onion whose cells grew rapidly in culture medium, going quickly through cycles of mitosis and interphase, for their study (40). The culture medium contained radioactive phosphorus (^{32}P) which was incorporated mostly into the newly synthesized DNA of the nucleus of the parent cell. The cells that incorporated the ^{32}P could be identified by a technique called autoradiography (32). After allowing cells to grow in a ^{32}P culture medium, they were covered with photographic emulsion in a darkroom and exposed in the dark for some days, during which the beta particles of the ^{32}P in the cells would be recorded by the overlying emulsion as they were emitted. Development of the emulsion revealed the radioactivity by the reduced grains of silver in the

and cytoplasm of cells (12,13). With the use of ultraviolet microscopy, histochemical staining, and enzymatic digestion of nucleic acids with ribonuclease or deoxyribonuclease, it was soon demonstrated that DNA was concentrated in the chromatin of the nucleus of the cell and RNA in the cytoplasm and nucleolus (7,12,13).

A pathway for protein synthesis whereby the information of the nucleotides of the DNA of the nucleus was relayed to the RNA of the cytoplasm, where the protein was synthesized at the nuclear-cytoplasmic membrane, was suggested by Caspersson (12). Caspersson had found an increase of RNA in the cytoplasm of every biological system tested that had an increase of protein synthesis. A. Claude at

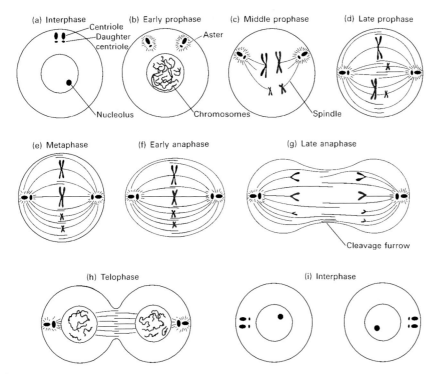

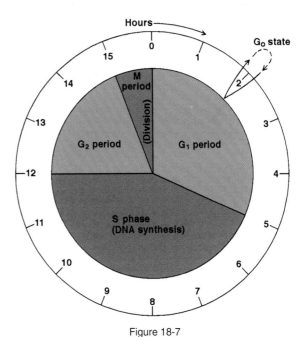

Figure 18-6

SCHEMATIC REPRESENTATION
OF THE CELL CYCLE OF
MITOSIS AND INTERPHASE

DNA is dispersed in irregular pieces of stainable chromatin material in the nucleus during interphase (a) and the amount of DNA is doubled. Mitosis begins with a condensation of DNA into discrete thread-like structures, the chromosomes (b), which split into pairs to form sister chromatids (c). These line up perpendicular to the equator of the cell (d,e,f). The chromosome pairs split apart and move towards opposite poles of the cell (g). After the chromosomes reach the poles of the cell there is division of the cell body into two daughter cells (h,i), each of which has a duplicate set of chromosomes and an equal normal amount of cytoplasm. One member of each pair of sister chromatids is derived from one parent. (Fig. 5.14 from Darnell JE, Lodish H, Baltimore D. Molecular cell biology. New York: Scientific American Books Inc., 1986:149.)

emulsion. The bonding of the emulsion and the histologic section of cells permitted the development of the emulsion and the staining of the biological material. One could thereby focus the microscope on either the emulsion to see whether reduced silver grains were present, or on the underlying histologic section to determine the localization of the radioactivity in different cells, in different parts of the cell, or in other structures.

Howard and Pelc showed that the grains in the emulsion were concentrated in the nuclei of the cells that were in the interphase period or had passed through it; no grains were seen over cells exposed to the isotope only during the mitotic period. Therefore, DNA was synthesized in the interphase period.

Howard and Pelc divided the cell cycle into four stages: the period of synthesis of DNA in interphase was called the S (synthesis) period; the mitotic period was labeled M; the time between the cessation of mitosis and the beginning of the S period became known as the G1 (gap 1) period; and the time from the cessation of DNA synthesis in interphase to the beginning of mitosis was called G2 (gap 2) (fig. 18-7).

Cells of the body have different rates of mitosis (48). There are two types of cells: 1) those that appear never to divide, e.g., the neurons of the

Figure 18-7

THE CELL CYCLE OF HOWARD AND PELC

M = mitotic period, S = period of synthesis of DNA, G1 = period between mitosis and the beginning of DNA synthesis, and G2 = period between the end of DNA synthesis to the beginning of mitosis (40). Later, G0 was postulated as a standby position for some cells which ordinarily do not divide (neurons) or have a low rate of division (47). (Fig. 5.13 from Darnell JE, Lodish H, Baltimore D. Molecular cell biology. New York: Scientific American Books Inc., 1986:148.)

Table 18-1

GENERATION TIMES OF THE CELLS OF SOLID TUMORS
AND THEIR NORMAL COUNTERPARTS*

Tissue	Cell Cycle Time (hours)	Reference
Chemically induced rat hepatomas	14–16	Post and Hoffman (1964, 1965)
Normal rat liver	21.5	
Chemically induced mouse epidermoid carcinomas	32	Dormer et al. (1964)
Normal mouse skin	150	
C_3H mammary tumors	33	Bresciani (1968)
Normal C_3H mouse alveoli	64	
Chemically induced hamster cheek pouch carcinomas	11	Reiskin and Berry (1968)
Normal cheek pouch epithelium	130–155	Brown and Berry (1968)
SPV-induced rabbit papillomas	21	Rashad and Evans (1968)
Normal rabbit epidermis	125–750	
Squamous cell carcinomas of mouse forestomach	8–12	Frankfurt (1967)
Normal forestomach epithelium	28–55	
Squamous cell carcinomas of human cervix	15	Bennington (1969)
Normal cervical epithelium (*in vitro* incubation)	100–600	Iliya and Azar (1967)

*Table 10.1 from Travis EL. Medical radiobiology, 2nd ed. Chicago: Year Book Medical Publishers, 1989:220.

brain and 2) other cells that normally have different rates of mitosis. Cells not going through mitosis, other than neurons, were designated by Lajtha et al. as being in a zero standby stage (G0) (47). These cells could be stimulated to enter mitosis. Cells with a normally low rate of mitosis such as those of the liver could be stimulated after partial hepatectomy to an increased rate of mitosis (8); after ethionine toxicity the pancreas acinar cell could also be stimulated to regenerate with a relatively high rate of mitosis (33). The compounds that stimulated some cells to enter mitosis were called mitogens (62).

Cells such as those of the duodenum could turn over a complete cycle of cell renewal in about a day (48). Bacteria had a very rapid rate of division, completing a cell cycle about once every 20 minutes. The small lymphocytes had a very long cycle time of many months (46).

Labeling Index. Prior to the Pelc-Howard study, the author, Eidenoff, and colleagues at Sloan-Kettering Institute had introduced tritium (^{3}H) as a radioactive label for autoradiography. Tritium's low energy gave relatively high resolution by localizing the isotope to areas of a micron or less (31). Later, Hughes and coworkers at Brookhaven Labora-

tories in New York labeled thymidine with tritium (41). For subsequent studies of the cell cycle, ^{3}H-thymidine was used as an indicator of DNA synthesis since thymidine was incorporated into DNA. The percentage of cells taking up ^{3}H-thymidine into DNA as seen in autoradiograms, was used as a labeling index, which measured the rate of mitosis (Table 18-1) (3,4,16,70).

In dividing cells, the synthesis of RNA and proteins also occurred during interphase. Nuclear DNA-associated proteins, such as the histones, which are present in an amount approximately equal to that of DNA, were also synthesized in the interphase (S) period (76).

Extensive studies of cell mitosis were carried out in normal and neoplastic tissues in animals and humans, as well as other studies of metabolism and disease. In general, neoplastic cells had a higher rate of labeling with ^{3}H-thymidine than normal cells and malignant cells had a higher rate than benign cells (4), but there were exceptions (16).

Control Mechanisms of the Normal Cell Cycle. In order to transmit genetic information from one generation to another there must be an accurate duplication of the DNA of the parent cell so that after

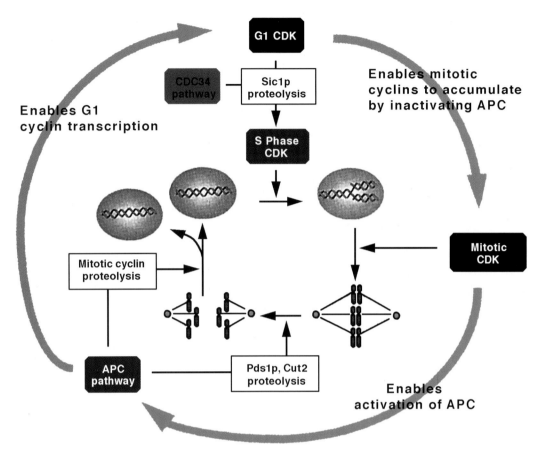

Figure 18-8

CHEMICAL ASPECTS OF THE CELL CYCLE

The cyclins drive mitosis and the anaphase promoting complex (APC) degrades the cyclins; in turn, the mitotic cyclins accumulate and inactivate APC (pink large arrows). Proteolysis is an important part of the process, which has been likened to the cycles of a reciprocating steam engine (60). The chromosome cycle is depicted in the center of the figure; the mitotic figures are below. G1 cyclin-dependent kinases (CDKs) trigger DNA replication by activating S-phase CDKs through proteolysis and also enable mitotic cyclins to accumulate by inactivating APC. Mitotic CDKs trigger chromosome condensation and spindle assembly, and also enable the activation of APC which initiates anaphase by ubiquitinating anaphase inhibitors such as Cut2 and Pds1p. The APC catalyzes destruction of cyclin B, resulting in exit from mitosis, and enabling G1 cyclins to be resynthesized. The destruction of mitotic CDK activity is required to allow formation of prereplication complexes (44). (Fig. 4 from King RW, Deshaies RJ, Peters JM, Kirschner MW. How proteolysis drives the cell cycle. Science 1996;274:1652–9.)

mitosis each daughter cell has the same amount of DNA as that present in the parent cell. In addition, the complicated process of mitosis must be strictly controlled. A series of authoritative review articles has discussed in detail recent advances in the study of the cell cycle (26,27,44,60,73,77).

There are two highly regulated transition points in the cell cycle. One is called START, in which the cell begins to replicate its DNA, and the other, called RESTRICTION (R), occurs when the cell initiates mitosis (35,54). These two important events have to be carefully regulated. The process has been compared to a two-phase reciprocating engine.

From studies of frog eggs (35,54), yeasts (15, 38,59,63), and mammalian tissue cultures (77), there arose the concept that the engine driving the cell cycle is protein kinase, encoded by the *cdc2* gene, which is activated by binding to cyclin proteins to give the cyclin-dependent kinases (CDKs) (fig. 18-8). The cyclins D1, D2, and D3 combine with the kinases cdk4 and cdk6, are activated through the G1 period, and reach a maximum in late G1. The kinases cdk4 and cdk6 associate only with the D type cyclins and they bind exclusively with the kinase inhibitors cdk4 and cdk6 (58). The catalytic subunits of these kinases are active only when a complex is formed with the regulatory cyclin subunits. The S phase is induced by cdk2 complexed with E cyclins and the M phase is induced by cdk1 complexed with the B cyclins. Additional kinases are necessary for both the initiation of DNA replication (44) and mitosis (60).

There are specific surveillance mechanisms that detect mistakes or damage to DNA and inhibit key cycle transitions (60). Human suppressor genes, such as p53 or ATM, prevent or slow cell entry into the S phase to permit repair when DNA is damaged or block rereplication when mitotic spindles are damaged (27).

Initiation of duplication of DNA depends on prior assembly at the points of origin of a prereplication complex (pre-RC), composed of three sets of proteins: ORC, Cdc6p, and Mcms. After duplication of DNA the cell must generate a bipoplar mitotic spindle and align each pair of sister chromatids on the metaphase plate. These events depend upon activation of the M-phase cdks. At anaphase, the separation of sister chromatids to opposite poles is accompanied by inactivation of M-phase cdks by degradation (proteolysis) of the associated cyclins.

A very large, multisubunit complex, called the anaphase promoting complex (APC), is important in chromosome splitting, and degradation of the M-phase cyclins and many other proteins (44). APC remains active for much of the subsequent G1 period and is not turned off until the accumulation cdks of G1 ensures that M-phase cyclins and other proteins needed for mitosis do not accumulate prematurely (44).

The Cell Cycle and Cancer. In cancer the cells remain in a proliferative state abandoning the normal regulatory controls, including those that cause cells to exit from the cell cycle. Genetic alterations affecting a protein, $p16^{INK4a}$, and the cyclin D1 protein, are frequent in cancers and these may affect the phosphorylation of a protein RB, the retinoblastoma protein (see Chapter 21). RB protein can inhibit cell cycle progression and control the exit of cells from the G1 phase. Inactivation of this pathway may be important in tumorigenesis (44).

Translocations or amplifications of the D1 locus in human chromosome 11q13 leads to overexpression of cyclin D1 in many human carcinomas. Homozygous deletions in the INK4a inhibitory locus of chromosome 9p21 also occur in some cancers (73).

It has been suggested that hyperphosphorylation of RB and its physiologic inactivation are parts of a pathway in which $p16^{INK4a}$, cyclin D1, and RB may

contribute to restrictive point control in the passage of cells through the cycle. Phosphorylation of RB during G1 relieves its inhibitory influence and allows cells to proceed into the S phase (73).

The cell cycle is not only important in cell division (67,84), but it is a key process by which a cell is committed to continue to proliferate or cease to proliferate. Sher (73) has pointed out the special role that p16, D1, and RB play in somatic cell division after birth and in cancer.

THE DOUBLE HELIX STRUCTURE OF DNA

The story of the discovery of the structure of DNA by James Watson; American biologist, Francis Crick of the Cavendish Laboratory, Cambridge University (fig. 18-9), a physicist who became a biologist; and Maurice Wilkins, a physicist at Kings College, London (82,88), is well known (43,64,69).

Watson wrote a book, *The Double Helix,* which became a best seller in the United States and led to a number of other books about the personal characteristics of the scientists involved in various projects. The book popularized the term "double helix" (80). Crick published a book, *What Mad Pursuit,* much later (19).

The discovery that the structure of DNA was that of a double helix (34,82,88) was monumental, ranking as one of the great scientific achievements, on a par with Darwinian evolution, Newton's gravitation, Einstein's relativity, the quantum theory of Max Planck, and a few other fundamental discoveries. Its influence on biology has been profound (43,59,64,69).

It was known in the 1950s that DNA was composed of four nucleotide bases, two purines, adenine (A) and guanine (G), and two pyrimidines, thymine (T) and cytosine (C); a sugar, deoxyribose; and a phosphate (PO_4) group. Erwin Chargaff, a biochemist at Columbia University in New York City, made the significant discovery that in DNA the number of adenine nucleotides equaled the number of thymidine nucleotides and the number of guanine nucleotides equaled the number of cytosine nucleotides. This relationship was shortened to the formulae A=T and G=C, meaning that the total number of purines (A+G) equaled the total number of pyrimidines (T+C) (14). This finding was important in the determination of the structure of the Watson-Crick model of DNA.

Using their own X ray diffraction studies of DNA and those of Maurice Wilkins and Rosalind Franklin

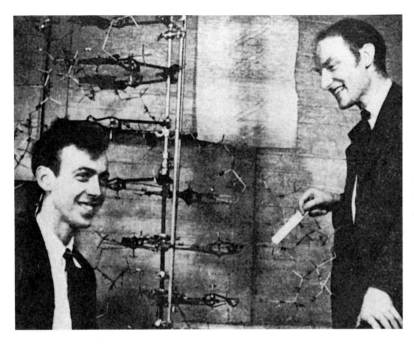

Figure 18-9
JAMES WATSON
AND FRANCIS CRICK
James Watson (left) and Francis Crick
(right), at Cambridge University, England, in
1953 with their model of DNA (69). (From
Watson JD. The double helix. New York:
Atheneum, 1968:215.)

of Kings College, London (88), Watson and Crick built physical models of DNA, testing their models by determining if they satisfied chemical and stero-physical requirements. Their successful model was that of two parallel anticomplementary strands of DNA wound around an axis in a double helical manner (83). The model arranged the nucleotide pairs on top of each other like steps in a spiral staircase on the inside of the strands. The nucleotide adenine (A) was attached to thymine (T) by two hydrogen bonds while guanine (G) was attached to cytosine (C) by three hydrogen bands (fig. 18-10) (82).

The nucleotides in the two helices were complementary, i.e., A in one strand was opposite to T in the other strand and G in one strand was opposite to C in the other strand. This complementarity was an important feature of the double helix pattern (Note 5).

THE REPLICATION OF DNA

After the structure of DNA was verified, the two major functions of DNA, the mechanism by which it is replicated and how its genetic information was expressed, were of most concern. Crick suggested that in the replication of DNA the two strands separated and each became a template so that enzymes could synthesize a duplicate strand of DNA (18). This model was labeled the semiconservative model (fig. 18-11).

Proof of the semiconservative model was furnished by J. H. Taylor, a geneticist of Columbia University and colleagues at the Brookhaven Laboratory, New York by an ingenious experiment using the division of chromosomes in *Vicia faba* seedlings, ^{3}H-thymidine, and high resolution autoradiography (78). The latter could resolve the location of the ^{3}H-thymidine to a part of a chromosome or to one of two sister chromatids (31).

Taylor's autoradiographic study illustrated the uptake of ^{3}H-thymidine in cells growing in a medium containing the isotope. During the first division of cells, both sister chromatids of each chromosome took up ^{3}H-thymidine from the medium. During the second division of cells, the cells were grown in nonradioactive thymidine and only one of

Note 5: Much has been written about the relationship between Watson and Crick of Cambridge and Wilkins and Rosalind Franklin of Kings College University of London, the Watson-Crick model, and the relationship between Wilkins and Franklin in the same department at Kings College, London. In regard to the latter, Sayre has written a book in which she states that Franklin's contributions to the solution of the problem had not been fully recognized and she writes of the personal differences between Wilkins and Franklin (72). Judson (43), Portugal and Cohen (69), and Olby (64) discuss the matter in detail. Franklin died in 1958; Watson, Crick, and Wilkins shared a Nobel prize in chemistry in 1962.

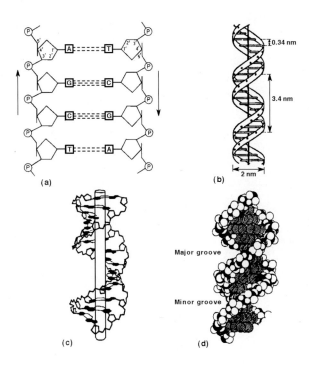

Figure 18-10
DOUBLE HELIX DNA MODEL

The double helix model of DNA shows: (a) polarity, sugars, phosphates, and base pairing but no helical twist; (b) helical twist and helix parameters; (c) helix and base pair combination; and (d) a space-filling representation with major and minor grooves. (Fig. 2.15 from Adams RL, Knowler JT, Leader DP. The biochemistry of the nucleic acids, 11th ed. London: Chapman & Hall, 1992:16.)

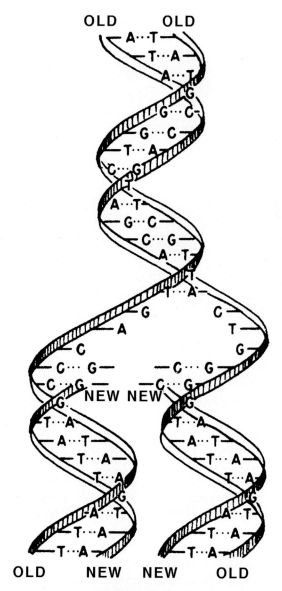

Figure 18-11
A PROPOSED MODEL FOR
SEMICONSERVATIVE REPLICATION OF DNA

Each of the two strands of DNA is a template for the synthesis of new DNA. (Fig. 11.15 from Portugal FH, Cohen JS. A century of DNA: a history of the discovery of the structure and function of the genetic substance. Cambridge: The MIT Press, 1977:270.)

the two sister chromatids was labeled (fig. 18-12). This could have happened only if in the second cell division one strand of the DNA double-stranded helix was used as a template for the synthesis of the new DNA of the second division: the semiconservative model of duplication.

J. Cairns of the phage group provided autoradiographic measurements with ^{3}H-thymidine that suggested that the chromosomes of bacteria and bacteriophages known to replicate conservatively had the proper mass per unit length expected for the double helix structure of the Watson-Crick model of DNA (9).

Confirmation of the semiconservative model of replication of DNA was also provided by an equally ingenious experiment performed by M. Meselsohn and F.W. Stahl, biochemists at California Institute of Technology (55). They used the bacterium *Escherichia coli* grown in culture medium containing normal nitrogen ^{14}N, and heavy nitrogen labeled with the stable isotope nitrogen, ^{15}N, as sources of

nitrogen. Both ^{14}N and ^{15}N were incorporated into the DNA of the growing bacteria. Extracts of DNA labeled with both could be separated by ultracentrifugation because of their different densities.

Similar to Taylor's experiment, bacteria were grown in a medium containing ^{15}N for replication and then grown in a medium containing normal nitrogen for a second replication. Centrifugation

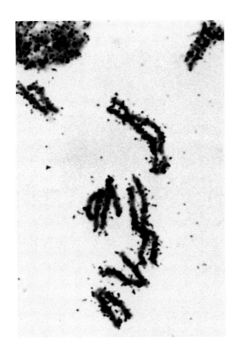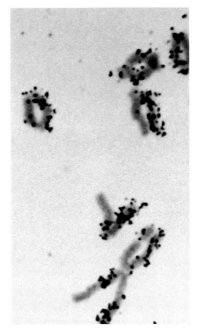

Figure 18-12
J.H. TAYLOR'S
AUTORADIOGRAPHIC STUDY
OF PROLIFERATING VICIA
FABA CELLS DURING
TWO CELL CYCLES

The first cycle occurred in a culture medium containing thymidine labeled with tritium (^{3}H-thymidine). Both sister chromatids show evidence of incorporation of ^{3}H-thymidine into the DNA by the presence of reduced emulsion grains over each chromosome (left panel). Cells were then grown for another cell cycle in a medium containing nonradioactive thymidine. Generally, only one sister chromatid was labeled with the ^{3}H-thymidine, indicated by the presence of emulsion grains over one sister chromatid (right panel). Results indicated that the semiconservative model of replication was probably the correct model (78). (Courtesy of National Academy of Science, Washington, D.C.)

analysis showed one band of DNA containing ^{15}N after replication. Following the second replication two bands appeared, ^{14}N and ^{15}N. This indicated, as with Taylor's experiment, that one strand of DNA acted as a template for replication in the second division (55). The model for DNA synthesis thereby was a semiconservative one (Note 6), confirming Taylor's findings.

CELL BIOLOGY—THE ULTRASTRUCTURE OF THE CELL

Electron Microscopy

In the 1930s, two physicists, Max Knoll and Ernst Ruska of the Technical University of Berlin, invented an electron microscope, a microscope that used electrons instead of light rays as the agent by which to examine a specimen (71). Electrons have a much narrower band width than light rays and they may be focused by magnetic lenses to a very small point. Electrons entering the specimen are stopped in proportion to the opacity of substance present; the emerging electrons are demonstrated on a fluorescent screen or recorded on film. The first commercial electron microscope was made available by Siemens Corporation in Germany in 1939.

Light microscopy has a theoretical resolution of about 0.25 μm, whereas the resolution of the electron beam is about 0.35 nm, a theoretical factor of about 1,000 times better resolution. The ultimate theoretical resolution is not reached with biological specimens but is from 100 to 1,000 times greater with the electron microscope.

A decade was spent developing the instrument and the techniques for processing the tissue in the 1940s. In 1945, Porter published a photograph of malignant cells, chick sarcoma cells in culture (68). W. Bernhardt of the Cancer Institute, Villejuife, France, made a search with the electron microscope for the presence of viruses in animal and human neoplasms (6); other such studies followed (28,65). The structure of viruses and bacteriophages was revealed (37), particularly in the pioneer studies of T. Anderson of Philadelphia (52).

A new world of ultrastructure was revealed to the biologist by the electron microscope (29,87). The demonstration of ribosomes in the cytoplasm of the cell by George Palade of the Rockefeller University showed the presence of organelles (ribosomes) that fit into a proposed model for the synthesis of proteins (fig. 18-13) (66). Small cytoplasmic bodies

---

Note 6: The same results obtained by two completely different techniques satisfied both the biochemists and the biologists that the semiconservative model was the correct model of DNA synthesis.

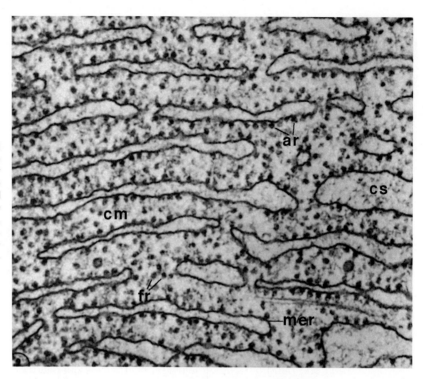

Figure 18-13
ENDOPLASMIC RETICULUM
AND RIBOSOMES OF
THE CELL CYTOPLASM

Ribosomes (round black bodies) stud the endoplasmic reticulum and some are free in the cytoplasm, as demonstrated by Palade (66). The ribosomes (rRNA) are the sites of protein synthesis (cs, cisternal space; cm, cytoplasmic matrix; fr, free ribosomes; ar, attached ribosomes; mer, membrane of the endoplasmic reticulum). (Fig. 2 from Palade G. Intracellular aspects of the process of protein synthesis. Science 1975;189:347–58.)

(mitochondria) whose existence was previously debated, were shown to be present in the cytoplasm of cells. The mitochondria furnished the energy required for the metabolic activity of the cell. They also contained DNA and genes. The existence of small vesicles in the apex of the cell was the subject of debate for many years. They were named by cytologists as Golgi bodies and electron microscopy revealed their ultrastructure, which aided in the understanding of their function. In the nuclear membrane of the cell nuclear pores were demonstrated, which implied that there were channels of communication between the nucleus and cytoplasm (Note 7). A discrete nucleolus in the nucleus, seen earlier by cytologists who had shown that it contained RNA, was better defined by electron microscopy.

The contrast between the depiction of the cell by Wilson in 1896 (fig.18-14) (89) and today's view of the anatomy of the cell (fig. 18-15) (29,87) is striking. Most other biologic disciplines, such as pathology, benefited greatly, directly or indirectly, from the information gained by electron microscopy.

Some cancers not well defined by light microscopy as to the cell of origin were clearly resolved by electron microscopy (28). Although there were no new definitive electron microscopic findings that distinguished benign and malignant tumors or normal cells and cancer cells, the differences seen by light microscopy were better defined by electron microscopy. If the electron microscopic findings were combined with histochemical, isotopic, immunocytologic, or biochemical techniques the scientific yield was enhanced over that of either alone (11,33,65,74).

PROTEIN SYNTHESIS

Proteins are vitally important constituents of biologic matter and enzymes that are essential to the function of the cell. Caspersson focused attention on protein synthesis in the 1930s and 1940s by suggesting that nucleotides with genetic information were transferred from within the nucleus to the cytoplasmic-nuclear membrane and that the proteins were synthesized there (12,13). In 1961, F. Jacob

---

Note 7: Günter Blobel, Rockefeller University, showed that newly synthesized protein carries a signal that determines whether it will pass through a membrane into an organelle, become integrated into a membrane, or be exported out of the cell. (Blobel G. Undirectional and bidirectional protein traffic across membranes. Cold Spring Harb Symp Quant Biol 1995;60:1–10.)

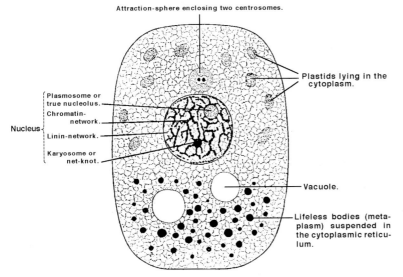

Attraction-sphere enclosing two centrosomes.

Plastids lying in the cytoplasm.

Plasmosome or true nucleolus.
Chromatin-network.
Nucleus
Linin-network.
Karyosome or net-knot.

Vacuole.

Lifeless bodies (meta-plasm) suspended in the cytoplasmic reticulum.

Figure 18-14
DEPICTION OF THE CELL IN 1896 FROM E.B. WILSON'S BOOK, *THE CELL*

Diagram of a cell. Its basis consists of a thread-work (*mitome* or *reticulum*) composed of minute granules (*microsomes*) and traversing a transparent ground-substance. (Fig. 5 from Wilson EG. The cell in development and inheritance. New York: Macmillan, 1896:14.)

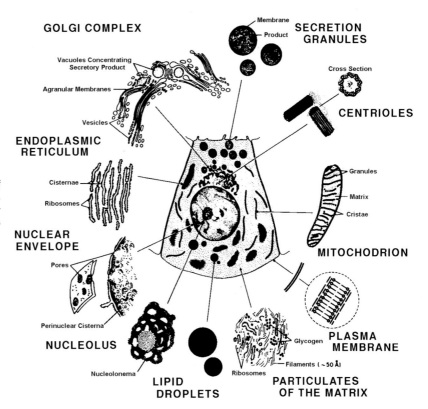

GOLGI COMPLEX

Membrane
Product

SECRETION GRANULES

Vacuoles Concentrating Secretory Product

Agranular Membranes

Vesicles

Cross Section

CENTRIOLES

Figure 18-15
MODERN (1993) STRUCTURE OF THE CELL

Modern version of the structure of the cell. (Fig. 1-1 from Fawcett DW. Bloom and Fawcett, a textbook of histology, 12th ed. New York: Chapman & Hall, 1994:2.)

ENDOPLASMIC RETICULUM

Cisternae

Ribosomes

Granules

Matrix

Cristae

NUCLEAR ENVELOPE

Pores

MITOCHODRION

Perinuclear Cisterna

NUCLEOLUS

Nucleolonema

LIPID DROPLETS

Glycogen

Ribosomes

Filaments (~50 Å)

PLASMA MEMBRANE

PARTICULATES OF THE MATRIX

and F. Monod of the Pasteur Institute of Paris proposed the existence of a short-lived messenger molecule (mRNA) which carried the genetic message from the nucleus to the cytoplasm (42).

Francis Crick suggested that for each of the 20 amino acids there might be a specific "adaptor" with which each would combine; the adaptor would also bind to the protein-synthesizing particle in the cytoplasm, the ribosome (rRNA). The specific messenger RNA and individual amino acid would be joined in the proper sequence in the protein being synthesized by the ribosome (18).

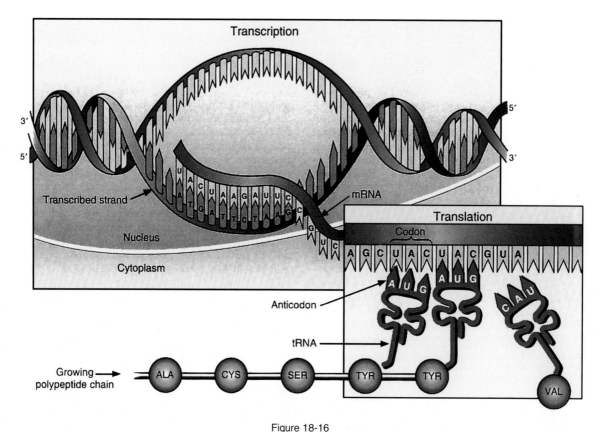

Figure 18-16
DRAWING OF TRANSCRIPTION (UPPER PORTION) AND TRANSLATION (LOWER PORTION) PROCESSES
In translation the ribosome (rRNA) is the synthesizer of amino acids into protein after the transfer RNA (tRNA) shepherds a specific amino acid with its specific anticodon into the ribosome. The messenger RNA (mRNA) provides the triplet code used by the ribosome to incorporate the proper amino acid into its correct position in the growing polymer peptide chain. (Modified from fig. 1 from Rosenthal N. DNA and the genetic code. N Eng J Med 1994;331:39–41.)

The "adaptor" of Crick was found to be a transfer RNA (tRNA) which combined with the specific nucleotides in messenger RNA and aligned the amino acids into the proper position in the ribosome (fig. 18-16). Messenger RNA was shown to be spliced into a truncated version of its original size before leaving the nucleus (79).

The ribosome is comprised of many fractions of RNA and protein; its complex metabolism has not yet been completely resolved. The newly synthesized protein, released from the ribosome, passes through the endoplasmic reticulum of the cell and moves to the Golgi apparatus, where additional biochemical changes may be made. Secretions are released through the apex of the cell (20). The process is unidirectional, from nuclear DNA to the ribosome of the cytoplasm.

Decipherment of the Gene—The Triplet Code

One of the great mysteries of biology was how the information of the gene was transcribed to give rise to the thousands of proteins necessary for life. The genetic code, which is composed of sequences of the four nucleotides of DNA, first expresses its information through a process called transcription. The first stage begins when the double strands of the DNA helix separate and unwind, and one strand acts as a template for the synthesis of a strand of RNA, messenger RNA (mRNA), complementary to the DNA of the strand. Messenger RNA carries within itself the coding nucleotide information necessary for the synthesis of a protein (fig. 18-16); it moves from the nucleus of the cell to the cytoplasm and there takes part in the complicated series of events called translation.

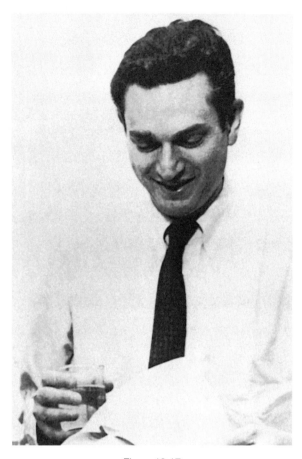

Figure 18-17
MARSHALL NIRENBERG
Marshal Nirenberg who, with Heinrich Mattaei, discovered the triplet code by which three nucleotides determine the amino acid to be incorporated into protein. (Courtesy of the National Institutes of Health, photography by R. Bredland.)

The genetic code*

First position (5' end)	Second position				Third position (3' end)
	U	C	A	G	
U	Phe	Ser	Tyr	Cys	U
	Phe	Ser	Tyr	Cys	C
	Leu	Ser	Stop (och)	Stop	A
	Leu	Ser	Stop (amb)	Trp	G
C	Leu	Pro	His	Arg	U
	Leu	Pro	His	Arg	C
	Leu	Pro	Gln	Arg	A
	Leu	Pro	Gln	Arg	G
A	Ile	Thr	Asn	Ser	U
	Ile	Thr	Asn	Ser	C
	Ile	Thr	Lys	Arg	A
	Met	Thr	Lys	Arg	G
G	Val	Ala	Asp	Gly	U
	Val	Ala	Asp	Gly	C
	Val	Ala	Glu	Gly	A
	Val (Met)	Ala	Glu	Gly	G

* Bases are given as ribonucleotides, so U appears in the table instead of T. "Stop (och)" stands for the ochre termination triplet, and "Stop (amb)" for the amber. AUG is the most common initiator codon; GUG usually codes for valine, but it can also code for methionine to initiate an mRNA chain.

Figure 18-18
THE TRIPLET GENETIC CODE
(Table 4.1 from Danell JC, Lodish H, Baltimore D. Molecular cell biology. New York: Scientific American Books, 1986:109.)

How the information contained in the nucleotides in the messenger RNA puts thousands of amino acids into the proper sequence in the building of a complex protein was unknown until 1961. At the National Institutes of Health in Bethesda, Marshall Nirenberg (fig. 18-17) and Heinrich Matthaei were testing a cell-free system by synthesizing proteins in vitro from amino acids (61). The addition or subtraction of various known substances necessary for the synthesis of proteins was being tested. They had received from Severo Ochoa, a master biochemist at New York University Medical School, a synthetic homopolymer made up entirely of uracil nucleotides, polyuridylic acid (poly U, UUUUUU etc.).

Surprisingly, they found that the polymer of poly U synthesized a chain of a single amino acid, phenylalanine (PHE), i.e., PHEPHEPHE etc. Uracil nucleotides (UUU) obviously coded for the amino acid phenylalanine (PHE). This suggested that proteins might be synthesized by three of the nucleotides in DNA (53,61). It was quickly found by a number of observers, particularly by Ochoa's group (50,75), that in general, the code was a triplet, i.e., three nucleotides were usually necessary to specify an amino acid to be incorporated into the protein being synthesized (fig. 18-18).

The triplet nucleotide AAA (adenine-adenine-adenine) coded for the amino acid lysine (LYS); the triplet nucleotide CCC (cytosine-cytosine-cytosine) coded for the amino acid proline (PRO); and similar nucleotide triplets coded for the other amino acids. The triplet code was not perfect because in some cases two nucleotides could specify for an amino acid, thus the description of the code as being degenerate. The first two letters of the triplet code were the

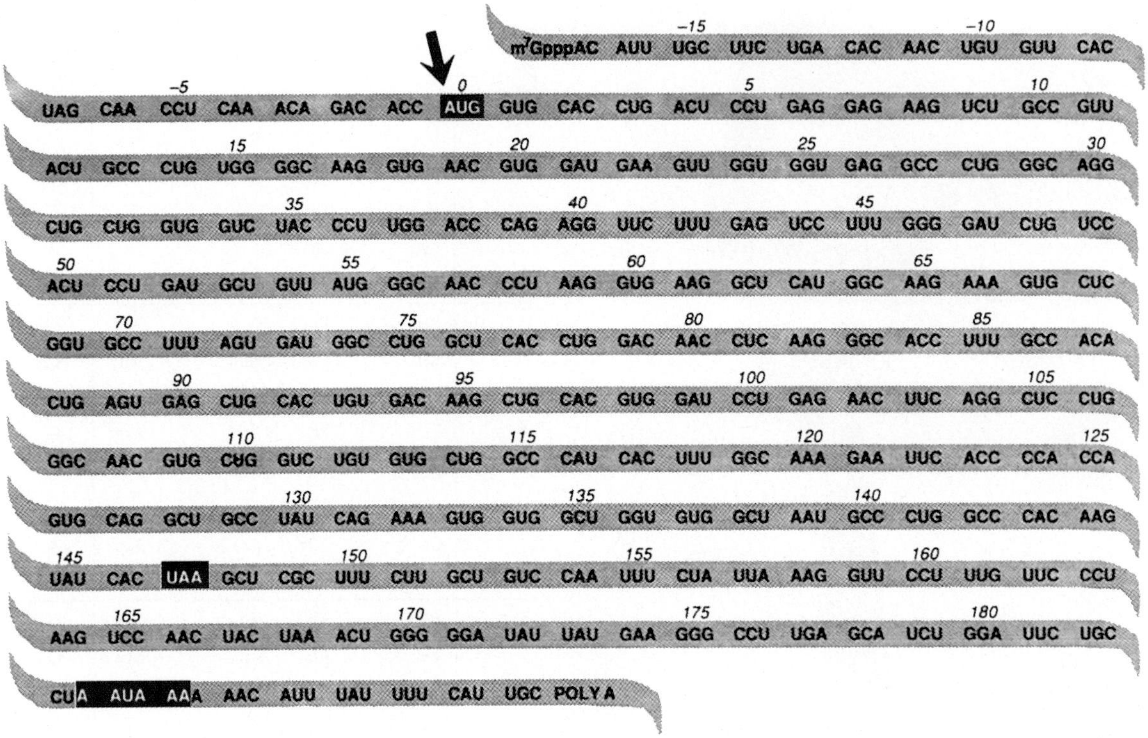

Figure 18-19

SCHEMATIC OF NUCLEOTIDE SEQUENCE OF HUMAN β-GLOBIN MESSENGER RNA

AUG initiates the process which begins at zero and ends at codon 147 with the terminating UAA signal. (Fig. 6.5 from Gelehrter TD, Collins FS. Principles of medical genetics. Baltimore: Williams & Wilkins, 1990:102.)

most important but there might be more than one nucleotide that made up the third letter. Some triplets acted as stop or start signals. Some transfer RNA (tRNA) responded to different nucleotide combinations, as shown by Bernard Weisblum and associates of Wisconsin University who found that there were two separate tRNAs for leucine, one responding to poly UC and the other to poly UG (86).

The 20 amino acids making up proteins require, at most, 60 nucleotide combinations. In a triplet code with 64 possible combinations, this would leave four extra triplets that could be used for punctuation marks to begin or stop the reading of the nucleotides or for other functions (fig. 18-19).

What had confounded experts for years, the mechanism of protein synthesis, turned out to be basically a relatively simple coding system using, at most, three nucleotides for each amino acid incorporated into protein. Much, of course, is still unknown about the details of the process.

The advent and achievements of molecular and cellular biology comprise truly revolutionary events. The demonstration of the double helix structure of DNA, the elucidation of the transcription and translation processes of DNA, the discovery of the triplet code for protein synthesis, plus the delineation of the finer structure of the cell set the stage for the development of new concepts concerning the mechanisms whereby normal cells function and how they transformed into cancer cells.

The birth of molecular biology was one of the great quantum leaps in the history of the biological sciences.

REFERENCES

1. Adams RL, Knowler JT, Leader DP. The biochemistry of the nucleic acids, 11th ed. London: Chapman & Hall, 1992.
2. Avery OT, McCleod CM, McCarty M. Studies on the chemical nature of the substance inducing transformation of pneumococcal types. I. Induction of transformation by a desoxyribonucleic acid fraction isolated from pneumococcus type III. J Exp Med 1944;79:137–58.
3. Baserga R. The biology of cell reproduction. Cambridge, MA: Harvard Univ. Press, 1985.
4. Baserga R. Multiplication and division in mammalian cells. New York: Marcel Dekker, 1976.
5. Beadle G. Genes and the chemistry of the organism. Am Sci 1946;34:31–53, 76.
6. Bernhard W. The detection and study of tumor viruses with the electron microscope. Cancer Res 1960;20:712–27.
7. Brachet J. La localisation des acides pentosenucleiques dans les Eissus animaux et les feuts des d'amphibiens envoie de développement. Arch de Biologie 1942;53:207–57.
8. Bucher NL, Malt RA. Regeneration of liver and kidney. Boston: Little Brown, 1971.
9. Cairns J. A minimum estimate for the length of the DNA of Escherichia coli obtained by autoradiography. J Molec Biol 1962;4:407–9.
10. Cairns J, Stent GS, Watson JD. Phage and the origins of molecular biology. Cold Spring Harbor, NY: Cold Spring Harbor Laboratory Press, 1969.
11. Caro L, Palade GE. Protein synthesis, storage, and discharge in the pancreatic exocrine cell. An autoradiographic study. J Cell Biol 1964;20:473–95.
12. Caspersson TO. Cell growth and cell function, a cytochemical study. New York: WW Norton Co, 1950.
13. Caspersson TO. Uber den chemischen Aufbau der Strukturen des Zellkernes. Skandinav Arch Physiol 1936;73:1–151.
14. Chargaff E. Chemical specificity of nucleic acids and mechanism of their enzymatic degradation. Experentia 1950;6:201–9.
15. Clarke PR, Karsenti E. Regulation of p34cdc2 and protein kinase: new insights into protein phosphorylation and the cell cycle. J Cell Science 1991;100:409–14.
16. Clarkson B, Ohkita BC, Ota K, Fried J. Studies of cellular proliferation in human leukemia. I. Estimation of growth rates of leukemic and normal hematopoietic in two adults with leukemia given single injections of tritiated thymidine. J Clin Invest 1967;46:506–29.
17. Claude A. Particulate components of normal and tumor cells. Science 1940;91:77–8.
18. Crick FH. On protein synthesis. Symp Soc Exp Biol 1958;12:138–63.
19. Crick FH. What mad pursuit: a personal view of scientific discovery. New York: Basic Books, 1988.
20. Darnell JE Jr. The origin of mRNA and the structure of the mammalian chromosome. The Harvey Lectures Series 1973;69:1–47.
21. Delbrück M. Experiments with bacterial viruses (bacteriophages). Harvey Soc Lectures, 1946;41:161–2.
22. DeRobertis ED, Nowinski WW, Saez FA. General cytology. Philadelphia: WB Saunders, 1954:175–214.
23. Dressler D, Potter H. Discovering enzymes. New York: WH Freeman, 1991.
24. Dubos RJ. The professor, the institute and DNA. New York: Rockefeller Univ Press, 1976:134–49.
25. Dulbecco R. In: Davis BD, Dulbecco R, Eisen HN, Ginsberg HS, eds. Microbiology. Philadelphia: JB Lippincott, 1990:795–832
26. Edgar BA, Lehner CF. Developmental control of cell cycle regulations: a fly's perspective. Science 1996;274:1646–52.
27. Elledge SJ. Cell cycle checkpoints: preventing an identity crisis. Science 1996;274:1664–72.
28. Erlandson RA. Application of transmission electron microscopy to human tumor diagnosis: an historical perspective. Cancer Invest 1987;5:487–505.
29. Fawcett DW. Bloom and Fawcett, a textbook of histology. New York: Chapman & Hall, 1993.
30. Fischer EP, Lipson C. Thinking about science: Max Delbrück and the origins of molecular biology. New York: WW Norton, 1988.
31. Fitzgerald PJ, Eidenoff MI, Knoll JE, Simmel EB. Tritium in radioautography. Science 1951;114:494–8.
32. Fitzgerald PJ, Simmel EB, Weinstein J, Martin C. Radioautography: theory, technic and applications. Lab Invest 1953;2:181–222.
33. Fitzgerald PJ, Vinijchaikul K, Carol B, Rosenstock L. Pancreas acinar cell regeneration. III. DNA synthesis of pancreas nuclei as indicated by thymidine-^{3}H autoradiography. Am J Pathol 1968;52:1039–65.
34. Franklin RE, Gosling RG. Molecular structure of nucleic acids–molecular configuration of sodium thymonucleate. Nature 1953;171:740–1.
35. Gerhart J, Wu M, Kirschner M. Cell cycle dynamics of an M-phase-specific cytoplasmic factor in Xenopus laevis oocytes and eggs. J Cell Biol 1984;98:1247–55.
36. Griffith F. The significance of pneumococcal types. J Hyg 1928;27:1113–59.
37. Gross L. Oncogenic viruses. New York: Pergamon Press, 1961.
38. Hartwell LH, Weinert TA. Checkpoints: controls that ensure the order of cell cycle events. Science 1989;246:629–34.
39. Hershey AD, Chase M. Independent functions of viral protein and nucleic acid in growth of bacteriophage. J Gen Physiol 1952;36:39–56.
40. Howard A, Pelc SR. Synthesis of desoxyribo-nucleic acid in normal and irradiated cells and its relation to chromosomal breakage. Heredity 1953;6:261–73.
41. Hughes WL, Bond VP, Brecher G, et al. Cellular proliferation in the mouse as revealed by autoradiography with tritiated thymidine. Proc Natl Acad Sci USA 1958;44:476–83.
42. Jacob F, Monod J. Genetic regulatory mechanism in the synthesis of protein. J Mol Biol 1961;3:318–56.
43. Judson JF. The eighth day of creation: makers of the revolution in biology. New York: Simon & Schuster, 1979:53, 72.
44. King RW, Deshaies RJ, Peters JM, Kirschner MW. How proteolysis drives the cell cycle. Science 1996;274:1652–9.
45. Kossel A. The protamines and histones. London: Longmans, Green & Co, 1928.
46. Kuby J. Immunology. New York: W.H. Freeman, 1992: 288–9.
47. Lajtha LG. On the concept of the cell cycle. J Cellular Comp Physiol 1963;62:143–5.
48. Leblond CP. Classification of cell populations on the basis of their proliferative behavior. Natl Cancer Inst Monogr 1964;14:119–50.
49. Lederberg J. Genetic recombination in bacteria: a discovery account. Am Rev Genet 1987;21:23–46.

50. Lengyel P, Speyer, JF, Ochoa S. Synthetic polynucleotides and the amino acid code. Proc Natl Acad Sci USA 1961;47:1936–42.

51. Levine PA. The structure of yeast nucleic acid. J Biol Chem 1917;31:591–8.

52. Luria SE, Anderson TF. The identification and characterization of bacteriophages with the electron microscope. Proc Natl Acad Sci 1942;28:127–30.

53. Martin RG, Matthaei JH, Jones OW, Nirenberg MW. Nucleotide composition of the genetic code. Biochem Biophys Res Comm 1962:6:410–4.

54. Masui Y, Markert CL. Cytoplasmic control of nuclear behavior during meiotic maturation of frog oocytes. J Exp Zool 1971;177:129–45.

55. Meselson M, Stahl FW. The replication of DNA in escherichia coli. Proc Natl Acad Sci 1958;44:671–82.

56. Miescher JF. Die histochemischen und physiologischen Arbeiten. Gesammelt und heraus geben von semen Freuden. Leipzig: FC Vogel, 1897;1:6.

57. Miescher F. Ueber die chemische Zusammensetzung der Eiterzellen. Hoppe-Seyler's Medizinish-Chemischen Unter-suchungen 1871;4:441–460.

58. Murray A, Hunt T. The cell cycle. New York: WH Freeman, 1993:42–65.

59. Murray AW, Kirschner MW. What controls the cell cycle? Sci Am 1991;264:56–3.

60. Nasmyth K. Viewpoint: putting the cell cycle in order. Science 1996;274:1643–5.

61. Nirenberg MW, Matthaei JH. The dependence of cell-free protein synthesis in E. coli upon naturally occurring synthetic polyribonucleotides. Proc Natl Acad Sci 1961;47:1588–602.

62. Nowell P. Phytohemagglutinin: an initiator of mitosis in cultures of normal human leukocytes. Cancer Res 1960;20:462–6.

63. Nurse P. Universal control mechanism regulating onset of M-phase. Nature 1990;344:503–8.

64. Olby RC. The path to the double helix. Seattle: Univ Washington Press, 1974.

65. Orenstein JM, Alkan S, Blauvelt A, et al. Visualization of human herpes virus type 8 in Kaposi's sarcoma by light and transmission electron microscopy. AIDS 1997;11:F35–45.

66. Palade G. Intracellular aspects of the process of protein synthesis. Science 1975;189:347–58.

67. Paterlini P, Suberville AM, Zindy F, et al. Cyclin A expression in human hematological malignancies: a new marker of cell proliferation. Cancer Res 1993;53:235–8.

68. Porter LR, Claude A, Fullam EF. A study of tissue culture cells by electron microscopy. J Exp Med 1945;81:233–46.

69. Portugal FH, Cohen JS. A century of DNA: a history of the discovery of the structure and function of the genetic substance. Cambridge: The MIT Press, 1977:3–30, 71–89.

70. Quastler H, Sherman FB. Cell population kinetics in the intestinal epithelium of the mouse. Exptl Cell Res 1959;17:420–38.

71. Ruska E; Mulvey T, trans. The early development of electron lenses and electron microscopy. Stuttgart: S. Hirzel Verlag, 1980.

72. Sayre A. Rosalind Franklin and DNA. New York: WW Norton, 1975.

73. Sherr CJ. Cancer cell cycles. Science 1996;274:1672–7.

74. Siekevitz P, Palade GE. A cytochemical study on the pancreas of the guinea pig. IV. Chemical and metabolic investigation of the ribonucleoprotein particles. J Biophysic Biochem Cytol 1959;5:1–10.

75. Speyer JF, Lengyel P, Basilio C, Ochoa S. Synthetic polynucleotides and the amino acid code, IV. Proc Natl Acad Sci USA 1962;48:441–8.

76. Stein G, Stein J, Chrysogelos S, et al. Cell cycle-dependent human histone genes: their organization and regulation. In: Huilica L, Stein GS, Stein JL, eds. Histones and other basic nuclear proteins. Boca Raton, FL: CRC Press, 1989:269–317.

77. Stillman B. Cell cycle control of DNA replication. Science 1996;274:1659–64.

78. Taylor JH, Woods, PS, Hughes WL. The organization and duplication of chromosomes as revealed by autoradiographic studies using tritium-labeled thymidine. Proc Natl Acad Soc USA, 1957;43:122–8.

79. Watson J. Involvement of RNA in the synthesis of proteins. Science 1963;140:17–26.

80. Watson JD. The double helix. New York: Atheneum, 1968.

81. Watson JD. Growing up in the phage group. In: Cairns J, Stent GS, Watson JD, eds. Phage and the origins of molecular biology. Cold Spring Harbor, NY: Cold Spring Harbor Laboratory Press, 1966:239–51.

82. Watson JD, Crick FH. Genetic implications of the structure of deoxyribonucleic acid. Nature 1953:171:964–7.

83. Watson JD, Crick FH. Molecular structure of nucleic acids. A structure for deoxyribose nucleic acid. Nature 1953; 171:737–8.

84. Watts CK, Wilcken NR, Hamilton JA, Sweeney KJ, Musgrove EA, Sutherland RL. Mechanism of cell cycle control in breast cancer. In: Pasqualini JR, Katzenellenbogen BS, eds. Hormone-dependent cancer. New York: M. Dekker, 1996;121–34.

85. Weaver W. Molecular biology: origin of the term. Science 1970;170:581–2.

86. Weisblum B, Benzer S, Holley RW. A physical basis for degeneracy in the amino acid code. Proc Natl Acad Sci USA 1962;48:1449–54.

87. Weiss L, Greep RO. Histology, 4th ed. New York: McGraw-Hill, 1977.

88. Wilkins MH, Stokes AR, Wilson HR. Molecular structure of nucleic acids. Molecular structure of deoxypentose nucleic acids. Nature 1953;171:738–40.

89. Wilson EB. The cell in development and inheritance. New York: Macmillan, 1896:14.

90. Zinder ND, Lederberg J. Genetic exchange in Salmonella. J Bacteriol 1952;64:679–99.

✳ ✳ ✳

19

THE GENE

HEREDITY

Although genetics as a scientific discipline developed late in the history of mankind, the inheritance of parental characteristics by progeny must have been recognized early in man's evolution. The "breeding true" of animals and plants from their forebears probably suggested to thoughtful observers that something was passed from generation to generation that was instrumental in keeping the form or shape of the organism intact.

Hippocrates (c. 400 BC) thought that each part of the body produced something which collected in the semen and was released at the moment of copulation. Aristotle criticized Hippocrates' view and pointed out that individuals sometimes resembled remote ancestors, not parents, and that what was inherited were not the characteristics as such but the potential for development of such characteristics (70).

Charles Darwin, one of the greatest biologists of all time, wrote of two types of heritable characteristics, which were later called "continuous" and "discontinuous." The former were gradual changes furthered by natural selection that gave rise to the survival of the fittest. Discontinuous characteristics were the "sports," the odd organisms, which were different from the average individual; Darwin thought they played a minor role in heredity. Hybrids were intermediate between parents and tended to keep populations uniform while inbreeding tended to lead to differences from the population average (13). Darwin's own theory of pangenesis, that germ cells were reservoirs of minute germs or gemmules derived from every part of the body, was an ingenious attempt to explain the transmission of acquired characteristics from generation to generation. It was abandoned after subsequent studies by Weissmann and others (80) (Note 1).

From the early speculations about the development of the embryo there appeared the concept of preformation: the fertilized egg contained the parts in miniature of the individual who was to be. The growth of the embryo consisted in the unfolding of these parts, similar to the development of a flower from a bud. From this concept there emerged two schools: the "ovists" who thought the preformed parts were contained in the unfertilized egg and that the sperm's function was merely to activate the egg, and the "spermists" who thought that the sperm was a complete animalcule that was only nourished by the egg (80). Some of the early microscopists were reported to have seen a fully developed small man, a homunculus, in spermatozoa (fig. 19-1) (33).

In the 1830s and 1840s, Schleiden and Schwann published their cell theory and in 1855 Virchow proclaimed his dictum that "All cells arise from other cells" (see chapter 10). These two major hypotheses, later theories, completed the chain linking inheritance to the orderly process of successive cell division from one generation to another.

Mitosis

Prior to about 1870, it had been thought that when the cell divided into two daughter cells, the nucleus divided in half just as the whole cell did, with each half of the nucleus going with a half of the cell body. Some thought, however, that the nucleus disappeared for a while during cell division and later a new nucleus appeared in each daughter cell. Many investigators had noted fragments of the nucleus and others had seen thread-like bits of nuclear material during cell division (2).

Van Beneden (74) and Fleming (19) illustrated the process of the division of the nucleus into the two daughter cells, a process called mitosis. The nuclear chromatin (the staining material) of the cell was observed to condense into thin thread-like units called chromosomes (Greek: colored bodies), which split longitudinally into halves and separated; each half of the chromosomal material went to one of the two daughter cells (fig. 19-2). Wilhelm Roux of Halle suggested in 1883 that the linear structure of the chromosomes and their division into longitudinal halves assured that each daughter cell would

---

Note 1: Evolutionists now debate whether the evolutionary changes occur precipitously, "punctuate evolution" (16), as well as gradually through a survival of the fittest.

Figure 19-1
SEVENTEENTH CENTURY
DRAWINGS OF
SPERMATOZOA

Spermatozoa from a dog as seen by Leeuwenhoek (a,b,c). Spermatozoa from man broken open to show the "homunculus," as seen by Hartsocker (d). The sperm as seen by Plantades (e) containing other sperm (f and g) also contain "humunculi." (Fig. 119 from Singer C. A short history of scientific ideas to 1900. Oxford: Clarendon Press, 1959:287.)

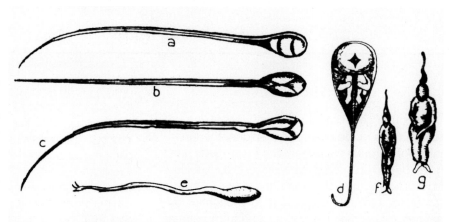

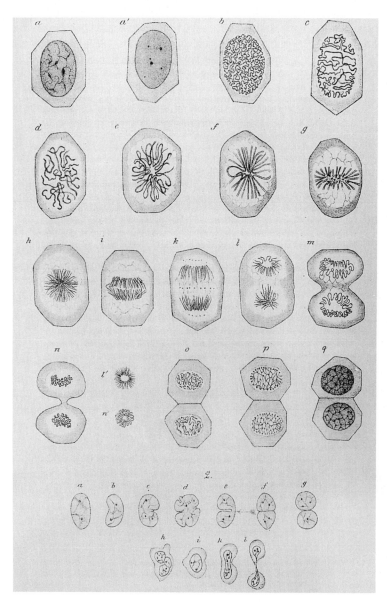

Figure 19-2
MITOSIS

Mitosis, from Walther Fleming's study of cells of the salamander. In 1879 there was a general understanding of how a cell divided into two daughter cells with division of chromosomes and an equal amount of chromosome material distributed to each cell. (Plate 1 from Fleming W. Ueber das Verhalten des Kerns bei der Zelltheilung, und über die Bedeutung mehrkerniger Zellen. Archiv für pathologishe Anatomie und Physiologie und für klinische Medicin. 1879; 77:1–29.)

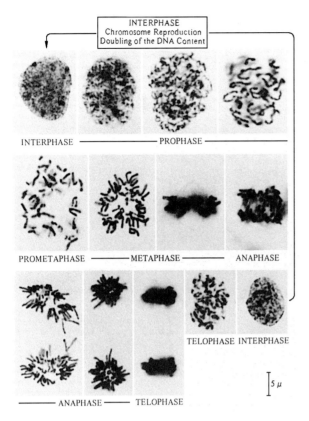

INTERPHASE
Chromosome Reproduction
Doubling of the DNA Content

INTERPHASE ———————— PROPHASE ————————

PROMETAPHASE ——————— METAPHASE ——————— ANAPHASE

TELOPHASE INTERPHASE

5 μ

———————— ANAPHASE ———————— TELOPHASE

Figure 19-3
MITOSIS, MODERN VIEW

Modern cytologist's view of the mitotic cycle and the period between mitoses, the interphase. (Fig. 3.1 from Therman E, Susman M. Human chromosomes, 3rd ed. New York: Springer-Verlag, 1993:27.)

receive an equal component of chromosomal material (61). Modern cytological studies have focused on the interphase, a period between mitoses (fig. 19-3) (see chapter 18).

August Weissman (1834–1914), professor of zoology at Freiburg, proposed a hypothesis concerning the role of the germ plasm from his study of the embryology of a fly (Diptera) (78). Early in embryogenesis, certain cells, called pole cells, were set aside. Some of these developed into germinal cells separate from the cells of the rest of the body, the somatic (Greek: body) cells. The pole (germ) cells were the continuous line of cells which carried the heritable substance of the organism from generation to generation. Germ cells of each generation came only from germ cells of the parent cells. The somatic or nongerminal cells were side branches that budded off from the zygote (egg) and were not transmitted to the progeny. This hypothesis decreased the earlier emphasis placed on the inheritance of acquired characters (Note 2). From the chromosomes of the egg and sperm cells came the heritable material, which was transmitted from the parents of one generation to the progeny of the following generation.

The Scientific Monk

In the 1860s, an Augustinian monk, Gregor Mendel, in a monastery in Brünn, Austria, became interested in the inheritance of plant characteristics and used the self-fertilizing garden pea plant (Pisum) as his test object (fig. 19-4). After 2 years of collecting and testing 34 different types of peas, he selected seven characteristics of a plant which bred true for his experiments. In 1865, he began to breed pea plants and test the inheritance of such single characteristics as seed color: plants with yellow seeds were crossed with plants with green seeds and the resultant plants were examined for the number and color of the seeds (31,49,70). In the first generation of plants, called the F1 (filial) generation, all the plants had yellow seeds. The yellow seeds were called dominant (fig. 19-5).

When Mendel interbred the plants expressing the dominant yellow seeds with each other, the second generation (F2) showed that 74 percent of the plants had seeds that were yellow and about 25 percent had green seeds (a 3:1 ratio). This indicated that the green seed trait was present in the plants of the previous F1 generation but was not expressed. Mendel reasoned that the color of the seeds was controlled by a unit factor, now called a gene, since there was no intermingling of the colors.

Further experiments were carried out to the third (F3) generation by the self-fertilization of the F2 generation. The dominant yellow seeds fell into two groups: one third bred true (all seeds were the dominant yellow), the remaining two thirds produced both yellow and green progeny seeds with a 3:1 ratio of dominant yellow to recessive green. Peas with the

Note 2: In a test of the concept of the inheritance of acquired characteristics, Weissmann cut off the tails of mice for 22 successive generations and found no decrease in tail length in the last generation (70). He was accused by a colleague of wasting time on such a trivial experiment.

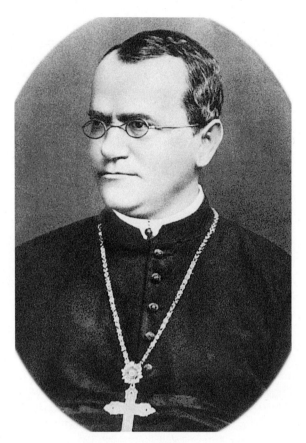

Figure 19-4
GREGOR MENDEL
Gregor Mendel, abbot of an Augustinian monastery at Brünn, Moravia, who showed that all peas in a pod are not identical and formulated some of the fundamental laws of genetics. (From Shimkin MB. Contrary to nature. Washington, D.C.: Department of Health, Education and Welfare, 1977:185.)

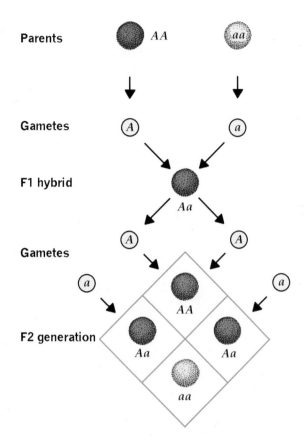

Figure 19-5
SEGREGATION OF ALLELES
(ALTERNATE FORMS OF THE GENES)
The parents are homologous (the alleles are identical). AA has two identical alleles and aa has two identical alleles; AA is dominant, aa recessive. The first generation are all the dominant red. In the second generation there are three dominant reds and one white. In the first generation the recessive white was present but not expressed. In the second generation the ratio of red to white was 3 to 1 because of the dominance of the red unit. (Fig. 1.3 from Lewin B. Genes, 3rd ed. New York: John Wiley & Sons, 1987:20.)

recessive green trait bred true, i.e., plants with green seeds that were interbred with each other gave progeny plants which had only green seeds.

Mendel then carried out a similar type of experiment but used two different characteristics per plant, i.e., plants with yellow round seeds versus plants with green wrinkled seeds. Figure 19-6 shows the results of the breeding of plants with two different characteristics.

Mendel's findings on the inheritance of pea plants led to generalizations that may be summarized as follows: units of inheritance, now called genes, are propagated from one generation to another; the units (genes) are not necessarily expressed in each generation but may exist in a masked or nonexpressed state; genes not ex-

pressed in one generation may be expressed in a subsequent generation; genes segregate as independent units, the law of independent segregation; and each unit of the gene—yellow, green, round, and wrinkled—is independently assorted and transmitted by the germinal cells, the principle of independent assortment (Note 3).

Mendel's findings, published in a respectable scientific journal (49), remained unknown to the biological world for about 31 years until 1900 when three plant biologists discovered the 1866 paper and made it widely known throughout the scientific world (31) (Note 4).

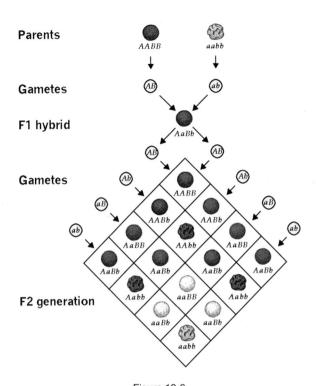

Figure 19-6

THE INDEPENDENT ASSORTMENT OF GENES

One parent is homozygous for two dominant genes (red and round). The other parent is homozygous for the recessive genes (no color and wrinkled shape). Independent assortment results in 9 colored-smooth, 3 colored-wrinkled, 3 noncolored-smooth, and 1 noncolored-wrinkled. (Fig. 1.4 from Lewin B. Genes, 3rd ed. New York: John Wiley & Sons, 1987:21.)

The name, "genetics" was coined from a Greek word meaning "to generate" by William Bateson, an English biologist (3). A Dane, W. L. Johannsen, suggested the term "gene" from the last syllable of Darwin's term, "pangene," used in his hypothesis of pangenesis (70), an explanation later given up.

Pairs of Like Chromosomes

In 1902, while studying the chromosomes of the somatic cells of the grasshopper, Walter Sutton, a graduate student at Columbia University, New York City, described different pairs of like chromosomes (48,70). He concluded: "I may finally call attention to the probability that the association of paternal and maternal chromosomes in pairs and their subsequent separation during the reducing division . . . may constitute the physical basis of the Mendelian law of heredity." He also described the pairing of the chromosomes at meiotic division as side by side, not longitudinal as believed earlier (70). This gave concrete form to units of heredity, the chromosomes, and suggested how heritable factors might be transmitted from parents to the progeny.

Mutation

In his studies of the evening primrose, *Oenothera lamarckiana,* which he found in an abandoned field in Hilversum, Holland, Hugo de Vries, a Dutch plant geneticist, found that the typical form of the flower produced a series of different types (mutants) which bred true generation after generation and differed from the parental form. de Vries thought the new forms were new species (mutants) and their sudden appearance meant that the Darwin hypothesis of selection of the fittest for survival did not apply in this case (15).

Sturtevant suggests that few of the original mutations observed by de Vries would be called mutations today (70). The concept of mutation, however, is most important; it suggests means by which variability might be introduced into inheritance.

Note 3: It is sometimes suggested that Mendel was a monk who had no training in science and who, somehow, from his studies of peas arrived at fundamental laws of genetics (31). Mendel's data have been questioned by the statistician R.A. Fisher, who has maintained that Mendel's ratios were consistently closer to expectation than sampling theory would predict (18).

Sturtevant, a geneticist, states that Mendel was a trained and practicing scientist in terms of the milieu of his time (70). He spent four terms at the University of Vienna between 1851 and 1853 studying physics, chemistry, mathematics, zoology, botany, and paleontology and had contact with at least two scientists at the University.

Apart from his experiments on peas, Mendel had scientific interests in other areas. He was a keeper of honey bees and attempted to cross different strains. Gray and white mice were kept, possibly for experimental studies. He was interested in meteorology and kept daily records of the rainfall, temperature, humidity, and barometric pressure of Brünn throughout his life. Several plants and their hybrids, mirabilis, maize, and stocks, were among those he tested.

Sturtevant describes Mendel as a ". . . man very actively and effectively experimenting, aware of the importance of this discovery, and testing and extending it on a wide variety of forms . . ." (70).

Note 4: Mendel submitted his results to a respectable scientific journal, *Proceedings of the Brünn Society,* in 1869 (49) but for 31 years they aroused very little interest until Hugo de Vries in Holland, Carl Corvens in Vienna, and Erich von Ischermak in Venice discovered and publicized them in 1900 (70).

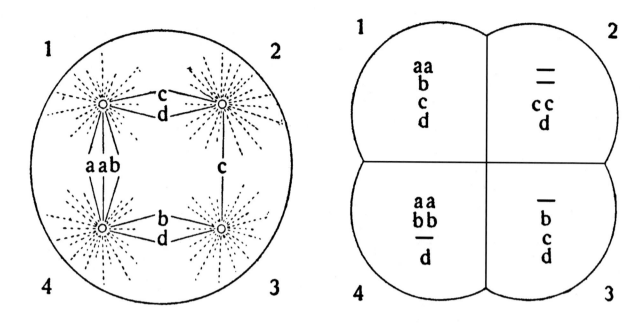

Figure 19-7

THE "SOMATIC MUTATION" HYPOTHESIS OF BOVERI

Boveri was concerned that multipolar mitoses would give rise to unequal distribution of chromosomes in the daughter cells. He suggested that this might disturb important functions in some cells and lead to abnormal events such as cancer. This suggestion was later called the "somatic mutation" hypothesis. (Figs. A and B from Boveri T; Boveri M, trans. The origin of malignant tumors. Baltimore: Williams & Wilkins, 1929:13.)

MITOTIC ANOMALIES AND CANCER

In 1902, T. Boveri, a zoologist in Würzburg, published a study of the fertilization of the egg of the sea urchin. If an excess of sperm was available, two sperm might enter a single egg and give rise to a three- or four-polar mitotic spindle (5). The egg would then divide, into three or four daughter cells, respectively. The result might be cells with an abnormal number of chromosomes, producing defective cells which had lost some of the qualities of normal cells, possibly leading to unchecked cell multiplication (6,7) (Note 5). His speculation that such chromosomal errors might cause cancer became known as the "somatic mutation" hypothesis (fig. 19-7) (5–7).

MORGAN'S "FLY ROOM"

T. H. Morgan, a professor of zoology at Columbia University, founded an American school of genetics in 1910 with two students, C. B. Bridges and A. H. Sturtevant. They began to investigate the chromosomes of the fruit fly, Drosophila (Greek: dew lover), which may have arrived in the United States with the importation of bananas. In a few years H. J. Mueller joined the group (70).

Note 5: Boveri suggested that in the normal cell there were chromosomes that inhibited cell division (6) and their inhibitory action could be overcome by external stimuli. Cells of tumors with unlimited growth would arise if these "inhibiting chromosomes" were eliminated. He also speculated that there were chromosomes that promoted division. The innate disposition of a chromosome, a disturbance by intercellular parasites, or external influences affecting chromosomes produced a "certain abnormal chromatin complex," which was important in producing tumors.

A zoologist who apologized for suggesting a mechanism of tumor formation, multipolar mitosis, even though he had no experience with tumors, Boveri nevertheless understood the importance of mitosis and how an error in mitosis might lead to serious consequences. He had a prophetic vision of what might be taking place in carcinogenesis. Later, Boveri looked at human cancer cells for multipolar mitosis but found none.

The Drosophila fly was chosen for study because it had only four chromosomes, a relatively short life span, and gave rise to a variety of characteristics (phenotypes) which could be easily recognized. Eye color, wing shape, anatomical anomalies, and lethal inheritance were among the characteristics that were studied.

Morgan, Bridges, Sturtevant, and Mueller worked for years in a small room, 16 x 23 feet, containing eight desks and a steady stream of doctoral and postdoctoral students. The four were to collaborate with their students on monumental studies that were to establish many fundamental principles of genetics derived from their interest in a household pest.

Among the genetic discoveries described by the Morgan group were (51): a linear map of the genes, including sex-linked genes, in the order and relative spacing that they occurred in the chromosome; the presence of sex-linked lethal genes; the phenomenon of nondisjunction of chromosomes (the failure of chromatids, duplicate chromosomes, to go to opposite poles during mitosis or meiosis); the "crossing over" phenomenon (the reciprocal exchange of chromosomal material between chromosomes during mitosis); the rearrangement of chromosomal material (recombination); the discovery that a female beetle had two X chromosomes (XX) whereas the male had one X chromosome and a different one called Y to give an XY pattern; the recognition of chromosomal abnormalities such as translocations (movement of a chromosome or part of a chromosome to another chromosome); deletions of a chromosome or part of a chromosome; and inversions of chromosomes. Many other important phenomena were also described. In 1927, Mueller demonstrated that X rays caused mutations in Drosophila and affected not only the irradiated sperm but its descendants as well (52).

By 1933, cytologic advances were combined with genetic studies so that T.S. Painter, a geneticist at the University of Texas, was able to present a drawing of the X chromosome from the salivary gland of *Drosophila melanogaster,* with discrete bands and points that were identified. Cytologically visible landmarks included deletions, translocations, and inversions of the chromosomes. Some gene loci were identified (59).

At about the time Mendel was observing the pea plants, a systematic study of genetics was initiated in 1865 by Francis Galton, an English biologist, who investigated natural inheritance in man and the inheritance of genius. He added the concept of quantitation of characteristics, even trying to quantify beauty and the effectiveness of prayer. Galton contributed the idea of correlation to genetics by studying the relationship between the height of the parents and their sons and daughters (20).

INBORN ERRORS OF METABOLISM

A. E. Garrod, professor of medicine at Oxford University, studied alkaptonuria, a disease in man in which an alternative pathway in the metabolism of nitrogenous wastes results in the excretion of homogentisic acid in the urine instead of the normal product, urea. His friend Bateson, a prominent geneticist, suggested that a ferment (enzyme) might be genetically absent in persons with the disease. Garrod decided that the disease was an inherited one. He later suggested that the diseases albinism, cystinuria, and porphyrinuria were also "inborn errors of metabolism," an apt phrase which has been used to characterize some diseases determined by genetic factors (4,22). Bearn points out that Garrod emphasized the biochemical individuality of each person (4).

CANCER FAMILIES

Medical investigators had noted certain cancer families in whom a higher incidence of cancer occurred than expected. Warthin, for one, had reported that an abnormal number of cases of cancer occurred in members of certain families (75). We know that such families exist, as do families in whom the occurrence of syndromes of specific cancers are inherited (38).

H. T. Lynch, of Creighton University, Nebraska, estimated that between 5 to 10 percent of all cancers in the United States have a hereditary origin (44). One or both parents of children with a cancer of the retina of the eye, retinoblastoma, have a defective chromosome which leads to the disease (35) (see chapter 21). In some families, there occurs a heritable high incidence of polyps and cancer of the colon (75), or a heritable gene that gives a higher risk for breast and ovarian cancers (see chapter 20). Many cancers are associated with a major or minor genetic factor(s) which may increase the risk of cancer in a patient. Victor McKusick of Johns Hopkins Medical School, a physician and a pioneer in the field of human genetics, has recorded over 4,000 diseases in which genetic factors are involved (47).

CANCER IN ANIMALS

The influence of heredity in cancer in animals was noted in 1911 by J.A. Murray of England who kept pedigrees of his mice. Female mice in whose ancestry (mother or grandmother) cancer of the breast occurred were more likely to develop breast cancer than female animals whose ancestors did not have cancer of the breast (53).

In 1916, C. C. Little and E. E. Tyzzer discovered that a tumor from waltzing mice of Japan could successfully be transplanted into mice of the same strain but not into mice of an unrelated strain. When the two strains, waltzing and nonwaltzing, were crossed, the progeny (the F1 generation) accepted the transplanted tumor of the waltzing mice, indicating that susceptibility to transplantation was dominant. Inbreeding of the F2 generation showed that only a few individuals were susceptible, suggesting that several independently segregating dominant genes must all be present in an individual to make it susceptible to tumor transplantation. This is true of many transplantable tumors in animals (39).

Tumors of lower forms of life including planaria, plants, and insects, have been described (30). Fish, amphibians, reptiles, birds, and mammals such as the horse, cattle, dog, cat, and especially the rodent, have all been shown to develop neoplasms (14,63,64,69). Some of these have been benign but most have been malignant, particularly those in rodents. The etiology of these tumors has been suspected to be viral in some cases, chemical in others, and many, particularly in the rodent, have been shown to be genetic in origin.

Maud Slye of the University of Chicago collected extensive pedigree data on mice and concluded in the 1920s that cancer in mice was inherited as a recessive gene. This opinion was debated throughout the cancer research establishment (68).

Mice have been inbred over many years to produce pure strains that produce cancers of specific organs in a high percentage of animals. The Jackson Memorial Laboratory of Bar Harbor, Maine, founded by C. C. Little, has provided millions of these mice for cancer researchers throughout the world (67).

Carcinogen-Produced Animal Cancers

Mice and rats are the animals most commonly used in studies of cancer produced experimentally by carcinogens. Other species have been susceptible to particular types of tumors and to different carcinogens. Cancers of most organs have been produced in animal models. Attempts to induce cancer of the pancreas were unsuccessful until recently when ductal cancer of the pancreas was produced in the hamster by nitrosamines (60) and acinar cell tumors of the pancreas by azaserine (43). Certain cancers were studied in animal models for long periods of time such as the sarcoma of rats introduced by C. O. Jansen of Denmark; this model was widely used through the early decades of the 20th century (32).

Radiation has produced most types of neoplasms (72) in animals (see chapter 14). Viruses have also caused some neoplasms (see chapter 15).

THE HUMAN GENOME

It has become apparent in recent years that the genes of the human cell may be involved in carcinogenesis (see chapters 20 and 21). Genes are units of heredity that are composed of strands of nucleotides organized into a double helical structure, the Watson-Crick model (77) (see chapter 18).

Bound to the DNA of the nucleus is about an equal amount of protein: five distinct histones and acidic and other proteins (27). The function(s) of the histones is not known in detail but they are part of a unit, the nucleosome, in which they are intimately linked with DNA. The nucleosome consists of a histone octomer, which forms a core, with DNA at the periphery (36,37). Marsh and the author found that one of the histones, a rich lysine fraction, may be involved in early pancreatic acinar cell division (45). Histones have been found as far back in the evolutionary trail as yeasts.

The DNA in the nucleus is densely compacted; if stretched out it would be about three yards in length. It is compressed into a volume said to be about two millionths of that of the head of a pin. Wells has calculated that the nucleus of a cell contains 240 million times as much information as a computer chip holding a million bits of information and the chip is 20,000 times larger (79).

There are about six billion nucleotides in the complete set of human chromosomes: about three billion pairs; around 130 million in each chromosome. It takes about 2,000 nucleotides to provide enough information to synthesize the average protein, a complex biological compound (79). The DNA of a bacterial chromosome such as from *Escherichia coli* contains about four million base pairs of nucleotides.

In the genome (the total amount of genes) of the normal human cell, there are 46 chromosomes: 22 pairs of somatic chromosomes and 1 pair of sex chromosomes. The sex pair of chromosomes contains two similar chromosomes labeled XX for females and two different chromosomes, one an X chromosome and the other labeled a Y chromosome (XY) for males. There are diseases associated with the inheritance of an abnormal number or alteration of sex chromosomes (47).

Alleles

A circumstance which gives further diversity to inheritance is that in the gene there are different forms or alternatives of each gene called alleles. A daughter cell would normally receive one copy of an allele from each parent, or there may be two copies of one allele from one parent, or one copy from one parent and none from the other. In some genes, there may be more than two alleles. Alleles are subject to mutation (21). Combinations of genes may be necessary to give rise to certain proteins, e.g., the important immunoglobulin compound is synthesized from the information furnished by three sets of mini-genes (28).

Intensive study has indicated that there are marked differences in function of individual chromosomes and between individual parts of each chromosome. Certain chromosomes or parts of chromosomes are associated with the normal functioning of the organism and some with disease states (23,47).

Exons, Introns, and Splicing

In 1977, A. Sharp, then at the MIT Center For Cancer Research, and R. J. Roberts at Cold Spring Laboratory, found that the active genes of a virus they were studying, the adenovirus, were discontinuous, i.e., each active gene was present in DNA segments that were separated from other DNA segments that were inactive. Previously, it was thought that all genes were continuous bands of functioning nucleotides. The genes with the information used to code proteins were later named exons, while the inactive DNA segments separating the exons were called introns (66). The introns were thought to be irrele-

vant nucleotides, nonactive in the synthesis of proteins, and were even called "junk DNA." The introns make up a very high percentage of the DNA, a far larger share of the total DNA than the exons.

The average gene is composed of segments of 15 to 20 exons separated by long strings of introns. During the processing of nucleic acids in the nucleus for protein synthesis, the introns of the RNA are cut out and the exons are stitched together into a continuous strand of nucleotides which provides the coding information for the synthesis of protein. The process is called splicing (12).

During evolution, introns have been added to the DNA of higher forms of life (the bacteria have none), possibly because the exons can thereby be shuffled about more easily and increase the variety of genetic expression.

Gene Injury and Repair

The genes of an individual are not fixed, immobile structures, but are subject to many forms of injury, deletion, breakage, reformation, translocation, and other alterations (21) (see chapters 20, 21). Injury to a gene can be repaired. Broken parts of one chromosome can be united with the broken ends of other chromosomes and various recombinations of parts of a chromosome may occur. Radiation damage can be repaired by enzymes which excise the defects and other enzymes which repair damage to one or even both strands of DNA (21) (see chapter 14). A defect in the DNA repair mechanism may be involved in some types of carcinogenesis (42).

Mutations

One of the most important processes affecting the genome is mutation, defined as a change, an alteration, in the nucleotides of the DNA. Mutations generally are deleterious to the cell but there are exceptions. Mutations are usually irreversible but very rarely there may be a back mutation, or revertant, to the original gene structure (21).

"Spontaneous" mutations are those occurring without any known factor causing them. Mutations may occur as the result of agents such as viruses, radiation, or chemicals; changes in the position of nucleotide(s); or other factors. In most cases, in order to transform a normal cell to a cancer cell it appears that at least two mutations are required (40,41). In some cancers, specific mutations have been found. If one or two mutations are necessary to

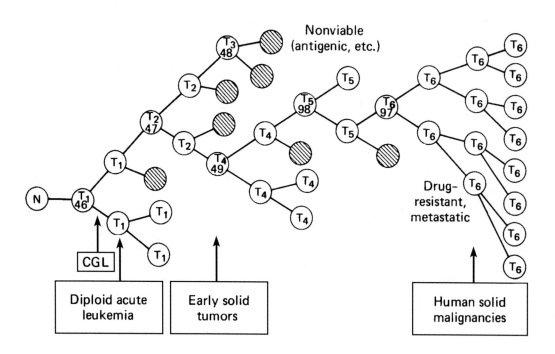

Figure 19-8
THE CLONAL HYPOTHESIS OF NOWELL

When a cell develops a mutation that gives it a growth advantage over other cells it multiplies and grows into a clone. The clone may become dominant and form a tumor. With continued growth more mutations in the tumor give rise to other clones, some of which die and while others have a factor(s) that allows them to persist and outgrow the other clones. In most human tumors at the time of diagnosis there is, usually, only one predominant clone present. (Fig. 1 from Nowell PC. The clonal evolution of tumor cell populations. Science 1976;194:23–8.)

produce a cancer, the rate of spontaneous mutations must be high enough to cause the cancer. If many mutations are required for transformation, "spontaneous" mutations could account for only a rare cancer. However, if early in carcinogenesis there was a mutation of the gene(s) involved in genomic stability, there would be a greater probability of a higher number of mutations later in the process (41). The latter theory seems the most reasonable since the number of known mutations in various cancers has been reported to be multiple, at least five in rectal cancers (17) and five in human breast cancer (8).

The Clonal Hypothesis

In 1976, Nowell suggested how a transformed cell may have acquired mutations that conferred a selective advantage to a subline of cells. The transformed cell had escaped the controls of a normal cell to give rise to a group of similar transformed cells called a clone. In the subsequent cloning of

cells there might develop a cell with an additional mutation, or mutations, which in turn favored proliferation so that a new distinctive clone of cells developed. Some clones might die, but others might persist because of a mutation(s) which gives the cell an advantage, permitting it to grow and survive. Eventually, as illustrated in figure 19-8, a surviving clone could contain the cells of an expanding tumor, a cancer. The tumor genome is increasingly unstable as the clones progress along the carcinogenesis pathway (55).

Susceptibility to Mutations

It is likely that mutations have been occurring throughout biological history at different rates in different organisms. Mutations are an important means by which variations of the genome occur.

In bacteria, the mutation rate per gene is about 1 in 100,000 to about 1 in 10 million per cell generation. For fruit flies, the rate is about 1 in 100,000 per gamete (either type of reproductive gene cell, sperm or egg). Genes associated with human diseases such as intestinal polyposis and muscular dystrophy have been estimated to mutate in about 1 in 10,000 to 100,000 people (21).

The measurement of mutation rates in cancer cells has led to discordant results. In some rodent cells, there has been no difference between the rates of mutation in transformed and normal cells. In a non-tumorigenic Chinese hamster cell line, there was no change in mutation rate when the same cell was transformed with the polyoma virus. However, S. Goldberg and V. Defendi of New York University Medical School found that when cells are super-infected with a second virus, the SV40 virus, the doubly-infected cells have a mutation rate of up to 25 times greater than that of the control cells (24).

Seshadri et al. compared the mutant gene *hqprt,* (hypoxanthine-guanine phosphoribosyl transferase) in human normal lymphocytes with the genes of malignant lymphocytes in cell culture. The rate of spontaneous mutations in the *hqprt* gene was 6 to 25×10^{-8} mutants per generation while in the malignant cells it was much greater, 53 to 666×10^{-8} mutants/generation (65).

Mutator Phenotype

L.A. Loeb of the University of Washington, Seattle, believes that hundreds of genes are required to stabilize the genome of somatic cells and that mutations in some of these genes could result in genetic instability and contribute to the multiplicity of mutations present in cancers. Because the "spontaneous" mutation rate in normal cells was thought to be inadequate to account for the high frequency of mutations in cancer cells, Loeb suggested that there is present in early carcinogenesis a mutator phenotype, i.e., a mutation(s) in genes involved in genomic stability. The resultant instability generates the multiple mutations found in cancer cells (40,41).

Transposable ("Jumping") Genes

Early in the study of genetics, it was believed that the genome was relatively inflexible, a fixed string of units that could be changed only by strong external factors. It is now recognized that the genome is far more flexible and susceptible to many influences.

Barbara McClintock of Cold Spring Harbor Laboratory, studied in the 1940s the colored and spotted kernels of Indian corn (maize) and observed that some of the genetic loci that produced the various patterns of the corn caused the kernels to appear in different places on the cob at various times (46). This pattern variation was the result of the movement of a transposable element (gene); the chromosomes of corn contain many of these mobile genes (34). A transposable gene is one that may move from place to place in the genome of the cell. It may disappear from one site and be inserted at another site in the same chromosome or on a different one, resulting in many mutations or chromosomal rearrangements.

The movement of the genes was activated by other genes. These activities resulted in a change in the rate of mutation in parts of the plant. A mutation in the gene locus which ordinarily gives rise to the synthesis of a red-orange pigment in the kernels of corn interfered with the synthesis of the pigment so that the kernels were white. But the mutation causing the change in color was unstable and reverted back and forth so that in the development of the kernel there were alternate streaks of pigmented and nonpigmented cells. The concept of McClintock's "jumping genes" was hard to accept for many geneticists but when they were found in bacteria and plants, her findings were accepted.

Insertion Sequence

Another form of gene motility is called an insertion sequence (IS) (79). It is a short piece of bacterial DNA that can make copies of itself and the copies may then be inserted into other parts of the genome. If a copy of an IS is inserted in the middle of a gene, it can destroy the expression of the gene because it interferes with the synthesis of the messenger RNA needed for the synthesis of the protein called for by that gene. If an IS occurs in the area of a regulatory gene, it might nullify its regulatory function and turn the gene inappropriately off or on (Note 6).

The existence of movable genes would seem to be unsettling to the genome. About 1 to 2 percent of the genome of *E. coli,* a bacterium residing in the human gastrointestinal tract, and about 15 percent of the genome of the fruit fly are composed of IS units. But mobile genes can't be permitted to move too often because they might kill the host. Only rarely do they duplicate themselves, about once in every 10 million generations. The human genome is relatively resistant to such disturbances, e.g., the rate of mutation in the human genome is one hundredth of that of the mouse per unit of absolute time (79). Many of the mobile genes survive because a symbiotic relationship has evolved, a live-and-let-live arrangement that insures the survival of both the host cell and the parasitic invader.

The presence of mobile genes illustrates the fact that the genome of even primitive organisms is not irretrievably fixed. The movement and action of promoters, inducers, and insertions that may affect other parts of the genome indicate a degree of flexibility that permits mutations to occur. Wells suggested that over time the genome has learned to adapt more efficiently to changes than in previous ages and that there is present a structure that facilitates the evolutionary process itself (79).

Position Effects

If there is no change in the amount of genetic material but only a change in the order of genes, the term "position effect" is used to describe the expression of the altered phenotype characteristics of the organism. Classic studies in the Drosophila fly have shown that mutational disturbances have resulted in the same expression of phenotype as a positional effect causing chromosomal structural changes in the same area. Induced structural changes have led to the same effects as X ray induced disturbances in the same area (21).

Insertion of proviral complexes that have no viral genes for replication and no genes for transformation may still cause transformation. The proviral complex in different lymphomas is located at a different position within a single cellular locus. It appears that because of its proximity to the oncogene (see chapter 16), the proviral complex may give the cell a growth advantage over neighboring cells, and clonal expansion and further mutations may give rise to neoplastic growth (11).

HUMAN CYTOGENETICS

In the late 19th century, pathologists had noted abnormalities in the chromosomes of cancer cells (1,25). As the cancer progresses clinically in the human, more abnormal changes in the chromo-

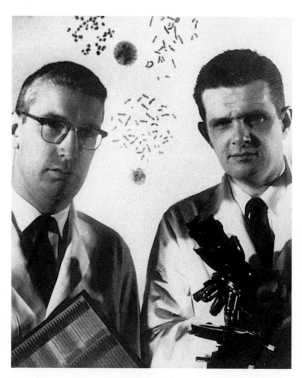

Figure 19-9
PETER NOWELL AND DAVID HUNGERFORD
Peter Nowell (left), then an assistant professor of pathology at the University of Pennsylvania Medical School and David Hungerford (right), a graduate student at the Cancer Research Institute, Fox Chase, Philadelphia. They discovered, in 1960, the Philadelphia (PH) chromosome defect of chronic myelogenous leukemia (58) and revolutionized the cytogenetic study of human cancer. (Courtesy of Dr. Nowell.)

somes were noted (50). The predominant opinion had been that the changes were secondary to the carcinogenic process.

Philadelphia (Ph^1) Chromosome

A seminal discovery was reported in an abstract in 1960 by Peter Nowell, a young pathologist at the University of Pennsylvania and David Hungerford, a graduate student at the Institute for Cancer Research, Philadelphia (fig. 19-9). In a smear of mitotic chromosomes of leukemic cells from patients with chronic myelogenous leukemia (CML), Nowell and

---

Note 6: A Mu bacteriophage may infect the common bacterium *Escherichia coli* of the human intestinal tract, insert itself into the host DNA in multiple sites, and cause mutations in about 3 percent of the bacteria. This is a mutation rate that is about 10,000 times greater than the normal rate in bacteria (79).

Another type of moving gene is the transposon which is able to move big pieces of DNA about the genome. The pieces have an insertion sequence (IS) at either end of the DNA. One large transposon, called Tr10, has mutations in the IS elements that can increase or decrease the rate at which it moves (79).

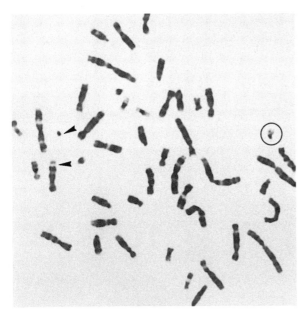

Figure 19-10
PHILADELPHIA CHROMOSOME

Illustration of the smaller chromosome 21 from a patient with chronic myelogenous leukemia. Arrowheads indicate the 9q+ and the Ph[1] chromosome (the smaller of the two). The circle contains the normal chromosome, originally assumed to be chromosome 21. (Fig. 1 from Heim S, Mitelman F. Cancer cytogenetics. New York: Alan R. Liss, 1987:43.)

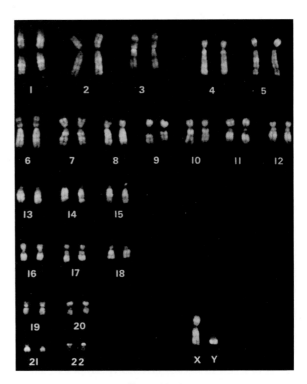

Figure 19-11
BANDING OF HUMAN CHROMOSOMES

The bands in human chromosomes discovered by Caspersson and Zech are stained with quinacrine mustard and fluoresced with ultraviolet light (9,10). (Fig. 3 from Caspersson T, Zech L, eds. Chromosome identification: technique and application in biology and medicine. Proc. 23rd Nobel Symposium. Stockholm, Sweden, Nobel Foundation, New York: Academic Press, 1973:29.)

Hungerford found one chromosome that was smaller in the leukemic cells than the comparable chromosome in normal cells in six of seven patients studied (58). The smaller chromosome was later named the "Philadelphia chromosome," abbreviated first as Ph[1], then as PH, in honor of the city in which it was discovered (fig. 19-10) (29,56,57).

Nowell and Hungerford stated that the smaller chromosome was specific and causal for chronic myelogenous leukemia since it did not occur in cases of acute myelogenous or lymphatic leukemia. The technique of chromosome preparation at that time did not permit them to decide whether the small chromosome was the result of a translocation or a deletion (56). Advances in the technique for preparing chromosomes permitted Tio and Levan (72) to count correctly the number of normal human chromosomes; the number was 46 and not the 48 that had been generally accepted for years.

The discovery of the Philadelphia chromosome was most seminal; it gave great impetus to the field of human cytogenetics: the study of the chromosomes in health and disease of humans. Cancer became the focus of much of the discipline.

Chromosomal Banding Techniques

Another major achievement in the study of chromosomes was the discovery in 1968 of the distinct banding patterns of individual chromosomes by Torbjörn Caspersson, a Swedish leader in the field of nucleic acids and genetics and his colleague L. Zech (9,10). They found that when quinidine mustard was combined with DNA and fluoresced by ultraviolet light, the stained chromosomes revealed discrete banding patterns (fig. 19-11). This revolutionized the field of human cytogenetics. Other stains and procedures were soon found that confirmed the existence of the banding patterns and were easier to use.

A schematic diagram of the human chromosomes evolved in which regions and bands are numbered consecutively from the centromere outward along each chromosome arm. The short arm of the chromosome is called p, the long arm is named q (fig. 19-12) (26).

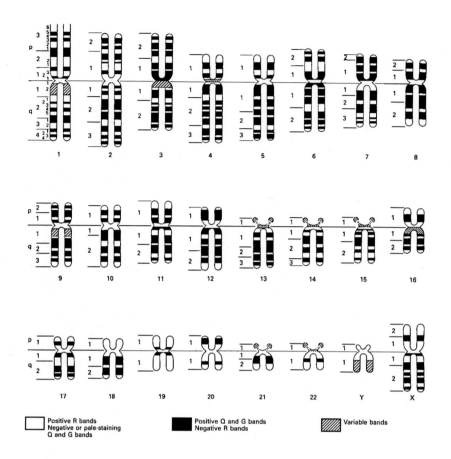

Figure 19-12
SCHEMATIC PRESENTATION
OF G-BANDED
CHROMOSOME
(IDIOGRAM)

Diagram of Q, G, and R bands in human chromosomes. The male sex chromosome is represented by XY and the female by XX. This is a standardized system of cytogenetic representation of chromosomes and their subdivisions. (Fig. 10.5 from Darnell J, Lodish H, Baltimore D. The discovery of splicing in the formation of adenovirus late mRNA. In: Molecular cell biology. New York: Scientific American Books, 1986:378.)

The cytogenetic stains for chromosomal banding quickly demonstrated that in animal and human cancers certain chromosomes were translocated, rearranged, lost, amplified, or otherwise altered. Many genes have been identified and localized to certain chromosomes or to a band of a chromosome, and associated with a specific function and/or disease.

Janet Rowley, a hematologist-cytogeneticist at the University of Chicago, used the new banding techniques in 1973 to show that the PH chromosome, chromosome 22, was not a simple deletion but the result of two translocations involving chromosomes 9 and 22 (fig. 19-13) (62). Breaks in the chromosomes occurred near the end of the long arm of chromosome 9 (band 9q34) and in the upper half of chromosome 22 (band 22q11); there was movement of part of chromosome 9 to chromosome 22 and part of chromosome 22 was translocated to chromosome 9.

Advancing the concept that there was a causal relationship between chromosomal abnormalities and cancer was the report by German, of the Rockefeller University, and associates (23), of a greater risk of leukemia and other neoplasms with the inherited clinical syndromes of Bloom's disease, ataxia telangiectasia, Fanconi's anemia, and xeroderma pigmentosa. Nowell has presented a thorough review of the history of human cytogenetics (54).

THE GENE

The normal gene may be visualized as depicted in fig. 19-14. The exons and intervening introns (the latter not expressed) are shown at the uppermost level. Promoter and enhancer locations are indicated. Transcription produces a pre-mRNA which is then spliced; further processing leads to the mRNA which is used in the translation of protein (19).

Since the revolutionary finding of Nowell and Hungerford that there was a consistent chromosomal change in chronic myelogenous leukemia, there has been a flood of studies showing that genes are involved in many neoplastic diseases: changes in gene structure may cause some types of human neoplasia. This is a reversal of a previous consensus that chromosomal changes were secondary to other causal factors.

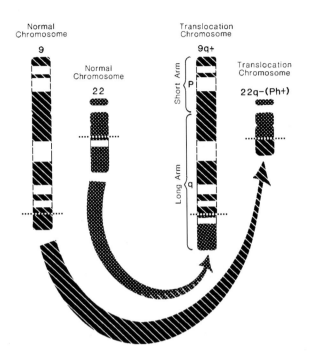

Figure 19-13
CHROMOSOME TRANSLOCATION IN
CHRONIC MYELOID LEUKEMIA

Using the chromosome banding techniques, Janet Rowley, a hematologist-cytogeneticist of the University of Chicago Medical School, recognized the correct defect in chronic myelogenous leukemia. There were reciprocal translocations between chromosomes 9 and 22. (Fig. 4.3 from Rowley JD. Principles of cancer biology: chromosomal abnormalities. In: DeVita VT Jr, Hellman S, Rosenberg SA, eds. Principles and practice of oncology, 2nd ed. Philadelphia: JB Lippincott 1985:69.)

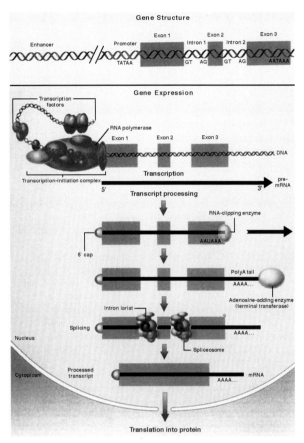

Figure 19-14
SCHEMATIC DEPICTION OF A NORMAL GENE

The uppermost panel shows exons, introns, and enhancer and promoter locations. Successively lower panels indicate the changes that occur during gene expression, including transcription and processing of the transcript (including splicing) which is then ready as mRNA for the translation of protein in the ribosomes of the cytoplasm. (Fig. 1 from Rosenthal N. Molecular medicine. Regulation of gene expression. N Eng J Med 1994;331:931–3.)

The emphasis in cancer research has changed from the search for a universal chemical agent or a panvirus giving rise to all cancers, to a realization that genetic factors may be important in the causation of some human neoplastic diseases. Genetic changes might also occur as ancillary factors. Many diseases, including neoplasia, have been localized to discrete chromosomes, to bands in a chromosome, to a particular locus in the genome, to a mutated gene, or to a combination of genes.

The focus was now on the gene.

REFERENCES

1. Arnold J. Beobachtungen uber Kerntheilungen in dem Zellender Geschwulste. Virchows Arch 1879;78:279–301.

2. Baker JR. The cell theory: a restatement, history and critique. Collection of articles, 1948–1955. New York and London: Garland Publishing, 1988.

3. Bateson W. Mendel's principles of heredity: a defense. Cambridge: Cambridge Univ. Press, 1902.

4. Bearn AG. Archibald Garrod and the individuality of man. New York: Oxford Univ Press, 1993.

5. Boveri T. Über mehrpolige Mitosen als Mittel zur Analyse des Zellkerns. Verh Phys-Med Gesellsch zu Würzburg, 1902;35:67–90.

6. Boveri T. Zur Frage der Entstehung maligner Tumoren. Jena: Fischer, 1914:1–64.

7. Boveri T; Boveri M, trans. The origin of malignant tumors. Baltimore: Williams & Wilkins, 1929.

8. Callahan R. Genetic alterations in primary breast cancer. Breast Cancer Res Treat 1989;13:191–203.

9. Caspersson T, Zech L, eds. Chromosome identification: technique and application in biology and medicine. Proc. 23rd Nobel Symposium. Stockholm, Sweden, Nobel Foundation, New York: Academic Press, 1973.

10. Caspersson T, Zech L, Johnasson C. Differential binding of alkylating fluorochromes in human chromosomes. Exp Cell Res 1970;60:315–9.

11. Cooper GM. Oncogenes. Cellular oncogene targets for retroviral integration. In: Oncogenes. Boston: Jones and Bartlett, 1990:83–95.

12. Darnell J, Lodish H, Baltimore D. The discovery of splicing in the formation of adenovirus late mRNA. In: Molecular cell biology. New York: Scientific American Books, 1986:337–56.

13. Darwin C. The descent of man, and selection in relation to sex. 2 vols. New York: Appelton, 1871.

14. Dawe CJ, Harshbarger JC, eds. Neoplasms and related disorders of invertebrate and lower vertebrate animals, monograph 31. Bethesda: National Cancer Institute, 1969.

15. de Vries H. Die Mutationstheorie, vol. 1. Leipzig: Veit, 1901.

16. Eldredge N, Gould SJ. Punctuated equilibria: an alternative to phyletic gradualism. In: Schopf TJ, ed. Models in paleobiology. San Francisco: Freeman, Cooper, 1972:82–115.

17. Fearon ER, Vogelstein B. A genetic model for colorectal tumorigenesis. Cell 1990;61:759–67.

18. Fisher RA. Has Mendel's work been rediscovered? In: Stern C, Sherwood ER, eds. The origins of genetics: a Mendel source book. San Francisco: WH Freeman, 1966.

19. Fleming W. Zellsubstanz, Kern und Zelltheilung. Leipzig: Vogel, 1882.

20. Galton F. Natural inheritance. London: Macmillan, 1889.

21. Gardner EJ, Simmons MJ, Snustad DP. Principles of genetics. New York: John Wiley & Sons. 1991:16, 22, 288–317, 488–99.

22. Garrod AE. Inborn errors of metabolism. London: Oxford Univ. Press, 1963.

23. German J. Patterns of neoplasia associated with chromosome breakage syndromes. In: German J, ed. Chromosome mutation and neoplasia. New York: Liss, 1983:97–134.

24. Goldberg S, Defendi V. Increased mutation rates in doubly viral transformed Chinese hamster cells. Somat Cell Genet 1979;5:887–95.

25. Hansemann D. Ueber asymmetrische Zelltheilung in Epithelkrebsen und deren biologische Bedeutung. Arch Path Anat Physiol 1890;119:199–326.

26. Heim S, Mitelman F. Cancer cytogenetics. New York: Alan R. Liss, 1987:14–5.

27. Hnilica LS, Stein GS, Stein JL. Histones and other basic nuclear proteins. Boca Raton, Florida: CRC Press, 1989.

28. Hozumi N, Tonegawa S. Evidence for somatic rearrangement of immunoglobulin genes coding for variable and constant regions. Proc Natl Acad Sci USA 1976;73:3628–32.

29. Hungerford DA. Some early studies of human chromosomes, 1879–1955. Cytogenet Cell Genet 1978;20:1–11.

30. Huxley J. Cancer biology: comparative and genetic. In: Fox HM, ed. Biological reviews of the Cambridge Philosophical Society. Cambridge: Univ Press, 1956;474–514.

31. Iltis H. Gregor Johann Mendel, Leben, Werk, und Wirkung. In: Iltis H; Eden P, Cedar P, trans. Life of Mendel. New York: WW Norton, 1932.

32. Jensen CO. Uebertragbare Rattensarkome. Ztsch Krebsforsch 1909;7:45–54.

33. Keele KD. William Harvey: the man, the physician, and the scientist. London: Nelson, 1965.

34. Keller EF. A feeling for the organism. The life and work of Barbara McClintock. San Francisco: Freeman, 1983.

35. Knudson AG. Mutation and cancer: a statistical study of retinoblastoma. Proc Natl Acad Sci USA 1971;68:820–3.

36. Kornberg RD, Klug A. The nucleosome. Sci Amer 1981; 244:52–64.

37. Lewin B. Genes, 3rd ed. New York: John Wiley & Sons, 1987:519–37.

38. Li FP, Fraumeni JF. Soft-tissue sarcomas, breast cancer and other neoplasms. A familiar syndrome? Ann Intern Med 1969;71:747–52.

39. Little CC, Tyzzer EE. Further experimental studies on the inheritance of susceptibility of a transplantable tumor. J Med Res 1916;33:393–453.

40. Loeb LA. Microsatellite instability: marker of a marker phenotype in cancer. Cancer Res 1994;54:5059–63.

41. Loeb LA. Mutator phenotype may be required for multistage carcinogenesis. Cancer Res 1991;51:3075–9.

42. Loeb LA, Springgate CF, Battula N. Errors in DNA replication as a basis of malignant changes. Cancer Res 1974;34:2311–21.

43. Longnecker DS, Crawford BG. Hyperplastic nodules and adenomas of exocrine pancreas in azaserine-treated rats. JNCI 1974;53:573–7.

44. Lynch HT, Tautu R, eds. Recent progress in the genetic epidemiology of cancer. New York: Springer Verlag, 1991.

45. Marsh WH, Fitzgerald PJ. Pancreas acinar cell regeneration. XIII. Histone synthesis and modifications. Fed Proc 1973;32:2119–25.

46. McClintock B. The discovery and characterization of transposable elements. In: Moore JA, ed. The collected papers of Barbara McClintock. New York: Garland Publishing, 1987.

47. McKusick VA. Mendelian inheritance in man. A catalog of human genes and genetic disorders, vol 2, 11th ed. Baltimore: Johns Hopkins Univ. Press, 1994:1483–4.

48. McKusick VA, Walter S. Sutton and the physical basis of Mendelism. Bull Hist Med 1960;34:487–97.

49. Mendel G. Versuche über Pflanzen-hybriden. Verh naturf Ver in Brunn, Abhandlungen, LV. In: Peters JA, ed; Royal Hort Soc London, trans. Classic papers in genetics. New Jersey: Prentice-Hall, 1959:1–20, 136, Chronology, appendix A.

50. Miles CP. Chromosome analysis of solid tumors. II. Twenty-six epithelial tumors. Cancer 1967;20:1274–87.
51. Morgan TH, Sturtevant AH, Muller HJ, Bridges CB. The mechanism of mendelian heredity. New York: Henry Holt, 1915.
52. Muller HJ. Artificial transmutation of the gene. Science 1927;66:84–7.
53. Murray JA. Cancerous ancestory and the incidence of cancer in mice. Proc Royal Soc. London. Series B. Biological Sciences 1911;LXXXIV:42–48.
54. Nowell PC. Chromosomes and cancer. The evolution of an idea. Adv Cancer Res 1994;62:1–17.
55. Nowell PC. The clonal evolution of tumor cell populations. Science 1976;194:23–8.
56. Nowell PC. From chromosomes to oncogenes: a personal perspective. In: Kirsch IR, ed. The causes and consequences of chromosomal aberrations. Boca Raton, FL: CRC Press, 1993:505–16.
57. Nowell P, Hungerford DA. Chromosome studies on normal and leukemic human leukocytes. JNCI 1960;25:85–110.
58. Nowell PC, Hungerford DA. A minute chromosome in human chronic granulocytic leukemia. Science 1960;132:1497.
59. Painter TS. A new method for the study of chromosome rearrangements and the plotting of chromosome maps. Science 1933;78:585–6.
60. Pour P, Kruger FW, Althoff J, Cardesa A, Mohr U. Cancer of the pancreas induced in the Syrian golden hamster. Amer J Pathol 1974;76:349–58.
61. Roux W. Über die Bedeutung der Kerntheilungsfiguren. Leipzig: Englemann, 1883:1–19.
62. Rowley JD. A new consistent chromosomal abnormality in chronic myelogenous leukemia identified by quinacrine fluorescence and Giemsa staining. Nature 1973;243:290–3.
63. Schlumberger HG. Tumors characteristic for certain animal species: a review. Cancer Res 1957;17:823–32.
64. Schlumberger HG, Lucké B. Tumors of fishes, amphibians and reptiles. Cancer Res 1948;8:657–753.
65. Seshadri R, Kutlaca RJ, Trainor K, Matthews C, Morley AA. Mutation rate of normal and malignant human lymphocytes. Cancer Res 1987;47:407–9.
66. Sharp PA. Biology, oncology and RNA splicing. Cancer 1987;59:1697–708.
67. Shimkin MB. Contrary to nature: being an illustrated commentary on some persons and events of historical importance of knowledge concerning cancer, Washington, D.C.: Department of Health Education and Welfare, Public Health Service, National Institutes of Health, 1977:196.
68. Slye M. The relation of heredity to cancer, with regard to the communication of President C.C. Little of the University of Michigan. J Cancer Res 1928;12:83–133.
69. Stewart HL, Snell KC, Dunham LY, Schlyen SM. Transplantable and transmissible tumors of animals. Atlas of Tumor Pathology, 1st Series, Fascicle 40. Washington, D.C.: Armed Forces Institute of Pathology, 1959.
70. Sturtevant AH. History of genetics. New York: Harper & Row 1965: 9–32, 45–7, 62.
71. Sutton WS. On the morphology of the chromosome group in *Brachystola magna*. Biol Bull 1902;4:24–39.
72. Tjio JH, Levan A. The chromosome numbers of man. Hereditas 1956;42:106.
73. Upton AC. Historical perspectives on radiation carcinogenesis. In: Upton AC, Albert RE, Burns FJ, Shore RE, eds. Radiation carcinogenesis. New York: Elsevier, 1986:1–10.
74. Van Beneden E. Recherches sur la maturation de l'oeuf et la fecondation. Archives de biologie 1883;4:26–83.
75. Vogelstein B, Fearon ER, Hamilton SR, et al. Genetic alterations during colorectal-tumor development. N Engl J Med 1988;319:525–32.
76. Warthin AS. Heredity with reference to carcinoma. As shown by the study of the cases examined in the pathological laboratory of the University of Michigan, 1895–1913. Arch Intern Med 1913;12:546–55.
77. Watson JD, Crick FH. Molecular structure of nucleic acids. A structure for deoxyribose nucleic acid. Nature 1953;171:737–8.
78. Weismann A. Evoluton, heredity, and reproduction, In: Shipley AE, Poulton EB, eds. Essays upon heredity and kindred biological problems, 2nd ed. Oxford: Clarendon Press, 1892:22–3, 124–30, 226, 276–87, 471.
79. Wills C. The wisdom of the genes: new pathways in evolution. New York: Basic Books, 1989:22–3, 124–130, 276–87.
80. Wilson EB. The cell in development and inheritance. New York: Macmillan, 1980:5–7, 10–2.

20

THE ONCOGENE

GENE AND VIRUS INTERACTION

In the 1950s and 1960s, after many viruses were found to cause tumors in animals, more credence was given to the hypothesis that viruses were involved in human carcinogenesis. Advances in virology, molecular biology, and microbial genetics made it possible to study how viruses infected cells and how some of them transformed normal cells into cancer cells (82).

It had been shown in 1963 by Y. Berwald and L. Sacks, investigators at the Weizmann Institute in Israel, that a layer of benign cells growing in a cell culture medium could be transformed by a virus into cells that expressed malignant characteristics (5). This approach stripped away much of the complexity of cancer research and implied that the relatively simple technique of growing cells in a culture medium would make them practical models in which to study carcinogenesis, leading to a deeper understanding of the process. Many types of cells, normal or malignant, can be grown in a culture medium and subjected to experimental manipulation.

Advances came rapidly in the 1970s with studies of the papova, SV40, and polyoma viruses which demonstrated that the viral genes became incorporated as a provirus into the genome of the cells that they transformed. The continued presence of these viruses in the genome was believed to be necessary for the perpetuation of the malignant change in the cells (see chapter 15).

When DNA from an adenovirus was introduced into normal cells growing in a culture medium, it was shown that the cells took up the viral DNA and were transformed into cancer cells (31). The power of the genes of transforming viruses was illustrated by the SV40 virus which had a genome of only 5,000 nucleotides and yet could control the growth rate of a cell with a one million times larger genome and transform the benign cell into a malignant cell (80).

In 1981, Robert Weinberg and associates of the Whitehead Institute, Massachusetts Institute of Technology (MIT) (51) and Geoffrey Cooper and colleagues of the Dana-Farber Cancer Institute at Harvard (41), showed that the DNA extracted from cells that had been transformed by the Harvey sarcoma virus was able to transform normal mouse recipient cells in culture (fig. 20-1). This occurred even when the viral gene was present only as a single copy within the donor cell's genome.

The *src* Gene

An important advance in nucleic acid research was the development of the chemical hybridization technique. This technique was based on the fact that two antiparallel, complementary, single-stranded nucleic acid molecules recognize one another and bind (anneal) to each other when heated because of hydrogen bonding . Adenine will bind to thymine and guanine to cytosine whether they are in DNA or RNA. Thus it is possible to have DNA-DNA, RNA-RNA, or RNA-DNA duplexes. One could identify a series of nucleotides by determining whether they annealed to a complementary strand of known nucleotide sequence of DNA or RNA. The technique became a probe, a means of identifying a sequence of nucleotides (2).

A transforming retrovirus that is a powerful carcinogen, such as the Rous sarcoma virus (RSV), can produce a sarcoma in chickens in a week or two; it is called an "acutely transforming virus." Other retroviruses, such as the avian leukosis virus (ALV), which take months to induce tumors, are called the "weakly transforming viruses" (fig. 20-2) (21). The weakly transforming virus does replicate but cannot transform the cells as rapidly as the Rous sarcoma virus does.

A significant physical difference between the Rous sarcoma virus (RSV) genome and the avian leukosis virus (ALV) genome was noted by P. Duesberg and P. Vogt of the University of California, Berkeley, in 1970 (27). The genome of the RSV was about 10 kb long while that of the ALV was 8.5 kb in length (fig. 20-3). Duesberg and Vogt et al. found that the Rous transforming gene was present in the extra length (1.5 kb) of the genome, near the 3' (amino) end of the RSV and it was called the *src* gene (28)

With the use of RSV mutants it was shown that the wild type RSV contained information that was required for transformation but not for virus replication (83).

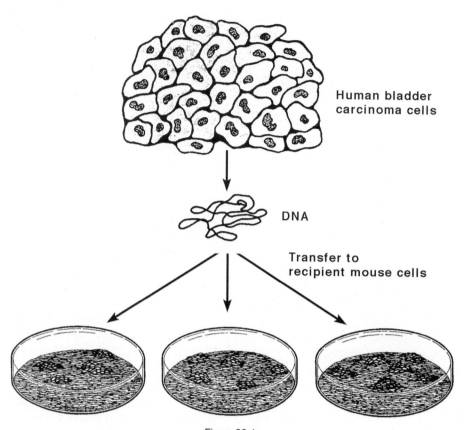

Figure 20-1

DETECTION OF THE FIRST HUMAN ONCOGENE

DNA was extracted from EJ human bladder carcinoma cells and transferred to a culture medium in which mouse fibroblasts were growing. The extracted DNA caused transformation of the fibroblasts. (Fig. 5.2 from Cooper GM. Oncogenes. Boston: Jones & Bartlett, 1990:70.)

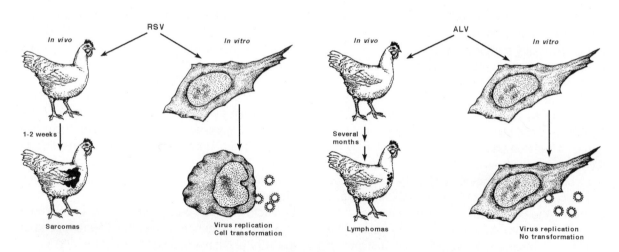

Figure 20-2

ROUS SARCOMA VIRUS VERSUS AVIAN LEUKOSIS VIRUS

Comparison of the ability of the Rous sarcoma virus (RSV), left, and the avian leukosis virus (ALV), right, to produce tumors and transform normal cells in culture mediums. The Rous sarcoma virus gave rise to sarcomas in a few weeks. The avian leukosis virus did not produce tumors for some months. (Fig. 3.1 from Cooper GM. Oncogenes. Boston: Jones & Bartlett, 1990:36.)

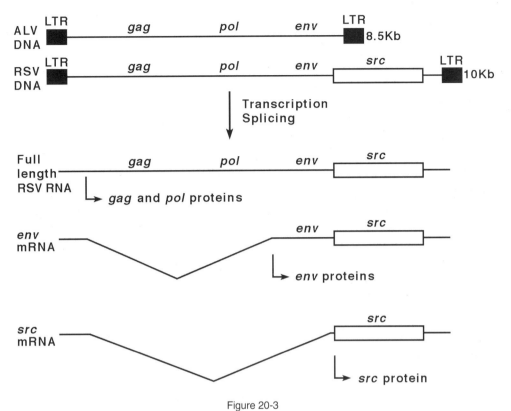

Figure 20-3

COMPARISON OF THE GENES OF THE AVIAN LEUKOSIS VIRUS (ALV) AND THE ROUS SARCOMA VIRUS (RSV)

The longer *RSV* gene contains the *src* gene, the first recognized transforming gene, called an oncogene. *qaq, pol* and *env* are genes that encode proteins involved in noncarcinogenic functions. The RSV primary RNA transcript is spliced to yield successively three mRNAs (lower 3 figures); two are involved on the nontransforming proteins and the third (lowermost) is for expressing the src oncoprotein. (Fig. 3.5 from Cooper GM. Oncogenes. Boston: Jones & Bartlett, 1990:43.)

With other techniques it was shown that the *src* gene could cause and was necessary for, the transformation of cells. The letters *src* were used in recognition of the fact that the sarcoma was produced by the Rous virus.

The *src* gene, the first transforming gene identified, was called an oncogene (see below). It contained about 1,500 nucleotides and encoded a cytoplasmic protein, the src protein, of 60 kD (kilodaltons; pp60^{v-src}). The src protein proved to be a protein kinase, an enzyme that added phosphate to compounds (17,43). The kinase was a protein tyrosine, a class of enzymes that has been proven to be involved in signal transduction, a process that regulates the proliferation of cells (39). An increase or decrease in the activity of the enzyme increases or decreases, respectively, the signal that determines the rate of proliferation of the cell; proliferation is a necessary step in carcinogenesis.

The identification of the *src* gene as an encoding gene for a protein that was involved in the transmission of a signal for cell proliferation demonstrated how a transforming gene might act in the carcinogenesis process (39).

THE ONCOGENE (BISHOP-VARMUS) HYPOTHESIS

The original oncogene hypothesis of Huebner and Todaro postulated that C-type retroviruses, known to cause cancer in animals, did so by inserting their viral RNA into the DNA of normal cells by the enzyme reverse transcriptase (see chapter 15). This gene complex of normal and viral DNA became an integral part of the normal cell's genome and was called a proviral complex. It could remain unexpressed in the cell genome, or it could be activated through viral, radiation, chemical, or other

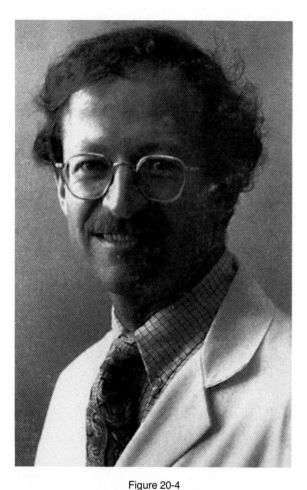

Figure 20-4
HAROLD VARMUS
Dr. Harold Varmus who with Dr. Bishop formulated the Bishop-Varmus oncogene hypothesis (82). (From the cover of Cancer Research 1990;50:2.)

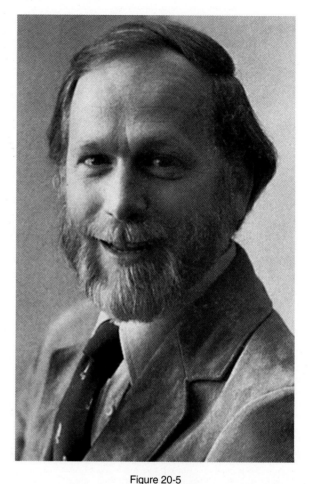

Figure 20-5
MICHAEL BISHOP
Dr. Michael Bishop, cofounder of the Bishop-Varmus oncogene hypothesis (6). (From the cover of Cancer Research 1990;50:2.)

means, and cause the transformation of normal cells into cancer cells. These C-type viral complexes with the host DNA were called oncogenes (Greek: tumor genes). When the oncogene was activated it would transform normal cells to cancer cells (38) (see chapter 15).

In 1970, two physicians who decided not to pursue a career in clinical medicine but to enter a basic science research field, collaborated on studies in the field of virology. Dr. Harold Varmus (fig. 20-4) became associated with Dr. J. Michael Bishop (fig. 20-5) in the latter's laboratory at the University of California Medical School in San Francisco where Bishop was studying animal viruses (8).

In 1976, Bishop and Varmus in collaboration with Stehelin and Vogt used a probe of the nucle-

otide sequence of the DNA of the *src* transforming agent of the Rous sarcoma virus to show, unexpectedly, that those nucleotides were also present in the normal avian cell DNA (73). That the nucleotide sequences of the DNA of the cells of normal, unaffected chickens were essentially the same as those present in the virus *src* that transformed cells was surprising and raised important questions (72).

The finding, in one sense, was in accord with the hypothesis that in the evolution of the acutely transforming viruses, such as the Rous sarcoma virus, some material from the DNA of normal cells might be picked up and incorporated into the viral genome. Experiments with other acutely transforming viruses gave results similar to those with the src probe: in all cases the transforming nucleotide sequences of the retroviruses of the acutely transforming type were homologous (very similar) to the nucleotide sequences of the DNA found in normal cells of the same species. These cellular homologs of the virus *src* transforming nucleotides were conserved throughout vertebrates (72) and were present in other species earlier in the evolutionary trail, such as the fruit fly Drosophila (37). It appeared, therefore, that retroviral oncogenes originated from nucleotide sequences of normal cells by a combination of the DNA of the cells and the viral DNA genes.

Oncogene and Transformation

A more significant question arose, an unanticipated possibility: Might the genome of normal cells contain genes vulnerable to change that might subsequently cause them to act as transforming agents? The amazing answer to the question was found to be, "Yes."

Certain cellular genes (or viral genes) could induce one or more characteristics of neoplastic transformation when introduced either alone or in combination with another gene of the appropriate type into a culture of normal cells. A gene capable of this transforming ability was called an oncogene by Varmus and Bishop (82). The same term, oncogene, had been used by Huebner and Todaro for their hypothesis that a C-type virus complex caused the transformation. It was used by Varmus and Bishop to indicate that a normal cell might contain a gene, an oncogene, that was involved in the transformation. The cellular oncogene was indicated by the prefix c (*c-src*); a viral oncogene was designated by the prefix v (*v-src*).

Weinberg (51) and Cooper (41) had shown that when the DNA of cells that had been transformed by the Rous sarcoma virus was extracted and the extract transferred to a culture of chicken embryo normal fibroblasts, transformation of the fibroblasts to fibrosarcoma cells occurred. From this important finding there followed a corollary: a single oncogene containing the *src* sequence of nucleotides could be detected in a nearly millionfold excess of normal cellular DNA (35). The ability to detect oncogenes by the transfer of DNA from experimentally transformed cells to noninfected cells could now be used as a means of detecting biologically active cellular oncogenes. The oncogene encoded protein is called an oncoprotein (7).

A single oncogene alone rarely causes transformation of a normal cell; two or more oncogenes are usually necessary for transformation to take place (42).

Retroviral oncogenes have been identified in over 40 viruses of the acute transforming retrovirus type. They have been isolated from chickens, turkeys, mice, rats, cats, and monkeys (21). At least 25 retroviral oncogenes are known as models for major forms of neoplasia. Oncogenes have been demonstrated in DNA viruses as well as in RNA retroviruses (21).

NOMENCLATURE

There is no universal convention for naming genes, mutations, and gene products. Genes and mutant genes are italicized and consist of a three-letter abbreviation that is followed by a letter or number. The same subscript is used as for other organisms. Gene products are designated by the same abbreviation as for the gene but with italics and by capitalizing the first letter, e.g., *Cdc*10 is the product of the yeast gene *cdc*10.

Oncogenes are designated by three-letter names that in most cases refer to strains of animals, species of isolation, or type of neoplasm induced by the acutely transforming viruses, e.g., *src* for the transforming gene of the Rous sarcoma virus (21). Superscripts may be added to a designation as follows: + indicates a wild type; −, a recessive mutant; ts, a recessive temperature-sensitive mutant; and D, a dominant mutant.

PROTO-ONCOGENES

There are other genes, called proto-oncogenes, that may be involved in the transformation process. Proto-oncogenes (Greek: proto, first) are genes derived from normal components of the cellular genome. These cellular genes may be activated to oncogenes. Nine viral oncogenes (*abl, erb-B, ets, mos, myc, myb, H-ras, K-ras,* and *Sis*) have proto-oncogenes that may be incriminated in oncogenesis (6). Four of these, *myc, ras, abl,* and *erb-B* may play a significant role in human cancer. The proto-oncogenes encode proteins that are involved in normal growth and differentiation. They could be activated by mutation or another genomic alteration to become oncogenes, which in turn have the potential of being activated to transform cells.

Proto-oncogenes have been found in the Drosophila fruit fly (37) which implies that they have been involved in important cellular functions for a long period of evolutionary life. The proto-oncogenes are probably the sites of action of some external carcinogens, such as chemical carcinogens and radiation.

Oncogenes differ from proto-oncogenes in many respects, such as the loss of regulating sequences, differences in the proteins encoded, and the accumulation of point mutations. A difference between oncogenes and proto-oncogenes is illustrated by the effect of the Rous sarcoma virus (RSV) when its oncogene *src* acts on cells in culture. When the oncogene *src* is activated from the proto-oncogene, the levels of RNA and the protein concentration in the transformed chick fibroblast cells are increased 10 to 100 times more than in cells with a nonactivated proto-oncogene (21).

ONCOGENES IN NONVIRAL-INDUCED TUMORS

But what about the DNA extracted from chemically induced tumors in animals? No viruses are involved in this type of carcinogenesis. Could such an extract of DNA transform cells?

Robert Weinberg and colleagues at MIT found that of DNA extracted from 15 cell lines of chemically transformed rodent cells, 5 could induce transformation in NIH3T3 cells growing in culture. The efficiency of transformation was similar to that induced by the DNA of murine sarcoma viruses (67).

Allan Balmain of Scotland and colleagues reported in 1983 that skin cancer in the mouse produced by chemical carcinogens contained activated *H-ras* oncogenes (3). Later they reported that *ras* activation was present in benign skin papillomas (4), suggesting that activation of the cancer occurred early in the neoplastic process.

These and many other examples showed that chemical carcinogens could transform cells without the necessary presence of viruses or viral products.

ONCOGENES AND PROTO-ONCOGENES IN HUMAN TUMORS

Most of the genes involved in human cancer represent previously unknown genes. There are more than 50 involved with the leukemias and lymphomas alone. They are not related to viruses; many

are lineage specific and produce tumors in only one type of cell. Many code for nuclear proteins.

ras Genes

After it was shown that DNA extracted from a human bladder cancer cell line induced transformation of NIH 3T3 mouse cells in a culture medium (fig. 20-1) (41), it was found that the involved *ras* oncogene was a cellular homolog of the oncogene of the Harvey rat virus sarcoma (*H-ras*) (58,62). The human bladder cellular oncogene was then labeled the *c-ras* oncogene.

Another cellular oncogene, activated in human lung carcinoma, was identified as a human proto-oncogene corresponding to the Kirsten rat virus sarcoma oncogene, *K-ras* (25). *H-ras* and *K-ras* proto-oncogenes are members of a gene family that encodes similar proteins. A third member of the cellular *ras* virus family, *N-ras*, was originally isolated from a neuroblastoma (hence the designation *N-ras*) (68), but it has been found in other human tumors.

The protein encoded by the *ras* genes is a 21,000-dalton phosphoprotein, p21, found in normal untransformed cells. It was concluded that the gene encoding the p21 protein was the oncogene of the Harvey and Kirsten viruses and other closely related viruses. The genes encoding p21 proteins are now referred to as the *ras* genes (49). The proteins of the *ras* group are Ha-ras, Ki-ras 2B, and N-ras. They share many common properties. It has been postulated that p21 protein forms a complex in the plasma membrane with GTP (guanine triphosphate) and GAP (GPT-ase activating protein), i.e., a p21 • GTP • GAP unit that may send a signal for mitosis to the cell (49).

Activation of the *ras* oncogene has been found in many cancers but not in all. K-*ras* is present in about 90 percent of pancreas cancers (see below), in 10 percent of some of the leukemias, and in less than 5 percent of most cancer types. None has been found in lymphocytic leukemia or non-Hodgkin's lymphoma. It is present in polyps of the human colon—benign, potential precancerous lesions (49).

COMBINED ONCOGENE AND VIRAL ACTION

The Epstein-Barr herpes virus (EBV) has been discussed in chapter 15, particularly in regard to Burkitt's lymphoma in equatorial Africa. Burkitt's lymphoma is malignant and characterized by a latent viral (EBV) infection and a *c-myc* oncogene

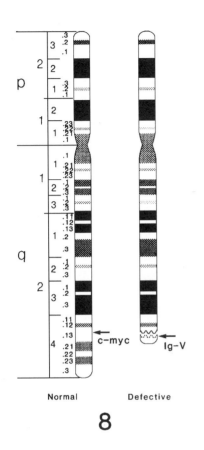
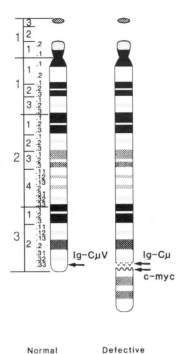

Normal   Defective   Normal   Defective

8   **14**

Figure 20-6
TRANSLOCATION IN
BURKITT'S LYMPHOMA

Translocation of *c-myc* from chromosome 8 to the immunoglobulin heavy chain locus on chromosome 14 in human Burkitt's lymphoma (21,40). The truncation of the *c-myc* gene may be important in triggering the transformation of the proliferating lymphocytes to a malignant lymphoma. (Fig. 29.2 from Therman E, Susman M. Human chromosomes, 3rd. ed. New York: Springer Verlag, 1993:315.)

translocation. The EBV virus "immortalizes" the B lymphocytes and contributes to the early stage of genesis of lymphoma, possibly by increasing the pool of proliferating cells. Immunosuppression permits further expansion of the lymphocytes and the truncation of the *c-myc* oncogene; recombination with immunoglobulin loci may produce Burkitt's malignant lymphoma (fig. 20-6) (40).

EXPERIMENTAL TRANSGENIC MICE

The ability to produce transgenic mice has many possibilities for future research. DNA generated by a molecular construct of the *c-myc* gene and the mouse mammary tumor virus gene (MMTV), when injected into the fertilized egg of a mouse, expressed the reactivation of the *c-myc* oncogene. If the eggs were injected into a foster mother mouse, a few of the progeny incorporated the foreign DNA construct into their DNA. These latter mice expressed the viral oncogene, as shown by the appearance of breast cancer several months after birth. Control mice of the same strain not given the viral oncogene construct did not develop breast cancer (69,74).

This experiment, as well as others, has led to the conclusion that oncogenes can contribute to tumorigenesis in intact animals. The activation of a single oncogene might initiate the process of transformation but other factors have to be present to complete the multiple stages of carcinogenesis. The transgenic technique is an important means by which the steps in the mechanism of carcinogenesis are delineated.

MULTIPLE ONCOGENES AND TRANSFORMATION

When the EJ bladder oncogene *H-ras* was introduced into relatively normal cells, transformation did not occur in contrast to when it was applied to the laboratory strain of test cells (NIH3T3) normally used for transformation purposes. The NIH3T3 strain represented cells that had already been immortalized, an early step in the transformation process. The *H-ras* oncogene by itself did not transform normal cells.

A combination of two oncogenes was shown to be necessary in order to obtain transformation in

	1	2	3	4	5	6	7	8	9	10	11	12	13		188	189
Normal	Met	Thr	Glu	Tyr	Lys	Leu	Val	Val	Val	Gly	Ala	Gly	Gly		Leu	Ser
Human *ras*H	ATG	ACG	GAA	TAT	AAG	CTG	GTG	GTG	GTG	GGC	GCC	GGC	GGT	......	CTC	TCC
												↓ GTC				
Activated EJ *ras*H	Met	Thr	Glu	Tyr	Lys	Leu	Val	Val	Val	Gly	Ala	Val	Gly	......	Leu	Ser

Figure 20-7

ACTIVATION OF THE *H-RAS* ONCOGENE BY POINT MUTATION

A single nucleotide change, which altered codon 12 from GGC (glycine) to GTC (valine), caused the transformation of the *H-ras* oncogene to produce the EJ bladder cancer. (Fig. 5.4 from Cooper GM. Oncogenes. Boston: Jones & Bartlett, 1990:73.)

some cases. Neither the *src* nor the *myc* gene alone could give rise to transformation of normal cells. When cells with the *myc* oncogene were added to the medium which contained the *src* oncogene, the combination of the two caused transformation (42) (Note 1).

Tumors occur in some strains of transgenic mice at several months of age. After the mating of a strain containing the *myc* oncogene with a strain containing the *ras* oncogene, the progeny showed an acceleration of tumor development (20). This need for cooperation of the two oncogenes implied that a complicated arrangement existed between oncogenes and transformation. It is consistent with the generally accepted belief that carcinogenesis is a multi-step process, and oncogenes may be involved in different steps of the process.

MECHANISM(S) OF ACTION IN TRANSFORMATION

The activation of proto-oncogenes and oncogenes is important in a significant number of types of carcinogenesis. Some proto-oncogenes have nucleotide sequences similar to those of the retrovirus oncogenes, e.g., the *ras* family. Other proto-oncogenes have sequences not found in retroviruses. Chemical, viral, radiation, and other carcinogens may activate proto-oncogenes to the oncogene stage. Following are some of the different methods by which activation may occur.

Point Mutation

***ras* Activation.** The EJ bladder transforming oncogene is not a viral gene, but arises from a normal cellular proto-oncogene, the first to be isolated from a human cancer. Comparison of the nucleotide sequence of the normal human *H-ras* proto-oncogene protein and the nucleotide sequence of the *H-ras* oncogene protein isolated from the EJ bladder cancer showed that there was a difference of only a single point mutation between them (21).

The normal *H-ras* proto-oncogene protein has, at one point (codon 12), a base sequence GGC (guanine-guanine-cytosine) that encodes the amino acid glycine (see chapter 14). The activated oncogene has thymine substituted for a guanine so that the

Note 1: Robert Weinberg and colleagues at the Whitehead Institute for Biomedical Research, Massachusetts Institute of Technology, Cambridge, MA, reported that normal human cells in cell culture were transformed into cancer cells by the presence of two oncogenes. This was said not to have been demonstrated previously (33a). The crucial part of the experiment was the addition of the telomerase enzyme catalytic subunit, known as hTERT, to the culture of human cells and the subsequent immortalization of the cells. The telomerase enzyme adds caps to the end of chromosomes which in humans appear to decrease in length with age and as cell divisions increase.

To the cell culture of human cells (fibroblasts or epithelial cells) were added the telomerase enzyme and two activated oncogenes: H-*ras* V12 and the simian virus 40 large-T oncoprotein allele, the latter known to inhibit two growth control factors, the suppressor p53 and the retinoblastoma proteins.

The experiment opened up new vistas of research (86a) indicating that the genetic mechanisms controlling carcinogenesis, although complex and difficult to unravel, can be profitably explored in cell cultures. An era of study of the interaction of gene and mutated gene products, growth factors, hormones, cytokines, and many other modifiers of genetic activity appears to be at hand.

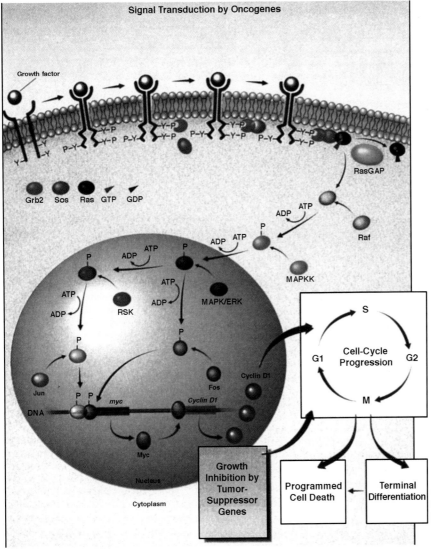

Figure 20-8
ACTION OF ONCOGENES
INVOLVED IN SIGNAL
TRANSDUCTION

There is the binding of the signal (upper left, a growth factor) to the transmembrane receptor (Y-shaped) on the cell membrane. The receptors phosphorylate each other, left to right, and the *ras* oncogene, which produces a ras protein to further the signal. The ras protein switches on another kinase, the oncogene *raf* which passes the signal through three proteins culminating in the activation of the transcription factors fos and jun in the nucleus. These transcription factors join, become phosphorylated, and bind to specific DNA sequences near the *myc* proto-oncogene, thereby activating it. The latter activates the gene for cyclin D1 which forwards the progression of cells through G1 to the S period of the cell cycle and to cell proliferation. (Fig. 1 from Krontirist TG. Molecular medicine. Oncogenes. N Eng J Med 1995;333:303–6.)

codon becomes a GTC (guanine-thymidine-cytidine) base sequence which encodes the amino acid valine (fig. 20-7). Later studies showed that additional sites, such as codon 61 and others, might be affected. Apparently, a single base substitution converted the gene from a normal component of the cell's growth apparatus into a transforming agent, resulting in the transformation of a normal bladder cell into a bladder cancer cell (21).

Point mutations leading to single amino acid substitutions are a characteristic feature of the activation of the *ras* genes and have probably occurred in the genome over the evolutionary period. The mechanism of action of the ras protein products seems to be related to their location in the cell's plasma membrane where they may act by binding to G (guanine) binding proteins (see below) and thereby affect the mitotic signals (fig. 20-8) (21,79) (Note 2).

Note 2: The *Ha-ras* oncogene acts by encoding the synthesis of a protein, called p21, which mediates the transformation. The *Ha-ras* proto-oncogene is present in organisms as low on the phylogenetic scale as the Drosophila fly, and is even in baker's yeast; the proto-oncogene has shown relatively little change in the 100 million years between the evolution of yeast and the human organism. The *ras* proteins couple surface receptors to second messengers such as cAMP (cyclic adenosine monophosphate) (79). Such a small change in the genome over this long period suggests that the proto-oncogene plays a part in some important function(s) of living organisms in order to have survived so long.

Deletion

The removal of one or more nucleotide sequences of DNA is termed a deletion and when this happens, the regions on the adjoining sides of the deletion can be joined together by an enzyme, a ligase. The best known deletions are those occurring in human retinoblastoma, in some childhood tumors, and in the loss of function of the oncoprotein p53. A repressor gene may be lost by deletion (see chapter 21); deletion of suppressor genes is a frequent occurrence in human cancers.

Recombination

Some oncogenes are activated by DNA rearrangements, e.g., the *met* oncogene from chemically transformed osteogenic sarcoma cells and the *trk* oncogene from human colon cancer cells. Both involve DNA rearrangements which give rise to deletion of the normal 5' nucleotide coding sequence in the proto-oncogene. The amino terminals are replaced by a coding sequence from a different cellular gene and the result is a recombinant fusion protein (21).

Other oncogenes, e.g. *mas, hst,* and *fgf*-5, appear to be activated by the increased expression of the gene. This is caused by the recombination of the proto-oncogene with an abnormal regulatory sequence of genes (21).

Insertional Mutation

Some rare retroviruses do not possess oncogenes yet induce transformation of normal cells, e.g., avian leukosis virus (ALV), mouse mammary tumor virus (MMTV), and leukemia viruses of various animals. The tumors contain defective proviruses which are integrated in the same region of cellular DNA—a target locus—that is present in many forms of leukemia. It has been postulated that the insertion of proviral DNA in the target locus is a mutagenic event, insertional mutagenesis, which initiates neoplasia by indirect perturbable means (fig. 20-8). This phenomenon probably does not involve site-specific incorporation of viral genes. Possibly the juxtaposition of promoters and enhancers in the LTR (long terminal repeat) of the retrovirus can augment expression of adjacent or nearby cellular genes (9).

The incorporation of viral genes into an arrangement with the normal genes of the cells adjacent to the proto-oncogene may trigger activation. Most commonly, cellular proto-oncogenes are activated by augmented transcription, as with *int*-1 and *int*-2, both mouse mammary tumor viruses, and *pim*-1, a T-cell mouse lymphoma. Over a dozen cellular oncogenes have been identified as having target proviral sites for such insertional mutagens (9).

Chromosomal Translocations

Chromosome translocations occur in human tumors and represent an important mechanism for oncogene activation. The discovery of the Philadelphia (PH) chromosome in chronic myelogenous leukemia by Nowell and Hungerford indicated that chromosomal translocation itself was responsible for the leukemia (56). The activation of the *myc* oncogene in Burkitt's lymphoma (23) and the activation of the novel oncogene *bcl-1* identified by the translocation between chromosomes 14 and 18 in follicular B-cell lymphoma (59) are other examples of this effect.

Gene Amplification

The oncogene *c-myc* was the first cellular oncogene found to be amplified in human neoplasms (19,24). Gene amplification results in increased expression of the oncogene in human tumor progression and has been noted in over a dozen human tumors. The *c-myc* gene is amplified about tenfold in the human promyelocyte leukemia cell line HL-60 (24); overexpression of *c-myc* has been detected in many other human tumors, particularly in breast cancers and small cell lung carcinomas (21). The oncogenes *N-myc* and *L-myc* have been shown to be amplified in human tumors; the amplification of *N-myc* has been correlated with tumor progression in neuroblastoma. The oncogene *erbB* has exhibited amplification and elevated transcription in many tumors, particularly in glioblastoma of brain and squamous cell carcinoma. A somewhat related oncogene, *erbB-2,* is found in about 25 percent of human breast and ovarian cancers (21). Amplification may be sporadic and secondary in tumors activated by other means (21).

GROWTH FACTORS

Many of the proteins encoded by oncogenes regulate normal cell growth and their overexpression or abnormal expression might lead to a neoplasm. A cell may produce a growth factor, which

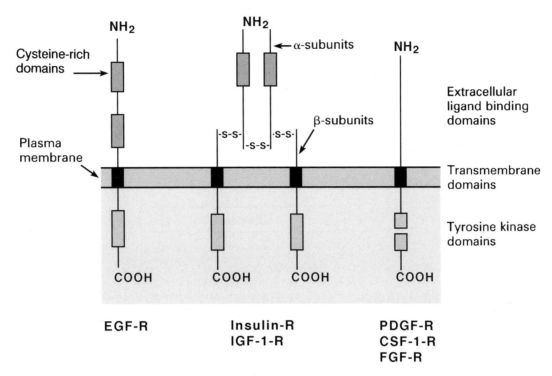

Figure 20-9
ORGANIZATION OF RECEPTOR PROTEIN–TYROSINE KINASES
There are extracellular, transmembrane, and intracellular domains. The tyrosine kinase catalytic domains are on the cytoplasmic side of the cell membrane. EGF-R = epidermal growth factor receptor; insulin-R = insulin receptor; IGF-1-R = insulin-like growth factor 1 receptor; PDGF-R = platelet-derived growth factor receptor; CSF-1-R = colony-stimulating growth factor receptor; and FGF-R = fibroblastic growth factor receptor. (Fig. 12.4 from Cooper GM. Oncogenes. Boston: Jones & Bartlett, 1990:181.)

after it has left the cell may be reabsorbed by the same cell and stimulate the cell to grow and proliferate, an autocrine response (21).

Some oncogenes express growth factors. The protein product of the *sis* oncogene, from the simian sarcoma virus of the wooly monkey, has been identified as being homologous with the platelet-derived growth factor (PDGF) β chain. The model for the action of sis/PDGF β chain-inducing transformation is that of an oncogene with continuous autocrine stimulation of the PDGF β chain growth factor response pathway (21).

Growth factors have been found experimentally to function as oncogenes. The epidermal growth factor (EGF) stimulates the proliferation of a variety of different epidermal cell types and there are other growth factors related to EGF (13). There is a family of oncogenes, *int*-2, *hst*, and *fgf,* which expresses polypeptides that are fibroblast growth factors (FGFs) (26).

The link between oncogene action and normal growth factors indicates how the regulation of cell proliferation may be affected in neoplastic cells.

Protein Tyrosine Kinases, Receptors, and Signal Transduction

Proteins are phosphorylated by the activity of enzymatic protein kinase, which adds phosphate to the protein. Protein phosphorylates are important in many regulatory mechanisms of the normal cell, particularly in signal transduction. In some systems, in order for an external signal to affect a cell it must bind to a receptor on the cell surface. The receptor then transmits the signal through the cell wall to intracellular biochemical components of the signaling network (fig. 20-9).

Stanley Cohen, a biochemist at Vanderbilt University, and colleagues, identified the receptor of the epidermal growth factor (EGF) and found that it exhibited protein kinase activity. The amino acid phosphorylated was tyrosine (13), not the usual amino acid to be affected since serine and threonine are more often affected.

Several oncogenes were found to have protein–tyrosine kinase activity, some requiring the involvement

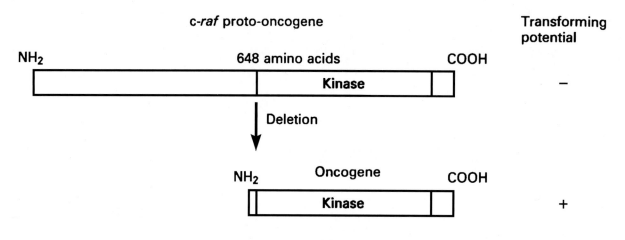

Figure 20-10
ACTIVATION OF A PROTO-ONCOGENE

The *c-raf* proto-oncogene has its normal amino-terminal regulatory domain deleted and thereby is converted to an active oncogene (21). (Fig. 14.2 from Cooper GM. Oncogenes. Boston: Jones & Bartlett, 1990:216.)

of a receptor (fig. 20-9), others functioning as non-receptor kinases (14). Many oncogenes encode the protein kinases that are involved in signal transduction. The cell surface receptor kinases carry information across the cell plasma membrane, coupling the binding of the external growth factor to a response inside the cell.

The nonreceptor protein–tyrosine kinases are intracellular proteins. Some, such as those of the *src* family, are not membrane spanning but are associated with the cytoplasm of the cell. The receptor and nonreceptor protein–tyrosine kinases transduce information within the cell cytoplasm by increasing the catalytic activity and transferring information to target molecules by phosphorylation. The cytoplasmic signal may then be transmitted to the nucleus. An increase in the signal may lead to increased mitosis and cell proliferation (21).

G (Guanine) Proteins

Another way in which receptors are bound to intracellular effectors is by guanine nucleotide binding (G proteins). The G proteins couple a variety of cell surface receptors to the metabolism of a second messenger system, cyclic adenosine monophosphate (cAMP), involved in the control of cell proliferation. The G proteins respond to the hormone activation of adenylate cyclase. Some hormones may bind to inhibitory receptors and lead to reduced cAMP-dependent protein kinase activity (21).

G proteins are also involved in other second messenger systems, e.g., in the retina, and in coupling receptors to other signaling systems, including phospholipid turnover and regulation of ion channel conductivity (21).

Protein Serine or Threonine Kinases

Abnormal expression or deletion of the regulatory domains of the normal genome may activate some protein serine or threonine kinases, kinases that are more common than protein tyrosine kinases. Over 50 protein serine or threonine kinases have been identified (21). The *raf* oncogene family of chicken and mouse retroviruses encodes soluble cytoplasmic proteins, which suggests that they are downstream effectors in signal transduction pathways initiated by a cell membrane oncogene and ultimately affect gene regulation in the nucleus. The *raf* oncogenes have deletions at their 5' terminals resulting in the loss of a few hundred amino acids from the amino terminal. The deletion presumably leads to activation of the *raf* protein kinase domain, unregulated catalytic activity, and transformation (fig. 20-10) (21).

Protein Kinase C

Protein kinase C has been shown to be an effector enzyme of the inositol phospholipid second messenger pathway, activated by diacylglycerol. The tumor promoter, phorbol ester (TPA) (see

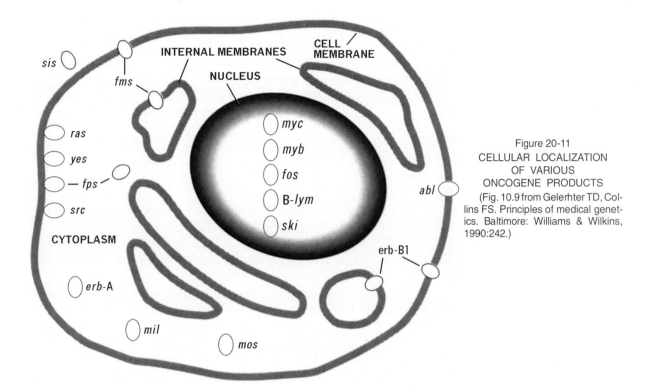

Figure 20-11
CELLULAR LOCALIZATION
OF VARIOUS
ONCOGENE PRODUCTS
(Fig. 10.9 from Gelerhter TD, Collins FS. Principles of medical genetics. Baltimore: Williams & Wilkins, 1990:242.)

chapter 13) activates protein kinase C, an intracellular target for carcinogenesis. The kinase consists of two distinct domains, a protein kinase catalytic area and a regulatory area. Proteolysis presumably removes the regulatory area and results in catalytic activity. Overexpression of protein kinase C has been found to induce cell transformation (21).

There is a correlation between the activation of the catalytic activity of protein kinase C by the proteolytic removal of the amino acid regulatory domain and the activation of the transforming potential of the *raf* oncogene (fig. 20-10).

Nuclear Oncogenes

While many oncogenes encode extracellular growth factors, signal transducing molecules on the cell surface membrane, or proteins in the cytoplasm, other oncogenes encode proteins localized to the cell nucleus. Some have been shown to function as transcriptional regulatory molecules or to bind to DNA (fig. 20-11) (21).

Transcription may be controlled by the interaction of proteins, called transcription factors, with specific regulatory DNA sequences, usually located upstream of the gene. Some of the nuclear oncogenes have been found to encode transcription factors, thereby controlling gene expression more directly.

In studying the relationship of oncogenes to transcription factors it was found that the *erbA* oncogene, the transforming retrovirus of avian erythroblastosis, had nucleotide sequences in common with steroid hormones. In addition, the *erbA* gene encoded a receptor for the thyroid hormone. The thyroid hormone receptor, encoded by the *erbA* proto-oncogene, regulates transcription by binding to the thyroid response element (TRE), preventing transcription (63).

Many oncogenes have been localized in the nucleus, e.g.,*myc, fos, myb, ski,* and B-*lym.* The *myb* oncogene is a sequence-specific DNA-binding protein that can function as a transcriptional activator (63), *sis* is a secreted growth factor, *erb*-B1 is a growth factor receptor, and *ras* is involved in the transmission of signals.

GENETIC CHANGES IN HUMAN CANCERS

Leukemias and Malignant Lymphomas

Leukemia, cancer of the blood cells, and malignant lymphoma, cancer of the lymphocytic line of cells, comprise about 10 percent of all cancers. With the advent of human cytogenetics increased attention has been paid to the involvement of the genome in these cancers. Nonrandom characteristic changes were noted in the genes of patients with acute leukemia by Rowley (61). A consistent alteration of chromosome 14 was found in patients with Burkitt's lymphoma (47), and shown to result from a translocation between chromosomes 8 and 14 (fig. 20-6) (88).

Since the 1960s the impetus for cytogenic studies was the discovery of the Philadelphia chromosome (Ph) in chronic myelogenous leukemia (CML) (54). In the latter disease Groffen et al. found that the translocation of the *c-abl* gene from a normal site on chromosome band 9q34 became associated with a previously unknown gene (*bcr*) on chromosome 22 (33). The product of this union was a fusion gene *bcr/abl* whose altered protein has a greatly elevated tyrosine kinase.

In some cases of CML, a progression to an acute blast phase, acute myelogenous leukemia (AML), occurs. The cytogenetic findings in this phase indicate that a subclone with additional chromosome changes has overgrown the original Ph chromosome population of cells. The development of a second clone during the carcinogenic process is consistent with Nowell's suggested clonal hypothesis and indicates an increase in genetic instability as the original disease persists (53).

An interesting contrast to CML is chronic lymphocytic leukemia (CLL) where genome stability is the rule and progression to a more aggressive acute lymphocytic leukemia state is uncommon (57). Survival is longer with CLL than with CML.

Other leukemias of the myeloid line exist. One, acute promyelocyte leukemia (APL), has abnormalities in the gene that codes for the alpha unit of the retinoic acid receptor (RARA) adjacent to the breakpoint on chromosome 17. Translocation in APL results in the formation of a fusion gene between the *RARA* gene and a gene on chromosome 15. The altered receptor acts abnormally to levels of retinoic acid and contributes to neoplastic growth (32).

Lymphocytic tumors, which comprise only about 5 percent of cancers, have contributed to an understanding of how genes are involved in cancer. Genetic changes in these tumors are usually nonrandom chromosomal translocations. B-cell lymphocytic tumors often involve immunoglobulin gene loci; in T-cell lymphocytic tumors, T receptor genes are associated with the translocations.

In about 75 percent of cases of Burkitt's lymphoma, tumor translocations occur when the *c-myc* proto-oncogene on band 8q24 is brought into jux-taposition with the immunoglobulin sequence on band 14q32 (8:14) (q24:q32) (fig. 20-6). This leads to the deregulation of the *myc* oncogene with the result that the normal action of the gene in regulating the growth of the cell is then deregulated, generating the rapidly expanding B-cell clone that is characteristic of the growing neoplasm (55).

New genes have been found in association with translocations in B-cell and T-cell lymphoid tumors. In low-grade human B-cell follicular lymphoma a translocation t(14:18)(q32:q21) is involved with the previously unknown gene *bcl*-2, which is moved from its position on chromosome 18 into juxtaposition with the immunoglobulin heavy chain locus on chromosome 14. This results in a deregulation of the *bcl*-2 gene, similar to the above described deregulation of *c-myc* in Burkitt's lymphoma (55). The *bcl*-2 gene is unusual; it is localized on mitochondrial membranes and acts to prevent programed death (apoptosis) of the cells (36). Translocations activate oncogenes in some tumors.

In T-cell lymphomas, at least eight new cancer genes have been described to be involved in translocations (55).

Solid Neoplasms

Advances in the study of solid tumors have been slowed by many technical difficulties. Tissue cells are not as readily available as blood cells. A prominent type of change in solid tumors has been a loss of genes or genetic function in contrast to the translocations found in leukemias and lymphomas (see chapter 21).

The K-*ras* Oncogene and Pancreatic Cancer

Indicative of the possible practical implications of advances in genetics is their effect on the diagnosis of pancreatic cancer. In 1987, an editorial by the author was published entitled, "Pancreatic Cancer. The Dismal Disease" (29). The term "dismal" was used because the 5-year survival rate was less than 10 percent (84), probably because metastases were present at diagnosis.

Within a decade, however, new genetic techniques led to the discovery of a mutation in the *K-ras* gene of patients with pancreatic cancer (1,70). This mutation was present in 70 to 90 percent of the cancers of the pancreatic duct system. The mutation also occurred in other cancers and in some benign lesions (10). Additional mutations were also present (10,60,65).

Mutation of the *K-ras* gene in cells obtained by needle aspiration of pancreatic tumors has been used as an aid in the diagnosis of pancreatic cancer. The cells from 48 of 60 patients with the cancer (72 percent) showed the presence of a mutation of the *K-ras* gene. All 23 patients (controls) who had noncancerous pancreatic lesions (chronic pancreatitis and benign tumors of the gland) were reported to have no evidence of the mutated gene (66,77,81).

Examination of the secretion of the pancreas, the pancreatic juice, also indicated the presence of a mutated *K-ras* gene in patients with pancreatic cancer (76,85). Mutated *K-ras* genes have been reported as well in the stool of patients with pancreatic cancer and pancreatic ductal hyperplasia (11). The mutated *K-ras* gene has also been found in the peripheral blood of patients with pancreatic cancer (71, 76). These findings stirred hope that an earlier diagnosis of pancreatic cancer could be made clinically.

Unfortunately, a recent study indicated that the mutation of the *K-ras* gene was present in the cells of the normal pancreatic ducts and in hyperplastic and metaplastic ductal epithelial cells (44). These findings decreased the value of a mutated gene as a diagnostic tool for pancreatic ductal cancer and indicated that the specificity and sensitivity of such findings need to be tested to be of diagnostic value.

Hereditary Familial Breast Cancer and *BRCA1* and *BRCA2* Genes

Oncologists have known for years that a family history of breast cancer in first degree relatives (mother, sister, or daughter) could be obtained in a small but significant percentage of women with breast cancer (45). A few percent of such women carry an inheritable mutated gene, *BRCA1* (breast cancer susceptibility gene), which is associated with the appearance of breast cancer at an earlier age. Some women with the mutation get the cancer in both breasts. The inherited gene acts in an autosomal dominant fashion; there is also an as-

sociated higher risk of ovarian cancer in those women carrying the mutated gene (46,52).

Hall et al. (34) of England first pointed out the link between the early onset of breast cancer and chromosomal changes; they mapped the *BRCA1* gene to chromosome 17q21. A second gene, *BRCA2,* also believed to be involved in familial breast cancer, has been mapped to chromosome 13q in the 12-13 region (87).

The *BRCA1* gene occurs in about half of the patients with familial breast cancer and there is a higher risk of ovarian cancer in this group. The *BRCA2* gene occurs in slightly less than half of the patients with familial breast cancer and it gives much less risk of ovarian cancer. There is the possibility that other genes are involved in the small fraction of patients with familial breast cancer. There is debate as to whether the *BRCA1* gene product is nuclear or cytoplasmic (16, 64). The mechanism of action of *BRCA1* is believed to be an increased proliferation of cells caused by the mutated gene (48).

Another genetic alteration has been described in familial breast cancer patients: a loss of heterozygosity (LOH) at a tumor suppressor locus on chromosome 17p which harbors the p53 suppressor gene (15,22,78,86).

As genetic tests are made available, women harboring the familial *BRCA1* or *BRCA2* gene may be diagnosed early in life as having a higher risk for breast cancer than women who do not have these genes and thereby could be carefully monitored for the appearance of breast cancer. Patients with the *BRCA1* gene are also at a high risk for ovarian cancer and could be alerted to this added risk (Note 3).

SIGNIFICANCE OF THE ONCOGENE AND PROTO-ONCOGENE

The discovery that normal cells have oncogenes and proto-oncogenes in their genome, that the latter have the potential to become activated to oncogenes, and that both may be involved in the transformation of normal cells into cancer cells, has

---

Note 3: A further development has been the discovery of a frame shift mutation at position 185 in exon 2 of the *BRCA1* gene. This involves the deletion of adenine and guanine (185delAG). A survey of Ashkenazi Jewish women without a family history of cancer revealed that about 1 percent carried this inherited mutation (75). Collins estimated that 7.5 percent of non-Jewish women and 38 percent of Jewish women with breast cancer under the age of 30 years would be expected to have germline *BRCA* mutations (18). A high frequency of the *BRCA1* 185delAG mutation (39 percent) was found in Jewish women in Israel who had ovarian cancer and a history of a first degree relative with breast or ovarian cancer. In Jewish women with ovarian cancer and a negative family history the incidence of the mutation was 13 percent (50).

been truly revolutionary. The long torturous trail from the discovery of the Rous virus, through the important chemical, viral, molecular biological, and genetic advances, has led to a detailed knowledge of the involvement of the genome in initiation and furtherance of the process of carcinogenesis. Pogo's dictum that, "the enemy is us," may, in one sense, apply to cancer in that a normal gene of a normal cell may undergo changes and become a transforming agent.

With the advent of the oncogene and proto-oncogene concepts there arose the hope that the final act in the drama of the long search for the mechanism of carcinogenesis was at hand. However, there are other mechanisms by which a normal cell may be transformed to a cancer cell. One such mechanism is the loss of the normal inhibitory effect of a gene which acts as a suppressor of the neoplastic process.

REFERENCES

1. Almoquera C, Shibata D, Forrester K, Martin J, Anheim N, Perucho M. Most human carcinomas of the exocrine pancreas contain mutant c-K-ras genes. Cell 1988;53:549–54.
2. Angerer LM, Stoler MH, Angerer RC. In situ hybridization: applications to neurobiology. Oxford: Oxford Univ. Press, 1987;42–70.
3. Balmain A, Pragnell IB. Mouse skin carcinoma induced in vivo by chemical carcinogens having a transforming Harvey ras oncogene. Nature 1983;303:72–4.
4. Balmain A, Ramsden M, Bowden GT, Smith J. Activation of the mouse cellular Harvey ras gene in chemically induced benign skin papillomas. Nature 1984;307:658–60.
5. Berwald Y, Sachs L. In vitro cell transformation with chemical carcinogens. Nature 1963;200:1182–4.
6. Bishop JS. The molecular genetics of cancer. Science 1987;235:305–11.
7. Bishop JM. Viruses, genes, and cancer. II. Retroviruses and cancer genes. Cancer 1985;55:2329–33.
8. Bishop MJ, Varmus HE. Cover. Cancer Res 1990;50:2.
9. Burck KB, Liu ET, Larrick JW. Oncogenes. An introduction to the concept of cancer genes. New York: Springer-Verlag, 1988;80–8.
10. Caldas C, Hahn SA, daCosta LT, et al. Frequent somatic mutations and heterozygous deletions of the p16 (MTSI) gene in pancreatic adenocarcinoma. Nature Gen 1994;8:27–32.
11. Caldas C, Hahn SA, Hruban RH, Redston MS, Yeo CJ, Kern SE. Detection of K-ras mutations in the stool of patients with pancreatic adenocarcinoma and pancreatic ductal hyperplasia. Cancer Res 1994;54:3568–73.
12. Caldas C, Kern SE. K-ras mutation and pancreatic adenocarcinoma. Int J Pancreatol 1995:18:1–6.
13. Carpenter G, Cohen S. Epidermal growth factor. Ann Rev Biochem 1979;48:193–216.
14. Carpenter G, King L Jr, Cohen S. Epidermal growth factor stimulates phosphorylation in membrane preparations in vitro. Nature 1978;276:409–10.
15. Chen LD, Neubauer A, Kurisu W, et al. Loss of heterozygosity on the short arm of chromosome 17 is associated with high proliferative capacity and DNA aneuploidy in primary human breast cancer. Proc Natl Acad Sci USA. 1991;88:3847–51.
16. Chen Y, Chen PL, Riley DJ, Lee WH, Allred DC, Osborne CK. Response. Science 1996;272:125–6.
17. Collett MS, Erikson RL. Protein kinase activity associated with avian sarcoma virus src gene product. Proc Natl Acad Sci USA 1978;75:2021–4.
18. Collins FS. BRCA1. Lots of mutations, lots of dilemmas. N Engl J Med 1996;334:186–8.
19. Collins S, Groudine M. Amplification of endogenous myc-related DNA sequences in a human myeloid leukaemia cell line. Nature 1982;298:679–81.
20. Compere SJ, Baldacci P, Sharpe AH, Thompson T, Land H, Jaenisch R. The ras and myc oncogenes cooperate in tumor induction in many tissues when introduced into midgestation mouse embryos by retroviral vectors. Proc Natl Acad Sci USA 1989;86:2224–8.
21. Cooper GM. Oncogenes. Boston: Jones & Bartlett, 1990;21–9, 35–42, 44–5, 59–60, 70–8, 97–112, 114–6, 144–8, 163–7, 197–201, 213–6, 225–36, 263–5.
22. Cornelisse CJ, Kuipers-Dijkshoorn N, van Vliet M, Hermans J, Devilee P. Fractional allelic imbalance in human breast cancer increases with tetraploidization and chromosome loss. Inter J Cancer 1992;50:544–8.
23. Dalla-Favera R, Bregni M, Erikson J, Patterson D, Gallo RC, Croce CM. Human c-myc oncogene is located on the region of chromosome 8 that is translocated in Burkitt lymphoma cells. Proc Natl Acad Sci USA 1982;79:7824–7.
24. Dalla-Favera R, Wong-Staal F, Gallo RC. Oncogene amplification in promyelocytic leukaemia cell line HL-60 and primary leukaemic cells of the same patient. Nature 1982;299:61–3.
25. Der CJ, Krontiris TG, Cooper GM. Transforming genes of human bladder and lung carcinoma cell lines are homologous to the ras genes of Harvey and Kirsten sarcoma viruses. Proc Natl Acad Sci USA 1982;79:3637–40.
26. Doolittle RF, Hunkapiller MW, Hood LE, et al. Simian sarcoma virus oncogene v-sis is derived from the gene (or genes) encoding a platelet-derived growth factor. Science 1983;221:275–7.
27. Duesberg PH, Vogt PK. Differences between the ribonucleic acids of transforming and non-transforming avian tumor viruses. Proc Natl Acad Sci USA 1970;67:1673–80.
28. Duesberg PH, Vogt PK. RNA species obtained from clonal lines of avian sarcoma and from avian leukosis virus. Virology 1973;54:207–19.
29. Fitzgerald PJ. Pancreatic cancer. The dismal disease. Arch Pathol Lab Med 1976;100:513–5.

30. German J. Patterns of neoplasia associated with chromosome breakage syndromes. In: German J, ed. Chromosome mutation and neoplasia. New York: AR Liss, 1983:97–134.

31. Graham FL, Vander Eb AJ, Heijneker HL. Size and location of the transforming region in human adenovirus type 5 DNA. Nature 1974;251:687–91.

32. Grignani F, Ferrucci PF, Testa U, et al. The acute promyelocytic-leukemia-specific PML-RAR alpha fusion protein inhibits differentiation and promotes survival of myeloid precursor cells. Cell 1993;74:423–31.

33. Groffen J, Stephenson JR, Heistercamp N, deKlein A, Bartram CR, Grosveld G. Philadelphia chromosomal breakpoints are clustered within a limited region, bcr on chromosome 22. Cell 1984;36:93–8.

33a. Hahn WC, Counter CM, Lundberg AS, Beijersbergan RL, Brooks MW, Weinberg RA. Creation of human tumor cells with defined genetic elements. Nature 1999;400:464–8.

34. Hall JM, Lee MK, Newman B, et al. Linkage of early-onset familial breast cancer to chromosome 17q21. Science 1990;250:1684–9.

35. Hill M, Hillova J. Production virale dans les fibroblastes de poule traités per l'acide désoxyribonucléique de celluies XC de rat transformées par le virale de Rous. Compt Rend Acad Sci 1971;272:3094–7.

36. Hockenbury D, Nunez G, Milliman G, Schreiber RD, Korsmeyer SJ. bcl-2 is an inner mitochondrial membrane protein that blocks programmed death. Nature 1990;348:334–6.

37. Hoffman-Falk H, Einat P, Shilo BZ, Hoffmann FM. Drosophila melanogaster DNA clones homologous to vertebrate oncogenes: evidence for a common ancestor to the src and abl cellular genes. Cell 1983;32:589–98.

38. Huebner RJ, Todaro GJ. Oncogenes of RNA tumor viruses as determinants of cancer. Proc Natl Acad Sci USA 1969;64:1087–94.

39. Hunter T. Oncogene production in the cytoplasm: the protein kinases. In: Cooper GM, ed. Oncogenes. Boston: Jones & Bartlett, 1990:147–55.

40. Kieff E, Liebowitz D. Oncogenesis by herpes viruses. In: Weinberg RA, ed. Oncogenes and the molecular origins of cancer. Cold Spring Harbor, NY: Cold Spring Harbor Press, 1989:263–6.

41. Krontiris TG, Cooper GM. Transforming activity of human tumor DNAs. Proc Natl Acad Sci USA 1981;78:1181–4.

42. Land H, Parada LF, Weinberg RA. Tumorigenic conversion of primary embryo fibroblasts requires at least two cooperating oncogenes. Nature 1983;304:596–602.

43. Levinson AD, Oppermann H, Levintow L, Varmus HE, Bishop JM. Evidence that the transforming gene of avian sarcoma virus encodes a protein kinase associated with a phosphoprotein. Cell 1978;15:561–72.

44. Lüttges J, Sohlehe B, Menke MA, Vogel I, Henne-Bruns D, Klöppel G. The K-ras mutation pattern in pancreatic ductal adenocarcinoma usually is identical to that in associated, normal, hyperplastic and metaplastic ductal epithelium. Cancer 1999;85:1703–10.

45. Lynch HT, Lynch JR. Breast cancer genetics in an oncology clinic: 328 consecutive patients. Cancer Genet Cytogenet 1986;22:369–71.

46. Lynch HT, Marcus JN, Watson P, Lynch J. Familial breast cancer, family cancer syndromes, and predisposition to breast neoplasia. In: Bland KI, Copeland EM, eds. The breast: comprehensive management of benign and malignant diseases. New York: WB Saunders, 1991:262–91.

47. Manolov G, Manolova Y. Marker band in one chromosome 14 from Burkitt lymphomas. Nature 1972;237:33–4.

48. Marcus JN, Watson P, Page DL, et al. Hereditary breast cancer: pathobiology, prognosis and BRCA1 and BRCA2 gene linkage. Cancer 1996;77:697–709.

49. McCormmick F. ras oncogenes. In: Weinberg RA, ed. Oncogenes and the molecular origins of cancer. Cold Spring Harbor, NY: Cold Spring Harbor Laboratory Press, 1989:125–45.

50. Modan B, Gad E, Sade-Bruchim RB, et al. High frequency of BRCA1 185delAG mutation in ovarian cancer in Israel. JAMA 1996;278:1823–5.

51. Murray MJ, Shilo BZ, Shih C, Cowing D, Hsu HW, Weinberg RA. Three different human tumor cell lines contain different oncogenes. Cell 1981;25:355–61.

52. Newman B, Austin MA, Lee M, King MC. Inheritance of breast cancer: evidence of autosomal dominant transmission in high-risk families. Proc Natl Acad Sci USA. 1988;85:3044–8.

53. Nowell PC. The clonal evolution of tumor cell populations. Science 1976;194:23–8.

54. Nowell PC. Foundations in cancer research. Chromosomes and cancer. The evolution of an idea. Adv Cancer Res 1994;62:1–17.

55. Nowell PC, Croce C. Chromosome, translocations and oncogenes in human lymphoid tumors. Am J Clin Pathol 1990;94:229–37.

56. Nowell PC, Hungerford DA. Chromosome studies on normal and leukemic human leucocytes. JNCI 1960;25:85–109.

57. Nowell PC, Moreau L, Growney P, Besa EC. Karyotypic stability in chronic B cell leukemia. Cancer Genet Cytogenet 1988;33:155–60.

58. Parada LF, Tabin CJ, Shih C, Weinberg RA. Human EJ bladder carcinoma oncogene is homologue of Harvey sarcoma virus ras gene. Nature 1982;297:474–8.

59. Pegoraro L, Palumbo A, Erikson J. A 14:18 and an 8:14 chromosome translocation in a cell line derived from an acute B-cell leukemia. Proc Natl Acad Sci USA 1984;81:7166–70.

60. Redston MS, Caldas C, Seymour AB, et al. p53 mutations in pancreatic adenocarcinoma and evidence of involvement of homocopolymer tracts in DNA microdeletions. Cancer Res 1994;54:3025–33.

61. Rowley J. Nonrandom chromosomal abnormalities in the hematologic disorders of man. Proc Natl Acad Sci USA 1975;72:152–6.

62. Santos E, Tronick SR, Aaronson SA, Pulciana S, Barbacid M. T24 human bladder carcinoma oncogene is an activated form of the normal human homologue of BALB and Harvey MSV transforming genes. Nature 1982;298:343–7.

63. Sap J, Muñoz A, Schmitt J, Stunnenberg H, Vennström B. Repression of transcription mediated at a thyroid hormone response element by the v-erb-A oncogene product. Nature 1989;340:242–4.

64. Scully R, Ganesan S, Brown M, et al. Location of BRCA1 in human breast and ovarian cancer cells. Science 1996;272:123–5.

65. Seymour AB, Hruban RH, Redston MS, et al. Allelotype of pancreatic adenocarcinoma. Cancer Res 1994;54:2761–4.

66. Shibata D, Almobuera C, Forrester K, et al. Detection of c-K-ras mutations in fine needle aspirates from human pancreatic adenocarcinomas. Cancer Res 1990;50:1279–83.

67. Shih C, Shilo BZ, Goldfarb MP, Dannenberg A, Weinberg RA. Passage of phenotypes of chemically transformed cells via transfection of DNA and chromatin. Proc Natl Acad Sci USA 1979;76:5714–8.

68. Shimizu K, Goldfarb M, Perucho M, Wigler M. Isolation and preliminary characterization of the transforming gene of human neuroblastoma cell line. Proc Natl Acad Sci USA 1983;80:383–7.

69. Sinn E, Muller W, Pattengale P, Teppler I, Wallace R, Leder P. Coexpression of MMTV/v-Ha-ras and MMTV/c-myc genes in transgenic mice: synergistic action of oncogenes in vivo. Cell 1987;49:465–75.

70. Smit VF, Boot AJ, Smits AM, Fieuren GI, Cornilisse CJ, Bos JK. K-ras-codon 12 mutations occur very frequently in pancreatic adenocarcinoma. Nucleic Acids Res 1988;16:7773–82.

71. Sorenson GD, Pribish DM, Valone FH, Memoli VA, Bzik DJ, Yao SL. Soluble normal and mutated DNA sequences from single-copy genes in human blood. Can Epidemiol Biomarkers Prev 1994;3:67–71.

72. Spector DH, Varmus HE, Bishop JM. Nucleotide sequences related to the transforming gene of avian sarcoma virus are present in DNA of uninfected vertebrates. Proc Natl Acad Sci USA 1978;75:4102–6.

73. Stehelin D, Varmus HE, Bishop JM, Vogt PK. DNA related to the transforming gene(s) of avian sarcoma viruses is present in normal avian DNA. Nature 1976;260:170–3.

74. Stewart TA, Pattengale PK, Leder P. Spontaneous mammary adenocarcinomas in transgenic mice that carry and express MTV/ myc fusion genes. Cell 1984;38:627–37.

75. Struewing JP, Abeliovich D, Peretz T, et al. The carrier frequency of the BRCA1 185delAG mutation is approximately 1 percent in Ashkenazi Jewish individuals. Nature Genetics 1995;11:198–200.

76. Tada M, Omata M, Kawai S, et al. Detection of ras gene mutations in pancreatic juice and peripheral blood of patients with pancreatic adenocarcinoma. Cancer Res 1993;53:2472–4.

77. Tada M, Omata M, Onto M. Clinical applications of ras gene mutation for diagnosis of pancreatic adenocarcinoma. Gastroenterology 1991;100:233–8.

78. Takita K, Sato T, Miyagi M, et al. Correlation of loss of alleles on the short arm of chromosomes 11 and 17 with metastases of primary cancer to lymph nodes. Cancer Res 1992;52:3914–7.

79. Toda T, Uno I, Ishikawa T, et al. Yeast, RAS proteins are controlling elements of adenylate cyclase. Cell 1985;40:27–36.

80. Tooze J. Molecular biology of tumor viruses, 2nd ed. Part 2. DNA tumor viruses. Cold Spring Harbor, NY: Cold Spring Harbor Laboratory Press, 1980:61–338.

81. Urban T, Ricci S, Grange JD, Detection of c-K-ras mutation by PCR-RFLP analysis and diagnosis of pancreatic adenocarcinomas. JNCI 1993;85:2008–12.

82. Varmus H. An historical overview of oncogenes. In: Weinberg RA, ed. Oncogenes and the molecular origins of cancer. Cold Spring Harbor, NY: Cold Spring Harbor Laboratory Press, 1989:3–44.

83. Vogt PK. Spontaneous segregation of non-transforming viruses from cloned sarcoma viruses. Virology 1971;46:939–46.

84. Warsaw AL, Castillo CF. Pancreatic carcinoma. N Engl J Med 1991;326:455–65.

85. Watanabe H, Sawabu N, Ohta H, et al. Identification of K-ras oncogene mutations in the pure pancreatic juice of patients with ductal pancreatic cancers. Jpn J Cancer Res 1993;84:961–5.

86. Weinberg RA. Tumor suppressor genes. Science 1991;254:1138–46.

86a.Weitzman JB, Yaniv M. Rebuilding the road to cancer. Nature 1999;400:401–2.

87. Wooster R, Heuhausen SL, Mangion J, et al. Localization of a breast cancer susceptibility gene, BRCA2, to chromosome 13q 12-13. Science 1994;265:2088–90.

88. Zech L, Haglund U, Nilsson K, Klein G. Characteristic chromosomal abnormalities in biopsies and lymphoid-cell lines from patients with Burkitt and non-Burkitt lymphomas. Int J Cancer 1976;17:47–56.

✳ ✳ ✳

21
SUPPRESSOR GENES

With the concept that proto-oncogenes and oncogenes had the potential of initiating the proliferation of normal cells, which might lead to the process of transformation (10), there arose the question: Are there any mechanisms present in cells that would prevent the uncontrolled, runaway activity of cell proliferation and the progression to other stages of carcinogenesis? Would not the lack of some safeguard lead to uncontrolled growth of cells, neoplasia, and even the possible extinction of life from such overgrowth of cells? Or a more fundamental question might be: What mechanism(s) causes normal cells to stop or slow down their multiplication? If such a mechanism were present in humans or animals why did it fail to prevent the occurrence of the continued multiplication of cancer cells? In the late 1960s and 1970s, some partial answers began to appear.

CELL FUSION

In the 1960s, it was discovered by Barsky and colleagues of L'Institut Gustave-Roussy, Villejuif, France, that when two different cell types were grown in a culture medium, some of the cells fused to form a large cell containing two nuclei, one from each cell, with a common cytoplasm containing the cytoplasms of the two cells (5,6). The hybrid cell grew, divided by mitosis, and formed daughter hybrid cells with two nuclei and two cytoplasms for many generations. The process was called somatic cell fusion. Bizarre cells containing many nuclei could be formed when different cell lines were grown in culture medium (fig. 21-1).

Animal Cell Fusion

Barski and Cornefert found that when cells from two separate cultured mouse cell lines, one malignant and the other less so, were fused together, there arose large cells which contained chromosomes from cells of both lines. However, the hybrid cell had the characteristics of the parent cell of the more malignant cell line (5). Fusion of cells from a malignant strain and normal fibroblasts (fig. 21-2) showed that such a hybrid cell expressed the properties of a malignant cell (77). Malignancy ap-

peared to be dominant over normalcy. When mouse sarcoma cells (HT1080) and normal fibroblasts were fused, the resulting hybrid cells when injected into an appropriate animal gave rise to malignant tumors, further suggesting the dominance of malignant cell characteristics (20).

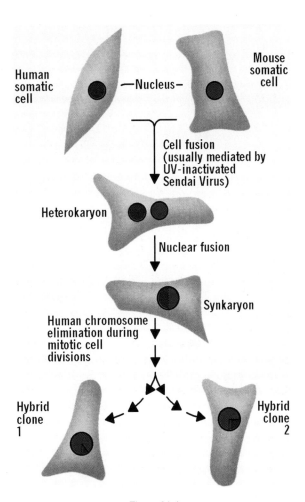

Figure 21-1

HETEROKARYON FORMATION

The fusion of a human cell and a mouse cell to form a heterokaryon with two nuclei and a common cytoplasm. The two nuclei fuse into one nucleus containing the chromosomes of both cells. After mitotic divisions the human chromosomes begin to drop out of the nucleus giving rise to cells with different numbers of human chromosomes. The cells can be cloned and the effect of the loss of chromosomes studied. (Fig. 7.21 from Gardner EJ, Simmons MJ, Snustad DP. Principles of genetics, 8th ed.. New York: John Wiley & Sons, 1991:184.)

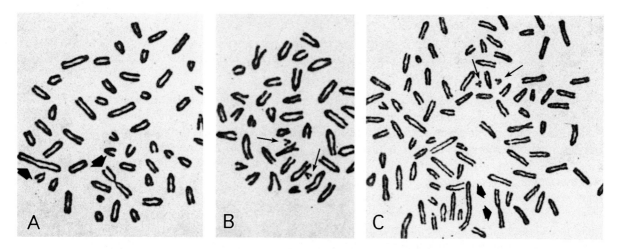

Figure 21-2
METAPHASE OF NORMAL AND HYBRID CELLS

A: Metaphase of a cell from the cancer line.

B: Metaphase of a normal fibroblast-like diploid cell from a skin culture of newborn CBA mice.

C: Metaphase of the hybrid cell formed by growth in culture of the two cell lines. Marker chromosomes permit identification of the chromosomes. The hybrid can be isolated by cloning techniques (77). (Figs. 1, 2, and 3 from Scaletta LJ, Ephrussi B. Hybridization of normal and neoplastic cells in vitro. Nature 1965;205:1169.)

Henry Harris of the Dunn school of Pathology at Oxford University (fig. 21-3); George Klein of the Karolinska Institute of Stockholm, who possessed many strains of mouse tumors; and O. J. Miller, a cytogeneticist, performed in 1969 an experiment utilizing cell fusion and cytogenetics (38). They fused cells from strains of highly malignant tumors of the mouse with cells from mice with normal fibroblasts. It was possible by cytogenetic techniques to identify in the hybrid cell the chromosomes of each cell line. If the hybrid cells were examined shortly after fusion, the unexpected finding was that they possessed the properties of the normal fibroblasts and they did not express the properties of the malignant cells. However, with the growth and further division of the hybrid cells, the latter quickly began to express the characteristics of the cells of the malignant parent cell line.

By careful cytogenetic analysis of the chromosomes of the hybrid cell, Harris and colleagues showed that as the hybrid cell grew and divided it began to lose some of the chromosomes of the normal fibroblast cell. The hybrid cells then began to express the properties of malignant cells (fig. 21-3). These findings were challenged by other observers (20,25), but were eventually shown to occur in some stable cell lines (26,37,47). Lymphocytic cell lines have not been successfully shown to display the same effects as other cell lines (37).

Originally, Harris, Klein, and colleagues suggested that a loss of just one particular chromosome from normal hybrid cells might lead to the expression of malignancy in the hybrid cell genome (25,38). It had been found subsequently that when a wide range of different malignant mouse tumor cells were fused with benign mouse fibroblast cells of the same strain, suppression of the malignant characteristics occurred only when a certain chromosome (or chromosomes) of the normal cells was retained in the hybrid. Chromosome 4 of the normal mouse fibroblast had to be retained in the genome of the nucleus of the hybrid cell in order for the hybrid cell to exhibit benign characteristics (37,47). In hybrid human cell lines the presence of chromosome 11 is necessary for the prevention of malignancy in the hybrid cells (8,80).

Loss of Heterozygosity (LOH)

Different forms of a gene are called alleles. They determine alternate traits or characteristics of a gene. The different colors of a flower, white or red, are used as an analogy for alleles. One allele of a pair usually comes from each parent, however, both alleles may come from one parent and none from the other. When a cell contains two identical alleles, it is said to be "homozygous"; those with different alleles are said to be "heterozygous." Loss

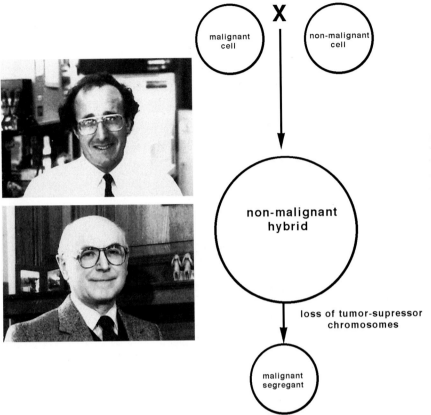

Figure 21-3
HENRY HARRIS AND
ERIC STANBRIDGE

Henry Harris, Director, Sir William Dunn School of Pathology, Oxford University (lower panel) who, with George Klein and colleagues, showed that hybrid cells of malignant and benign composition gave rise to malignant progeny only when certain chromosomes of the benign cells were lost.

Dr. Eric Stanbridge of Stanford University (upper panel) who with colleagues inserted the human chromosome 11 into a line of Wilms' tumor cells and prevented their malignant expression. (Cancer Research. Cover and legend. Cancer Research 1989;49:1620.)

of heterozygosity (LOH) has been noted in a wide variety of animal and human cancers.

If both alleles of chromosome 4 of the normal mouse fibroblasts, which were fused with malignant mouse tumor cells, were retained, the hybrid cell exhibited benign characteristics, i.e., no malignancy was expressed. Loss of one of the two alleles of chromosome 4 of the normal fibroblast in the hybrid cell permitted some limited malignant tumor growth. This suggested that suppression was dose-related, i.e., two normal alleles of chromosome 4 prevented the expression of malignant characteristics in the hybrid cell, whereas the presence of only one normal allele permitted some cells to produce tumors of limited malignant growth, but the number of tumors of the latter type was low (47).

Quantitative effects were also apparent when there was present one set of alleles from normal cells and two sets from malignant cells; the result was that the cells expressed malignant behavior (26). Fusion of two malignant strains of cells—HeLa and HT1080—produced nontumorigenic hybrid cells,

suggesting a genetic complementation between strains that carried different genetic lesions that produced malignancy and normal genes that prevented malignancy in the other strain (8).

From these studies it was apparent that in contrast to oncogenes which induce carcinogenesis, there are genes that act as negative regulators in normal cells, i.e., they inhibit carcinogenesis. If they are lost or decrease in function, the result might lead to decreased suppression and the emergence of cells lacking the normal restraints.

Human Cell Fusion

The findings from the fusion of animal cells have been duplicated in humans. When cells from malignant fibrosarcoma were fused with normal fibroblasts malignancy was suppressed. When chromosome 1 of the normal human fibroblast cell line was lost from the hybrid cells, the latter expressed the features of the malignant cell line (8).

Human chromosome 11 also seemed to have an effect of suppressing malignancy, analogous to the suppressor effects of mouse chromosome 4 and human chromosome 1. In a fusion of cells from carcinoma of the uterus (D98AH2) and normal human fibroblasts, the malignant behavior was suppressed in the hybrid cell. The eventual loss of chromosome 11 from the hybrid cell was followed by the appearance of malignant characteristics (52,80).

The loss of one allele from each of two chromosomes (11 and 14) of the normal human fibroblast cell line fused to the malignant human uterine cancer cell line, permitted the appearance of malignant tumorigenic properties in the hybrid cell. If both alleles of the chromosomes of the benign fibroblast cell line were present in the hybrid cell, the latter expressed benign behavior (80).

Replacement of a Lost Chromosome or Allele

The technique of cell fusion has been replaced by a microcell transfer method in which one or a few chromosomes within a reconstituted membrane are transferred by membrane fusion to recipient tumor cells (76). This simplified the identification of chromosomes carrying a suppressor gene.

Eric Stanbridge (fig. 21-3) and colleagues injected a single chromosome 11 from normal human fibroblasts directly into either a strain of human uterine carcinoma cells or Wilms' malignant kidney tumor cells and found that in both cases the ability of the cancer cells to express tumor growth was suppressed (76,88). Further studies in animals and humans indicated that there were chromosomes that exerted a suppressor effect in some types of cancers and their loss or decrease of function permitted the emergence of the malignant state.

LOSS OR MODIFICATION OF REPRESSOR ALLELE(S)

Retinoblastoma Gene

A clinical study of a rare tumor in children led Alfred Knudson (fig. 21-4), a pediatrician then at the MD Anderson Cancer Center in Houston, Texas, to formulate an important concept in tumorigenesis (53). He studied the retinoblastoma, a tumor of the retina of the eye, which occurs in children before the age of 5 years. At that age the retinal cells reach maturity. The cancer can be cured by surgical removal of the eye and the children may live to adulthood.

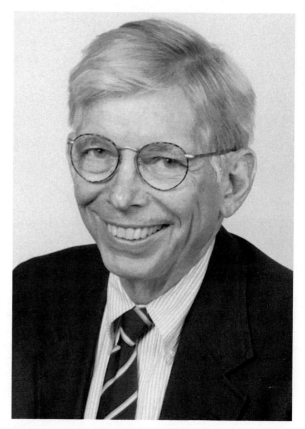

Figure 21-4
ALFRED G. KNUDSON, JR.
Alfred G. Knudson, Jr., Fox Chase Institute for Cancer Research. Author of the "two hit" explanation for retinoblastoma. (Courtesy of Dr. Knudson.)

There were genetic features to the disease: in about 50 percent of the patients the disease was familial, i.e., one or more parent had the tumor and transmitted susceptibility to about half of his or her children. In this group of cases the retinoblastoma was called the inherited type. In about 50 percent of patients no obvious genetic defect was detected in the parents; this was called the sporadic type. All patients with bilateral retinoblastomas seemed to have inherited (germline) disease since one parent was known to have the tumor.

Knudson developed the proposal that retinoblastoma was caused by two mutations, a "two hit" process (21,53). In the inherited type the first mutation was in the genes of the germline of a parent; the second mutation occurred after birth in the retina cells of the young child or adult. In the sporadic case both mutations occurred in the eye after the birth of the child (54).

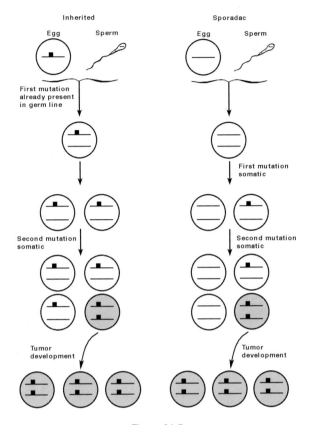

Figure 21-5

THE "TWO-HIT" HYPOTHESIS OF KNUDSON FOR INHERITED AND SPORADIC RETINOBLASTOMA

The first hit (a mutation) (small black square) in the inherited type occurs in the germline of an affected parent. The second mutation occurs in a somatic, retinal cell of the child (dark cell with two small black squares). In the sporadic type the necessary two mutations occur in the retinal cell after birth, usually in late adulthood—first mutation with small black square; second mutation is a dark cell with two small black squares. (Fig. 9.3 from Cooper GM. Oncogenes. Boston: Jones & Bartlett, 1990:125.)

The "two-hit" process is illustrated in figure 21-5. In the inherited type of retinobastoma, the first mutation (one small black square), occurred in the germline of the affected parent. The second mutation (a second small black square), occurred in the cells of the retina of the child after conception. The sporadic type occurred after two retinal cell mutations following birth; there was no familial factor involved. The mutations in the sporadic form caused the loss of function of both alleles.

The loss of function might be the result of a loss of one allele, the loss of an allele with duplication of one mutated allele, or a mitotic recombination with a fragment of a chromosome other than a retinoblastoma gene.

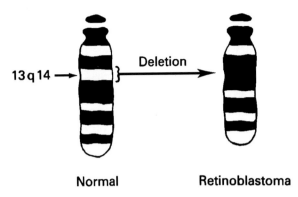

Figure 21-6

DELETION OF BAND 13q14 IN CHROMOSOME 13 OF A PATIENT WITH RETINOBLASTOMA

This deletion is detected in both inherited and sporadic retinoblastomas. (Fig. 9.4 from Cooper GM. Oncogenes. Boston: Jones & Bartlett, 1990:126.)

Cytogenetic studies by Francke showed that there was a deletion in one copy of chromosome 13 in the white blood cells of about 5 percent of the children with the inherited form of retinoblastoma (30). A band (13q14) of chromosome 13 was missing (fig. 21-6). The band was not missing in the majority of cases, but it was possible that the cytogenetic techniques might not have been sensitive enough to reveal the deletion in all cases. Studies employing linkage with an enzyme, esterase D, indicated that susceptibility to retinoblastoma was indeed inherited via a gene in the chromosome band 13q14 (79). This was labeled the *RB-1* gene. Its nucleotide sequence gave rise to a protein called the RB oncoprotein (16,59). When a *RB-1* gene was isolated, cloned, and introduced into a *RB-1* deficient cell line of human retinoblastoma cells, the gene exhibited a suppressive effect, suppressing the malignant behavior of the cells (43).

The *RB* gene is the prototype of the tumor suppressor gene. It is crucial to the appearance or nonappearance of the retinoblastoma tumor of humans, but it is also involved in other tumors and other activities. Its protein, the RB protein, is involved in the cell cycle during mitosis and in the apparatus that regulates gene activity. In G1 stage of the cell cycle, when the cell begins to replicate its DNA, RB protein lacks phosphate groups. When the cell is replicating DNA for cell division, the RB protein is phosphorylated and it remains so during mitosis. Unphosphorylated RB has growth suppressive activity.

Phosphates may be added to the RB protein by the specific kinases involved in the cell cycle, i.e., the cdc2 kinases (see chapter 18). This suggests the possibility that the build-up of phosphates in the RB protein may decrease its inhibitory action and lead to increased growth and proliferation of the cell (34).

In addition, the RB protein binds to proteins known to regulate gene transcription into messenger RNA (mRNA), an early step in gene expression. The RB protein may act as a negative regulator of transcription factors by binding to a transcription factor known as E2F (17).

Surviving patients with inherited retinoblastoma have a higher incidence of other cancers than normal persons or those who have had sporadic retinoblastoma; about 15 percent of such patients develop a second tumor. In nearly half of the latter, the cancer is an osteogenic sarcoma. In a high percentage of these cases the *RB* gene has been deleted or has mutated (32). Other types of cancer with changes in the *RB* gene are small cell lung cancer (33), breast cancer (58), and soft tissue sarcomas (87).

SUPPRESSOR GENES IN TUMORS OF CHILDHOOD

Analogous to retinoblastoma is a tumor of the kidney in children (Wilms' tumor) which shows a deletion in a chromosome, the short arm of chromosome 11 (11p). Wilms' tumor can be inherited or sporadic as well (55). When Stanbridge and colleagues introduced a single normal human chromosome 11 into a culture strain of Wilms' tumor cells, the cells lost their ability to produce tumors, indicating that the introduced chromosome suppressed the ability of the cells to form malignant tumors (74). Other childhood tumors, rhabdomyosarcoma (a malignant tumor of striated muscle) and hepatoblastoma (a malignant tumor of the liver) associated with Wilms' tumor, have also lost genes at the 11p locus (19).

SUPPRESSOR GENES IN OTHER CANCERS

There is a wide spectrum of cancers in which loss of heterozygosity (LOH) can be found. Colon cancer (discussed below) is illustrative of many cancers in which one or more chromosomes or alleles have been lost, modified, or mutated, so that their function is lost or diminished.

There may be multiple gene losses in a patient's tumor; these are believed to represent loci where suppressor genes had been present. It is not known whether these losses represent causal factors in carcinogenesis or were mostly associated with the process of tumor progression. Some LOHs have been verified as causally significant with confirmatory linkage studies that have indicated malfunction of the gene. Further studies are needed to determine the significance of many LOHs in carcinogenesis.

The *p53* Gene

The *p53* gene on chromosome band 17p13 was originally thought to be an oncogene but further study showed that it was a suppressor gene. It is the most common gene involved in human malignancies and has been found to be mutated in about 50 percent of all cases of cancer (35).

The protein expressed by the *p53* gene is a nuclear phosphoprotein involved in many functions such as cell cycle control, DNA synthesis, DNA replication, cell differentiation, genomic stability, and programmed cell death (apoptosis) (see below). The wild type *p53* gene is a recessive tumor gene whereas mutated forms can act as a dominant oncogene. The latter acts, uniquely, as a Figaro-like suppressor gene involved in many functions. C.C. Harris and colleagues of the National Institutes of Health, Bethesda, have made the most extensive studies of *p53* mutant genes (35). The p53 protein can induce transcription of several different genes and can also, in contrast, repress the transcription of other genes.

The *p53* gene itself can be repressed, or its repression modified, by the expression of an oncogene (*mdm2*) (fig. 21-7) (56) (Note 1). This occurs in about 30 percent of soft tissue sarcomas (35). The *p53* gene also tends to keep in check the inherent mutability of the genome (90).

Mutations of the *p53* gene are characteristic: a change occurs in the amino acid sequence, a single base change with one amino acid substituting for another, a missense mutation. Eighty percent of *p53* mutations are of the missense type; alterations in other tumor-suppressor genes are missense mutations in only a small percentage of cases (41).

In some cancers of the liver (hepatocellular cancers), there is a transversion of the usual CG-AT arrangement of nucleotides to a GC-TA arrangement in the *p53* gene. It occurs in codon 249. This

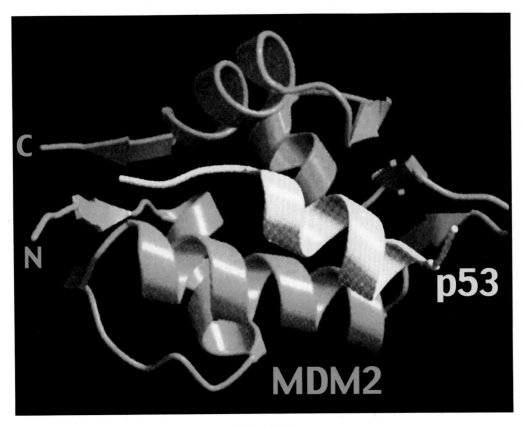

Figure 21-7

THE *mdm2* ONCOPROTEIN

The *mdm2* terminal domain (in cyan) forms a structure reminiscent of a twisted trough. It has a hydrophilic cleft where the p53 peptide (in yellow) binds as an amphipathic alpha helix. The *mdm2* oncoprotein may repress or modify the *p53* gene (56). (Fig. 2A from Kussie PH, Gorina S, Marechal V, et al. Structure of the *mdm2* oncoprotein bound to the p53 tumor suppressor transactivation domain. Science 1996;274:948–53.)

change has been attributed to dietary aflatoxin (AFB1) (see chapter 13), because the same pattern of change is also found in studies of aflatoxin mutagenesis (14,42). There has been a positive correlation between the frequency of *p53* mutations at codon 249 and the incidence of hepatocellular cancer. An exception is a patient with the cancer with the *p53* mutation at codon 249 and the absence of evidence of hepatitis B infection (89). Anaplastic and undifferentiated tumors are more likely to have a mutant *p53* allele; with loss of *p53* there is a shortened survival period in some patients (36).

Another mutation of the *p53* gene that gives a distinctive fingerprint in DNA is the damage caused by ultraviolet light on cells: unrepaired cytosine dimer-induced tandem mutations in which two adjacent cytosine residues (cytosine-cytosine) are replaced by two thymine bases (thymine-thymine) (see chapter 15). In squamous cell carcinoma of the skin (believed to be caused by the ultraviolet rays of the sun), mutations of the *p53* gene show this tandem substitution (13).

The *p53* protein is antigenic and antibodies to it can be demonstrated in the serum of about 20

Note 1: In a fundamental study, N. P. Pavletich of the Sloan Kettering Institute and colleagues portrayed the structure of *p53* and its binding to the oncoprotein *mdm2* which inhibits the tumor suppressor action of *p53* (56). Such a graphic portrayal aids in the attempt to understand the action of the *p53* suppressor gene, and how it, in turn, is inhibited. It should be of considerable value to the pharmacologist and the chemotherapist in their search for compounds to affect the action of the suppressor (fig. 21-7).

percent of patients with breast and lung cancers and malignant lymphomas (35). In many tumors immunocytochemical staining of cancer cells for the p53 protein antibody has been demonstrated; staining was more intense as the cancer became less differentiated and more malignant. In cancers of the breast and lung, the loss of p53 function was associated with a shortened survival time (36).

GENETIC CHANGES IN COLORECTAL CANCER

One of the most impressive applications of the advances in genetics has been in the study of colorectal cancer by B. Vogelstein and colleagues of the Oncology Center at Johns Hopkins University School of Medicine (4,27,28,86). Many cancers of the colon arise from preexisting benign tumors, polyps or adenomas. This presents an opportunity to study the pathogenesis of tumors from the normal epithelium lining the colon and rectum to the benign neoplastic lesions, polyps and adenomas, and then the full-blown cancer.

Sporadic Colorectal Cancers

The most prevalent type (about 80 percent) of colorectal cancer is the noninherited variety in which polyps or adenomas are few. Mutations are frequent, some appear significant, others do not, but in many cases their significance is uncertain. A description of the prominent genetic changes follows.

Oncogene Changes. In about 50 percent of colorectal cancers and in larger adenomas, there is a mutation in the *ras* gene. In small adenomas, the *ras* mutation has been identified in less than 10 percent of cases, suggesting that the mutation may play a part in the transition from adenoma to carcinoma. Mutation of the *ras* gene probably is not an initiating event in most tumors. Amplification or rearrangement of oncogenes does not play a major role in colorectal cancer (28).

Loss of Heterogeneity (LOH). The loss of a specific chromosomal region occurs frequently in colorectal neoplasms associated with polyposis. It usually involves the loss of one of the two alleles. Such LOH of an allele has been interpreted as evidence that the region of the loss contained a tumor suppressor gene(s).

Deletions in chromosome 5q are not seen in patients with adenomas of the colon, without the presence of polyposis, but deletions do occur in 29

percent of those with larger adenomas and 36 percent of those with cancer (86). In familial adenomatous polyposis deletion in chromosome 5q is rare (28).

Loss of a large portion of chromosome 17p has been noted in more than 75 percent of patients with colorectal cancer, but such loss is infrequent with adenomas. However, when the loss is present with adenomas, it is associated with a progression of the adenoma to carcinoma (4,28). Subsequently it was learned that the region of loss on chromosome 17 in colorectal tumors contained the *p53* gene.

Vogelstein's group has found that mutations in the p53 gene were present in several colorectal cancers in which there was also a loss of alleles in chromosome 17p (27,86). Point mutation of one allele of the *p53* gene and loss of the remaining wild type allele seemed to occur frequently (28). It was suggested that the wild type *p53*, as well as the mutated *p53*, could function as a tumor suppressor (29).

Another chromosome, 18q, sustained the loss of an allele in more than 70 percent of patients with carcinoma and in almost 50 percent of patients with a more advanced adenoma (28). A gene from this region, the *DCC* gene, coding for a member of the adhesion family of molecules (23), was present in normal colonic mucosa but its expression was reduced or absent in the majority of colorectal cancers. It has been suggested that it is also a suppressor gene (4). It has been postulated that loss of adhesion to normal adjacent cells contributes to the transformation of a cell by the loss of inhibitory substances in these adjoining cells.

It has been shown that the mutated *p53* gene can cooperate with the *ras* oncogene in mice to transform primary rodent cells in vitro, even though the rodent cells express the wild type *p53* (39). The mutant *p53* gene product may bind to the wild type, inactivate it, and prevent its association with other cellular constituents.

Fearon and Vogelstein have come to the following conclusions about their study of colorectal neoplasms (28): associated with the appearance of colorectal tumors is the activation of oncogenes and the mutational inactivation of tumor suppressor genes; mutations of four or five genes appear to be necessary to produce a cancer of colorectal tissues; the total number of mutations is important in the carcinogenetic process and there is some suggestion of a preferred sequence of mutations; in regard to the sequence of gene changes and the progression of carcinogenesis, the occurrence of any given gene

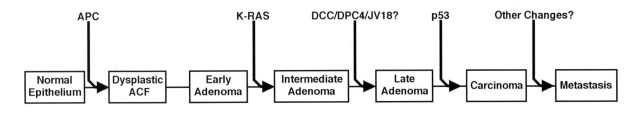

Figure 21-8
SUGGESTED SEQUENCE OF EVENTS IN COLORECTAL CANCER
A schematic suggestion of genetic events occurring in colorectal cancer. (Fig. 1 from Vogelstein B. Genetic testing for cancer: the surgeon's critical role. Familial colon cancer. J Am Coll Surg 1999;188:74–9.)

alteration is not restricted to a particular stage of carcinogenesis; and the progressive accumulation of changes in the genes is the most consistent feature of the neoplastic process (fig. 21-8) (4,27, 28,86).

There are losses in other chromosomes in colorectal cancer as well of those in chromosomes 5q, 17p, and 18q. Regions in chromosomes 1q, 4p, 6p, 6q, 8p, 9q, and 22q are lost in 25 to 50 percent of patients. There may be tumor suppressor genes in many different chromosomes.

Inherited Types of Colorectal Cancer

Much of the genetic information about colorectal cancers has come from studies of the inherited types of the disease by Vogelstein and colleagues (85). The recognized forms of this type of cancer follow.

FAP (familial adenomatous polyposis) is a rare, inherited disease characterized by the presence of a large number, even up to thousands, of polyps in the colon. There is a 90 percent chance that some of the polyps may become malignant. The cancer is caused by the mutation of a tumor suppressor gene, *APC* (adenomatous polyposis coli), which normally prevents the occurrence of the disease.

HNPCC (hereditary nonpolyposis colon cancer) is a rare hereditary type of colon cancer in which multiple polyps are not a characteristic feature (also called Lynch's syndrome after Henry Lynch of Creighton University, the discoverer of the syndrome). Defects in the DNA repair system, called DNA mismatched repair, cause the disease. There are six proteins involved in the system and four of these are mutated in the germline of HNPCC patients. Patients do not inherit polyps or adenomas at any greater incidence than the general population, but when benign adenomas or polyps

do occur, they relatively rapidly (3–5 years) change to colon cancer.

FCC (familial colorectal cancer) is the most common of the hereditary types, making up almost 20 percent of the total number of cases. It is difficult to recognize this type clinically, although in some cases there may be a family history of colon cancer. Recently, a mutation (I 1307 K) was found in the *APC* gene which causes a substitution of one nucleotide for another, e.g., substitution of a thymine by an adenine. The mutation was found in Ashkenazi Jews (about 6 percent). The I 1307 K mutation does not directly affect the *APC* gene but it makes a little segment of the gene more susceptible for additional mutation (85).

EPIGENETIC CHANGES

Methylation

Epigenetic changes are heritable alterations in gene function that are mediated by factors other than changes in primary DNA sequences. It has been suggested that the degree of methylation (hypermethylation or hypomethylation) as part of the genome is significant in aging, carcinogenesis, the cell cycle, hematopoietic diseases, genomic stability, genetic imprinting, and the development and silencing of tumor repressor genes. 5'methylcytosine is a common site of DNA methylation (50).

Leegwater and colleagues of Nijmegan, the Netherlands, found that 13 of 14 patients with hematopoietic diseases such as acute lymphatic leukemia (ALL) had an increased number of methylated CpG (cytosine-guanine) sites in the calcitonin gene region at initial diagnosis and at relapse of tumors compared to healthy individuals. There was a higher degree of methylation in patients with T-cell than

B-cell lineage ALL. The authors believed that methylation may play a role in tumor progression (60).

Hypermethylation within the promoters of selected genes appears to be common in all types of human hematopoietic neoplasms and is usually associated with inactivation of the involved genes. Such silencing of expression has been shown for several genes regulating growth and differentiation of hematopoietic cells. Issa of the Johns Hopkins group found that hypermethylation in the promoters of some genes is an early neoplastic event while in other genes it seems to occur during the progression of the leukemia (46).

Kay and colleagues from the University of Western Australia studied methylation in lymphomagenesis and have shown that in all cases of non-Hodgkin's lymphoma and leukemia studied, the myogenic development gene *Mgf*-3 was abnormally hypermethylated. In these cases the *PAX* family of genes associated with cell mobility and regional expression was controlled by DNA methylation. The authors suggest that the abnormal profiles of *PAX* methylation may be associated with transformation and metastasis (49).

Lenguar et al. of the Johns Hopkins Oncology Center found that when retroviral genes were exogenously introduced into colorectal cancer cell lines the expression of gene products was extinguished and this was associated with DNA methylation (61). The effect could be reversed by treatment with a demethylating agent, 5-azacytidine. The correlation between genetic instability and methylation capacity led the authors to suggest that methylation may play a role in chromosome segregation processes in cancer cells.

Kanai et al. of the National Cancer Center Research Institute in Tokyo studied the DNA methylation of chromosome 16 in both early and late stages of liver cell (hepatocellular) carcinogenesis. A loss of heterozygosity (LOH) has frequently been detected in this chromosome. Two precancerous hepatocellular lesions, chronic infectious hepatitis and cirrhosis of the liver, as well as cancer itself, revealed aberrant methylation of DNA, hypermethylation of some genetic loci and hypomethylation at another locus. Aberrant methylation of DNA was greater in the more advanced cancers. The incidence of DNA hypermethylation was higher than the loss of heterozygosity at one locus. The authors suggested that DNA hypermethylation might predispose a locus to alle-

lic loss and may also participate in the early stages of hepatocellular carcinoma (48).

More study is needed to determine how widespread in the tumor spectrum methylation changes are and how they correlate with the various stages of carcinogenesis.

MECHANISM OF ACTION IN TUMOR SUPPRESSION

Balance of Promoter and Inhibitor Influences

Hitotsumachi and colleagues from the Weitzman Institute, Israel, proposed a carcinogenesis model in which malignancy was determined by the balance within the cell between one set of chromosomes that favored the emergence of malignancy and a different set that favored its suppression (40). D. E. Comings of the City of Hope Medical Center, California, postulated that every cell contained structural "transforming" genes that were active during embryonic life but were suppressed during adult differentiation by suppressor or regulatory genes. With the loss of both copies of the alleles of the suppressor gene, the normal control mechanism of suppression was lost and there was renewal of the "transforming" ability of the embryo cells with the resulting appearance of tumor growth (18).

The Suppressor Gene Effect

The suppressor genes have a regulatory function(s) in the normal cell and play a role in the differentiation of a cell into its mature adult state, called terminal differentiation. The means by which suppressor genes inhibit cell proliferation are known in some cases but unknown in many more.

George Klein, of the Karolinska Institute, Stockholm, in a thoughtful discussion mentioned many means and pathways whereby tumor suppression could be brought about (51). Somatic hybridization of normal cells with malignant cells has shown that the normal genome may provide the tumor cell with the ability to respond to appropriate differentiation signals. Signals induced by physiological or chemical differentiation agents may down-regulate other highly expressed oncoproteins and thereby lift the maturation block. Even the increased expression of amplified *myc* oncogene may be overridden by such signals. The transformed and tumorigenic phenotype of *v-Ki-ras* oncogene-infected fibroblasts was reverted by a dominant-acting cellular gene or genes

Table 21-1

EXAMPLES OF TUMOR-SUPPRESSOR GENES INVOLVED IN HUMAN CANCERS*

Tumor-Suppressor Gene	Chromosomal Locus	Location/ Proposed Function	Somatic Mutations Major Types	Examples of Neoplasms	Inherited Mutations Syndrome	Heterozygote Carrier Rate Per 10^5 Birth	Typical Neoplasms
p53	17p13.1	Nucleus/ transcription factor	Missense	Most types of human cancer	Li-Fraumeni syndrome	~2	Carcinomas of breast and adrenal cortex; sarcomas; leukemia; brain tumors
RB1	13q14	Nucleus/ transcription modifier	Deletion and nonsense	Retinoblastoma; osteosarcoma; carcinoma of the breast, prostate, bladder, and lung	Retino-blastoma	~2	Retinoblastoma; osteosarcoma
APC	5q21	Cytoplasm/ unknown	Deletion and nonsense	Carcinoma of the colon, stomach, and pancreas	Familial adenomatous polyposis coli	~10	Carcinomas of colon, thyroid, and stomach
WT1	11p13	Nucleus/ transcription factor	Missense	Wilms' tumor	Wilms' tumor	~0.5–1	Wilms' tumor
NF1	17q11	Cytoplasm/ guanosine tri-phosphatase-activating protein	Deletion	Schwannomas	Neurofibroma-tosis type 1	~30	Neural tumors
NF2	22q	Cytoplasm/ cytoskeleton-membrane link	Deletion and nonsense	Schwannomas and meningiomas	Neurofibroma-tosis type 2	~3	Central schwannomas and meningiomas
VHL	3p25	Unknown/ unknown	Deletion	Unknown	von Hippel-Lindau disease	~3	Hemangioblastoma and renal cell carcinoma

*Table 1 from Harris CC, Hollstein M. Clinical implications of the p53 tumor-suppressor gene. N Eng J Med 1993;329:1319.

in spite of the continued presence of a wild-type transforming virus and full expression of the p21 ras protein. The same genes could also cancel the transforming action of some genes such as *src, fes,* and members of the *ras* family, but not the genes of *sis, fms, raf,* polyoma, or SV40. Normal genes may oppose oncogenes by controlling cell maturation or by acting at different levels of expression to overrule the transforming action of the oncoproteins.

Other types of suppressor action may occur: by the loss or alteration of a receptor for an activated growth factor oncogene; by an interference with the increase of signal transduction caused by an oncogene; by strong differentiation-inducing signals which would overpower the action of oncogenes; by bypassing differentiation blocks by down-regulation of oncogenes; or by exposure to strong differentiation signals (9).

Regulatory sequences in the immediate vicinity of an oncogene, e.g., *c-mos* and *c-fos* oncogenes, can prevent activation of the oncogene (51). Tumor growth can be inhibited by diffusible products released by surrounding normal cells and suppressor genes may act by increasing cell-to-cell communication (70).

Table 21-1 illustrates that several different genes can be deleted or mutated in the same tumor, the same genes may be mutated or lost in different kinds of tumor, and more than one suppressor gene may be lost during progression of the tumor.

Suppressor genes function in other areas than those of proliferation and transformation. In teratoma studies, suppressor genes have been shown to play a significant role in the differentiation of embryonic cells to normal adult cells. The blastocyst cells of the embryo have genes that inhibit some types of carcinogenesis (44,73).

As mentioned earlier, the phosphorylated RB retinoblastoma protein of the *RB* gene may act to inhibit progression of cells through the cell cycle (34,67) and thereby act as a repressor. But the RB complex may also bind to proteins involved in the transformation process and lead to the removal of the inhibitory action of RB and permit unrestrained multiplication of the cell.

Apoptosis in Neoplasms

As mentioned before (see chapter 13), there occurs normally and in neoplastic lesions a genetically programmed cell death process called apoptosis. Human neoplasms of the liver (15), prostate (22), hematologic neoplasms (3,75), colorectal cancer (83), and other tumors (78) have been examined for apoptotic changes. Large variations in the quantitative degree of apoptosis in different tumors has been found, possibly partly because of technical difficulties in determining an apoptotic index (78).

Radiation effects on tumors were investigated by Meyn et al. of the M.D. Anderson Cancer Center, Houston, Texas (66). They reported the results of the quantitative response of apoptosis in different types of murine tumors that were irradiated. Three of four mammary carcinomas, one ovarian carcinoma, and one lymphoma showed significant apoptosis in at least 10 percent of the tumor cells; five sarcomas, three squamous cell carcinomas, and one hepatocellular carcinoma did not reveal significant apoptosis. There was a significant relationship between the degree of radiation-induced apoptosis and the efficacy of the radiation treatment. Both intratumor and intertumor heterogeneity in apoptotic response was present. The authors believe that apoptosis may be a significant factor in the elimination of tumor cells in some types of irradiated tumors.

Bedi and colleagues from the Johns Hopkins Oncology Center have reported an extensive study of the susceptibility of human colorectal cancer to apoptosis (7). They examined normal colon mucosa, flat mucosa, and adenomas from patients with familial adenomatous polyposis, sporadic adenomas, and sporadic colorectal carcinomas. Transformation from colorectal epithelium to carcinoma was associated with progressive inhibition of apoptosis. Immunocytochemical techniques demonstrated the presence of bcl-2 protein, known to inhibit apoptosis, throughout the glands of the colon in carcinoma instead of being confined to the epithelium of the base of the colonic crypts in the normal mucosa. This illustrated the relationship of the gene product to the apoptotic process. The authors suggested that the inhibition of apoptosis may have contributed to tumor growth and progression.

An increase in both proliferative and apoptotic activities was noted in early invasive esophageal cancer in comparison to noninvasive carcinoma by Ohashi et al. of the University of Tokyo (69). Tsujitani and colleagues of the Tottori University, Japan, found an increase in the proliferative index and an inhibition of apoptosis in Japanese patients with cancer of the colon with adenoma and cancer de novo (83). They believed that a reduction in the rate of apoptosis might explain the rapid-growing nature of cancer de novo, particularly in nonpolyploid flat type cancers.

Nematode Apoptosis

The nematode *Caenorhabditis elegans* has provided a model of apoptosis that resembles that of the mammal and has aided in an understanding of the process in the latter (24,91). Genes *ced-3* and *ced-4* of the nematode have to be activated for apoptosis and the death of the nematode. The *ced-9* gene inhibits the products of *ced-3* and *ced-4* and thereby prevents apoptosis. The nematode requires both sets of genes to maintain an equilibrium between cell survival and cell death.

bcl-2 and Apoptosis

The mammalian homolog of the nematode gene *ced-9* is the proto-oncogene *bcl-2*, which is regarded as a suppressor of programmed cell death by its direct action in preventing apoptosis (11,65, 84). *bcl-2* was reported to be involved in the regulation of apoptosis in human follicular lymphoma and in non-Hodgkin's lymphoma (82). High levels of bcl-2 protein have been reported in several other types of human cancer, including prostate, colorectal, lung, gastric, renal, melanoma, neuroblastoma, thyroid, and acute and chronic leukemias (11).

bcl-2 Family of Genes

The *bcl-2* gene is found in mitochondria (inner membrane), endoplasmic reticulum, and the nuclear membrane. It is thought to act as an antioxidant, or as an inhibitor of the production of free radicals. It forms a fusion gene with the immunoglobulin heavy chain whose ultimate action is the inappropriate expression of high levels of bcl-2 protein (82,84).

The *bcl-2* family of genes contains *bcl-x* which codes for two proteins: the larger protein, *bcl-x,* acts similarly to *bcl-2,* i.e., it protects cells from entering apoptosis; the smaller protein, *bcl-xs,* suppresses *bcl-2* and leaves the cell susceptible to apoptosis. Gene *bax* dimerizes with *bcl-2* and its overexpression antagonizes the action of *bcl-2* (12).

Another mammalian homolog of the nematode gene *ced-3* is the gene encoding the interleukin 1β-converting enzyme (ICE) and four other proteins (12). ICE is a cysteine protease that converts prointerleukin 1ß to its active form. Ectopic expression of ICE triggers apoptosis in rodent fibroblasts. It has been suggested that ICE and homologues may activate each other and other proteases to initiate a protease cascade terminating in apoptosis (64).

Signals from the environment may trigger the process of cell death secondary to the appearance or withdrawal of hormones, cytokines, or changes in intercellular environment through control by cell surface receptors (31,68,78).

There is not, in general, a definite relationship between all neoplastic lesions and apoptosis. In malignant lymphoma and hormone-dependent epithelial tumors—breast, endometrial, or thyroid carcinomas—a high degree of apoptosis is associated with a high grade of malignancy. In other epithelial neoplasms the relationship is less evident. Apoptosis is not generally associated with the survival of patients. An increase of apoptosis is associated with the proliferative state of neoplasia in many

tumors but not in all (78); its exact role in many tumors is not yet clarified.

GENETIC INSTABILITY

Recently, a new phenomenon has been discovered in patients with a subset of human colorectal tumors called inherited colon cancer without polyposis or hereditary nonpolyposis colorectal cancer (HNPCC) (1,2,9,45,71,72,81). The finding was a genome-wide tendency for multiple replication errors (RER) in the genes that control this process. Shifts in the electrophoretic mobility of microsatellites, short repeat fragments of DNA (2), were found in about 70 percent or more of the colorectal tumors from patients of the HNPCC group (Note 2). In gastric and endometrial cancers, also part of the HNPCC syndrome, similar changes were noted in 18 percent and 22 percent, respectively, of the patients. No evidence of these abnormal findings were present in cancers of the lung, breast, or testis (72). The tendency to form microsatellite DNA alternatives can be inherited and may be directly related to a gene(s) causing genetic instability in the HNPCC syndrome (71). A gene predisposing to HNPCC has been mapped to chromosome 2p (9).

Thibodeau et al. found that microsatellite instability correlated directly with tumor location and patient survival, but inversely with the loss of heterogeneity in chromosomes 5q, 17p, and 18q (81). Aaltonen et al. suggested that genomic instability was part of the HNPCC syndrome (1). Bhattacharyya et al. believed that mutator genes involved in manipulating the rates of copying errors in other genes gave rise to hypermutation affecting different repair, or error-avoidance, pathways (9).

Loeb for many years suggested that since the number of mutations is low in normal cells and high in cancer cells that cancer is a mutator phenotype (62). The hypothesis proposes that the intrinsic instability of the cancer cells drives tumorigenesis by producing a pool of mutations, some of which confer a selective advantage permitting proliferation and survival of some cells. Both intrinsic genomic instability and clonal expansion driven by

---

Note 2: There is a fraction of DNA in the nucleus of the human cell that can be separated from most DNA by ultracentrification; it is called satellite DNA. It contains frequently repeated short sequences of nucleotides arranged in tandem arrays. There may be as many as a million copies per genome, many concentrating near the centromere of the chromosome. A subset of satellite DNA of short repeats is called a minisatellite and individuals have different numbers and sizes of copies of these minisatellites (2).

selective advantage are thought to be the major driving forces in tumorigenesis (62,63).

SIGNIFICANCE OF LOH AND SUPPRESSOR GENES

It is apparent from the loss of a specific repressor gene and the resultant appearance of retinoblastoma or some other childhood cancer, that loss of suppressor gene function is causative in some cancers. In many other cancers there is also a loss of homogeneity or chromosomal substance but the relationship of these findings to transformation is not clear. Loss of repressor gene function is not apparent in many cancers.

The relative significance of loss of homogeneity and suppressor genes in carcinogenesis will require much further investigation inasmuch as both appear to occur relatively frequently in many cancers. As in all mutations the problem will be to determine whether they are in the causal train of genetic events or are secondary to a more vital unknown process.

REFERENCES

1. Aaltonen LA, Peltomäki P, Leach, FS, et al. Clues to the pathogenesis of familiar colorectal cancer. Science 1993;260:812–6.

2. Adams RL, Knowler JT, Leader DP. The biochemistry of the nucleic acids, 11th ed. London: Chapman & Hall, 1992:48–50.

3. Allen PD, Bustin SA, Macey MG, Johnston DH, Williams NS, Newland AC. Programmed cell death (apoptosis) in immunity and haematological neoplasia. Br J Biomed Sci 1993;50:135–49.

4. Baker SJ, Fearon ER, Nigro JM, et al. Chromosome 17 deletions and p53 gene mutations in colorectal carcinomas. Science 1989;244:217–21.

5. Barski G, Cornefert F. Characteristics of "hybrid"-type clonal cell lines obtained from mixed cultures in vitro. JNCI 1962;28:801–21.

6. Barski G, Sorieul S, Cornefert F. Production dans des cultures in vitro de deux souches cellulaires en association de cellules de ceractère "hybride." Compt Rend Acad Sci 1960;251:1825–7.

7. Bedi A, Pasricha, PJ, Akhtar AJ, et al. Inhibition of apoptosis during development of colorectal cancer. Cancer Res 1995;55:1811–6.

8. Benedict WF, Weissman BE, Mark C, Stanbridge EJ. Tumorigenicity of human HT1080 fibrosarcoma X normal fibroblast hybrids: chromosomal dose dependency. Cancer Res 1984;44:3471–9.

9. Bhattacharyya NP, Skandalis A, Ganesh A, Groden J, Meuth M. Mutator phenotypes in human colorectal carcinoma cell lines. Proc Natl Acad Sci USA 1994;91:6319–23.

10. Bishop JM. Oncogenes. Sci Am 1982;246:80–92.

11. Blandino G, Strano S. BCL-2: the pendulum of the cell fate. J Exp Clin Cancer Res 1997;16:3–10.

12. Blank KR, Rudoltz MS, Kao GD, Muschell RJ, McKenna, WG. The molecular relation of apoptosis and implications for radiation oncology. Int J Radiat Biol 1997;71:455–66.

13. Brash DE, Rudolf FJ, Simon JA, et al. A role for sunlight in skin cancer. UV-induced p53 mutations in squamous cell cancer. Proc Natl Acad Sci USA 1991;88:10124–8.

14. Bressac B, Kew M, Wands J, Ozturk M. Selective G to T mutations of p53 gene in hepatocellular carcinoma from southern Africa. Nature 1991;350:429–31.

15. Bursch W, Grasl-Kraupp B, Ellinger A, et al. Active cell death: role in hepatocarcinogenesis and subtypes. Biochem Cell Biol 1994;72:669–75.

16. Cavenee WK, Hansen MF, Nordenskjold M, et al. Genetic origin of mutations predisposing to retinoblastoma. Science 1985;228:501–3.

17. Chellappan SP, Hiebert S, Mudryj M, Horowitz JH, Nevins JM. The E2F transcription factor is a cellular target for the RB protein. Cell 1991;65:1053–61.

18. Comings DE. A general theory of carcinogenesis. Proc Natl Acad Sci USA 1973;70:3324–8.

19. Cooper GM. Oncogenes. Boston: Jones & Bartlett, 1990:135.

20. Croce CM, Barrick J, Linnenbach A, Koprowski H. Expression of malignancy in hybrids between normal and malignant cells. J Cell Physiol 1979;99:279–85.

21. DeMars R. Discussion. In: genetic concepts and neoplasia, 23rd Ann. Symposium Funding Cancer Research, 1969. Baltimore: Williams & Wilkins, 1970:105–6.

22. Denmeade SR, Lin, XS, Isaacs JT. Role of programmed (apoptotic) cell death during the progression and therapy for prostate cancer. Prostate 1996;28:251–65.

23. Edelman GM. Morphoregulatory molecules. Biochemistry 1988;27:3533–43.

24. Ellis RE, Jacobson DM, Horvitz HR. Genes required for the engulfment of cell corpses during programmed cell death in Caenorhabditis elegans. Genetics 1991;129:79–94.

25. Ephrussi B, Davidson RL, Weiss MC, Harris H, Klein G. Malignancy of somatic cell hybrids. Nature 1969;224:1314–6.

26. Evans EP, Burtenshaw MD, Brown BB, Hennion R, Harris H. The analysis of malignancy by cell fusion. IX. Re-examination and clarification of the cytogenetic problem. J Cell Sci 1982;56:113–30.

27. Fearon ER, Hamilton SR, Vogelstein B. Clonal analysis of human colorectal tumors. Science 1987;238:193–7.

28. Fearon ER, Vogelstein B. A genetic model for colorectal tumorigenesis. Review. Cell 1990;61:759–67.

29. Finlay CA, Hinds PW, Levine AJ. The p53 protooncogene can act as a suppressor of transformation. Cell 1989;57:1083–93.

30. Francke U. Retinoblastoma and chromosome 13. Birth Defects Orig Artic Ser 1976;16:131–4.

31. Golstein P, Marguet D, Depraetere V. Homology between reaper and the cell-death domains of Fas and TNFRI [Letter]. Cell 1995;81:185–6.

32. Hansen MF, Koufos A, Gallie BL, et al. Osteosarcoma and retinoblastoma: a shared chromosomal mechanism revealing recessive predisposition. Proc Natl Acad Sci USA 1985;82:6216–20.

33. Harbour JW, Lai SL, Whang-Peng Jr, Gazdal AF, Minna JD, Kaye FJ. Abnormalities in structure and expression of the human retinoblastoma genes in SCLC. Science 1988; 241:353–7.

34. Harlow E. A research shortcut from a common cold virus to human cancer. Cancer 1995;78:558–65.

35. Harris CC. p53 mutational spectrum and molecular epidemiology of human cancer. In: Fortner JG, Rhoads JE, eds. Accomplishments in cancer research 1992. Philadelphia: Lippincott, 1993:179–88.

36. Harris CC, Hollstein M. Clinical implications of the p53 tumor-suppressor gene. N Engl J Med 1993;329:1318–27.

37. Harris H. The analysis of malignancy by cell fusion: the position in 1988. Cancer Res 1988;45:3302–8.

38. Harris H, Miller OJ, Klein G, Worst P, Tachibana T. Suppression of malignancy by cell fusion. Nature 1969;223:363–8.

39. Hinds PW, Finlay C, Levine AJ. Mutation is required to activate the p53 gene for cooperation with the ras oncogene and transformation. J Virol 1989;63:739–46.

40. Hitotsumachi S, Rabinowitz Z, Sachs L. Chromosomal control of reversion in transformed cells. Nature 1971;231:511–4.

41. Hollstein M, Sidransky D, Vogelstein B, Harris CC. p53 mutations in human cancers. Science 1991;253:49–53.

42. Hsu IC, Metcalf RA, Sun T, Welsh JA, Wang NJ, Harris CC. Mutational hotspot in the p53 gene in human hepatocellular carcinomas from Qidong, China. Nature 1991;350:427–8.

43. Huang HJ, Yee JK, Shew JY, et al. Suppression of the neoplastic phenotype by replacement of the RB gene in human cancer cells. Science 1988;242:1563–6.

44. Illmensee K, Stevens LC. Teratomas and chimeras. Sci Am 1979;240:120–32.

45. Ionov Y, Peinado MA, Malkhosyan S, et al. Ubiquitour somatic mutations in simple repeated sequences reveal a new mechanism for colonic carcinogenesis. Nature 1993;363:558–61.

46. Issa JP, Baylin SB, Herman JG. DNA methylation changes in hematologic malignancies: biologic and clinical implications. Leukemia. 1997;11:S7–11.

47. Jonasson J, Povey S, Harris H. The analysis of malignancy by cell fusion. VII. Cytogenetic analysis of hybrids between malignant and diploid cells and of tumors derived from them. J Cell Science 1977;24:217–54.

48. Kanai Y, Ushijima S, Tsuda H, Sakamoto M, Sugimura, T, Hirohashi, S. Aberrant DNA methylation on chromosome 16 is an early event in hepatocarcinogenesis. Jpn J Cancer Res 1996;87:1210–7.

49. Kay PH, Spagnolo DV, Taylor J, Ziman N. DNA methylation and developmental genes in lymphomagenesis–more questions than answers? Leuk Lymphoma 1997;24:211–20.

50. Klein CB, Costa M. DNA methylation, heterochromatin and epigenetic carcinogens. Mutat Res 1997;386:163–80.

51. Klein G. The approaching era of the tumor suppressor genes. Science 1987;238:1539–45.

52. Klinger HP. Suppression of human tumorigenicity. Birth Defects Orig Artic Ser 1982;32:68–84.

53. Knudson AG Jr. Mutation and cancer: statistical study of retinoblastoma. Proc Nat Acad Sci USA 1971;68:820–3.

54. Knudson AG Jr, Meadows AT, Nichols WW, Hill R. Chromosomal deletion and retinoblastoma. N Engl J Med 1976;295:1120–3.

55. Koufos A, Hansen MF, Lampkin BC, et al. Loss of alleles at loci on human chromosome 11 during genesis of Wilms' tumor. Nature 1984;309:170–2.

56. Kussie PH, Gorina S, Marechal V, et al. Structure of the mdm2 oncoprotein bound to the p53 tumor suppressor transactivation domain. Science 1996;274:948–53.

57. Leach FS, Tokinu T, Meltzer P, et al. p53 mutation and mdm2 amplification in human soft tissue sarcomas. Cancer Res 1993;53:2231–4.

58. Lee EY, To H, Shew JY, Bookstein, R, Scully P, Lee WH. Inactivation of the retinoblastoma susceptibility gene in human breast cancers. Science 1988;241:218–21.

59. Lee WH, Shew JY, Hong FD, et al. The retinoblastoma susceptibility gene encodes a nuclear phosphoprotein associated with DNA binding activity. Nature 1987;329:642–5.

60. Leegwater PA, Lambooy LH, Deabreau RA, Bokkerink JP, Vandenheuvel LP. DNA methylation patterns in the calcitonin gene region at first diagnosis and at relapse of acute lymphoblastic leukemia (ALL). Leukemia 1997;11:971–8.

61. Lengauer C, Kinzler KW, Vogelstein B. DNA methylation and genetic instability in colorectal cancer cells. Proc Natl Acad Sci USA 1997;94:2545–50.

62. Loeb LA. Cancer cells exhibit a mutator phenotype. Cancer Res 1998;72:25–56.

63. Loeb KR, Loeb, LA. Commentary. Genetic instability and mutator phenotype. Studies in ulcerative colitis. Am J Path 1999;154:1621–6.

64. Martin SJ, Green DR. Protease activation during apoptosis: death by a thousand cuts? Cell 1995;82:349–52.

65. McDonnell TJ, Marin MC, Hsu B, et al. Symposium: Apoptosis/programmed cell death. The bcl-2 oncogene: apoptosis and neoplasia. Radiat Res 1993;136:307–12.

66. Meyn RE, Stephens LC, Ang KK, et al. Heterogeneity in the development of apoptosis in irradiated murine tumours of different histologies. Int J Radiat Biol 1993;64:583–91.

67. Mihara K, Cao XR, Yen A, et al. Cell cycle-dependent regulation of phosphorylation of the human retinoblastoma gene product. Science 1989;246:1300–3.

68. Nagata S, Golstein P. The Fas death factor. Science 1995;267:1449–56.

69. Ohashi K, Nemoto T, Eishi Y, Matsamo A, Nakamura K, Hirokawa K. Proliferative activity and p53 protein accumulation correlate with early invasive trend, and apoptosis correlates with differentiation grade in oesophageal squamous cell carcinoma. Virchows Arch 1997;430:107–15.

70. Paul J. The role of oncogenes in carcinogenesis. In: Iverson OH, ed. Theories of carcinogenesis. Washington, D.C.: Hemisphere, 1988:45–60.

71. Peltomäki P, Aaltonen LA, Sistonen P, et al. Genetic mapping of a locus predisposing to human colorectal cancer. Science 1993;260:810–2.

72. Peltomäki P, Lothe RA, Aaltonen, LA, et al. Microsatellite instability is associated with tumors that characterize the hereditary non-polyposis colorectal carcinoma syndrome. Cancer Res 1993;53:5853–5.

73. Pierce GB, Aguilar D, Hood G, Wells RS. Trophectoderm in control of murine embryonal carcinoma. Cancer Res 1984;44:3987–96.

74. Reid LH, West A, Gioelli DG, et al. Localization of a suppressor gene in 11p15.5 using the G401 Wilms tumor assay. Hum Mol Genet 1996;5:239–47.

75. Sachs L, Lotem J. Apoptosis in the hemopoietic system. In: Gregory CD, ed. Apoptosis and the immune response. New York: Wiley, 1995.

Loeb, LA, 136, 199
Loss of heterozygosity (LOH), 226
    with colorectal cancer, 232
Lucke, Baldwin, 124
Lusitanus, Zacutus, 79
Lymphocyte, 139
Lymphokine-associated lymphocytes (LAK), 144

MacMahon, Harold, 109
Macrophages,141
Maggee, P, 90
Major histocompatibility complex (MCH), 139, 141, 142, 147
Malignant neoplasm, 4, 83
Marsh, HC, 103
Matthaei, Heinrich, 184
Mayneord, WV, 85
McCarty, Maclyn, 169, **170**
McCleod, Colin, 169, **170**
McClintock, Barbara, 199
McKusick, Victor, 195
Mdm2 oncoprotein, 230, **231**
Membron concept, 92
Mendel, Gregor, 191, **192**
Mesopotamia, ancient, 9
Metaplasia, 67
Metastasis, 4, 68, 89
Metchnikoff, Ely, 136
Methylation, 97, 233
Michelangelo, 42
Microscope, 59
    compound, 61
    simple, 59
Microtome, 62
Miescher, Friedrick, 172
Miller, Elizabeth, 93, **93**
Miller, James, 93, **93**
Miller, OJ, 226
Minerals and cancer, 161
Mitochondria, 182, **182**
Mitosis, 174, **175**, 189, **190, 191**
    assymetric, 69, **70**
Molecular correlation concept, 93
Monoclonal antibodies, 139, 144, **145**
Morgagni, Giovanni Battista, 47, **47**, 48
Morgan, TH, 194
Mortality, cancer, 3, 154
Mouse mammary tumor virus (MuMTV), 129
Müller, Johannes, 65, 66
Mummy, 11, **11, 12**
Murine leukemia virus (MLV), 124
Murine mammary tumor virus (MMTV), 124
Mutagens, 96
Mutation, 193, 197, **198**
    insertional, 216
    somatic, 194, **194**
Mutator phenotype, 199
Myc oncogene, 234
Mycotoxin, 127

N-methyl-N-nitrosurea, 95
N-nitroso compounds, 90

Nagasaki, 105, 109
National Cancer Act, 133
National Cancer Survey, 151
Natural killer (NK) cells, 139, **140**
Nei Ching, 17
Neoplasm, 4
    classification and definition, 83
Nirenberg, Marshall, 184, **185**
Nitrogen mustard and cancer, 95
Nitrosamines, 90, 158
Nowell, Peter, 198, **200**
Nucleic acids, 172, **173**
Nucleic acid adducts, 97
Nucleotide excision repair (NER), 118
Nucleus, 64, **65**
Nude mice, 96

Odds ratio, 153
Omnis cellula e cellula, 67
Oncogene, 130, 207, **208**, 212, 221
    K-ras, 220, 232
    myc, 234
    nuclear, 219
    transformation, 243
Oncogene hypothesis, 129, 209
One gene, one enzyme hypothesis, 169
Oral contraceptives and cancer, 156
Ord, MG, 116

p53 gene, 230
Pack, George, 68
Painter, TS, 195
Paleopathology, 5
Papyrus, 12
Paracelcus, 39, **39**, 45, 85
Parasites and cancer, 79
Pavletich, NP, 231
Pelc, Stephan, 174
Peruvian Indians, ancient, 19
Phage group, 170, **171**
Phagocytes, 136
Philadelphia chromosome, 200, **201**, 220
Physician's Health Study, 161
Pitot, Henry, 89, 92
Pituitary gland, 157
Pneumatists, 27
Point mutation, 214, **214**
Poirier, CG, 118
Polonium, 107
Polycyclic aromatic hydrocarbons, 95
Polynuclear aromatic hydrocarbons, 159
Polyomavirus, 125, **129**
Position effect, 200
Potter, V, 93
Procarcinogen 94, **94**
Protein deletion hypothesis, 93
Protein kinase C, 97, 218
Protein serine kinase, 218
Protein synthesis, 182
Protein threonine kinase, 218
Protein tyrosine kinase, 217
Proto-oncogene, 211, 221